Pathophysiology
Second Edition

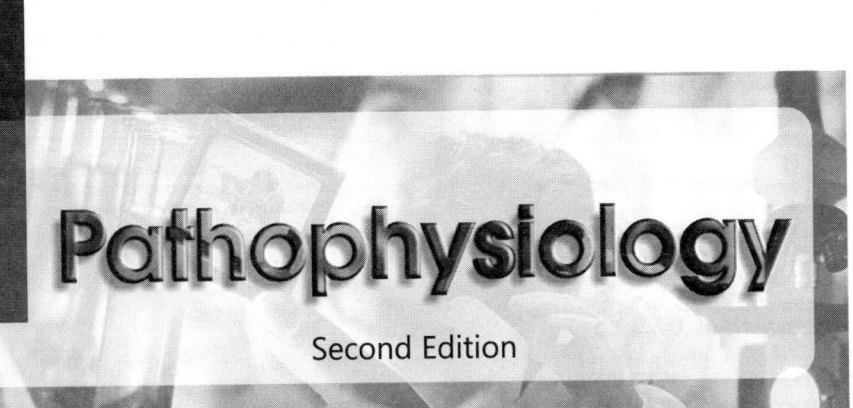

Pathophysiology
Second Edition

RK Marya MD PhD
Professor and Head
Department of Physiology
Faculty of Medicine
Quest International University of Perak
Plaza Teh Teng Seng
Jalan Raja Permaisuri Bainun
30250 IPOH, Perak Darul Ridzuan
Malaysia

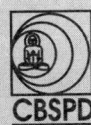

CBSPD

CBS Publishers & Distributors Pvt Ltd

New Delhi • Bengaluru • Chennai • Kochi • Kolkata • Lucknow • Mumbai
Hyderabad • Jharkhand • Nagpur • Patna • Pune • Uttarakhand

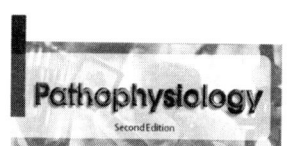

Disclaimer

Science and technology are constantly changing fields. New research and experience broaden the scope of information and knowledge. The author tried his best in giving information available to them while preparing the material for this book. Although, all efforts has been made to ensure optimum accuracy of the material, yet it is quite possible some errors might have been left uncorrected. The publisher, the printer and the author will not be held responsible for any inadvertent errors, omissions or inaccuracies.

ISBN: 978-81-239-2470-0

Copyright © Author and Publisher

Second Edition 2014
Reprint: 2016, 2018, 2020, 2024
First Edition 2006

All rights reserved. No part of this book may be reproduced or transmitted in any form or by any means, electronic or mechanical, including photocopying, recording, or any information storage and retrieval system without permission, in writing, from the author and the publisher.

Published by **Satish Kumar Jain** and produced by **Varun Jain** for
CBS Publishers & Distributors Pvt Ltd
4819/XI Prahlad Street, 24 Ansari Road, Daryaganj, New Delhi 110 002, India.
Ph: 011-23289259, 23266861
Website: www.cbspd.com
e-mail: delhi@cbspd.com

Corporate Office: 204 FIE, Industrial Area, Patparganj, Delhi 110 092
Ph: 011-4934 4934   Fax: 011-4934 4935 e-mail: publishing@cbspd.com

Branches

- **Bengaluru:** Seema House 2975, 17th Cross, K.R. Road, Banasankari 2nd Stage, Bengaluru 560 070, Karnataka, India
  Ph: +91-80-26771678/79   Fax: +91-80-26771680   e-mail: bangalore@cbspd.com
- **Chennai:** 7, Subbaraya Street, Shenoy Nagar, Chennai 600 030, Tamil Nadu, India
  Ph: +91-44-26680620, 26681266   Fax: +91-44-42032115   e-mail: chennai@cbspd.com
- **Kochi:** 42/1325, 1326, Power House Road, Opp KSEB, Ernakulam 682 018, Kochi, Kerala, India
  Ph: +91-484-4059061-67   Fax: +91-484-4059065   e-mail: kochi@cbspd.com
- **Kolkata:** 147, Hind Ceramics Compound, 1st Floor, Nilgunj Road, Belghoria, Kolkata 700 056, West Bengal, India
  Ph: +91-33-25633055/56   e-mail: kolkata@cbspd.com
- **Lucknow:** Basement, Khushnuma Complex, 7-Meerabai Marg (Behind Jawahar Bhawan), Lucknow 226 001, UP, India
  Ph: +0552-4000032   e-mail:tiwari.lucknowi@cbspd.com
- **Mumbai:** PWD Shed. Gala no. 25/26, Ramchandra Bhatt Marg, Next to JJ Hospital Gate no. 2, Opp. Union Bank of India, Noorbaug, Mumbai 400 009, Maharashtra, India
  Ph: 022-66661880/89   e-mail: mumbai@cbspd.com

Representatives

• Hyderabad	0-9885175004	• Jharkhand	0-9811541605	• Nagpur	0-8692091830
• Patna	0-9334159340	• Pune	0-9664372571	• Uttarakhand	0-9716462459

Printed at: Glorious Printers, Delhi, India

Preface to the Second Edition

Readers would appreciate that the book *Pathophysiology* still remains the only book of its kind being published in India. The second edition of the book is being released eight years after release of the first edition. During this period, the knowledge of pathophysiology of various clinical disorders has expanded to the extent that practically all the chapters had to been rewritten. A prominent change in the 2nd edition is that the chapters of the book have been reduced from a total of 52 to 30. This change has been brought about by elimination of chapters which dealt with only physiologic or clinical aspects and had a little discussion of pathophysiology. Examples of the chapters excluded are electrophysiology of the heart, cardiomyopathies, pneumothorax, cerebral edema, neuromuscular disorders, autonomic nervous system, properties of hormones, physiology of the kidneys, urinary tract obstruction, nephrotic syndrome, etc. Some of the chapters of the 1st edition have been clubbed, e.g. obstructive lung disease and interstitial lung disease. As a result, pathophysiological aspects of disorders could be discussed in greater depth and detail. Moreover, a large number of figures have been changed and many new figures are added to provide better understanding of the text.

In Chapter 1 (*anemias*), new topics include details of iron metabolism, and pathophysiology of transfusional hemosiderosis, primary hemochromatosis, anemia in elderly population, anemia of renal insufficiency and unexplained anemia. Chapter 2 (*inflammation and repair*) has been brought uptodate. In Chapter 3 (*disorders of hemostasis*), new topics include pathophysiology of immune thrombocytopenic purpura and disseminated intravascular coagulation, whereas topic of fibrinolytic system has been rewritten. In Chapter 4 (*disorders of esophagus*), pathophysiology of dysphagia and gastroesophageal reflux disease has been rewritten and a new topic, pathophysiology of hiatus hernia, has been added. In Chapter 5 (disorders of stomach), role of *H. pylori* in causation of peptic ulcer has been rewritten and a new topic, pathophysiology of infantile hypertrophic pyloric stenosis, has been added. In Chapter 6, discussion on pathophysiology of small intestine and large intestine has been clubbed. Rewritten topics include pathophysiology of malabsorption syndrome, small bowel syndrome, bacterial overgrowth syndrome, irritable bowel syndrome and Hirschsprung's disease. A new topic, pathophysiology of inflammatory bowel syndrome, has been added. Pathophysiology of acute and chronic pancreatitis has been discussed in detail in Chapter 7. In Chapter 8 (disorders of liver), liver function tests and pathophysiology of alcoholic cirrhosis and hepatic encephalopathy has been rewritten. Moreover, a new topic, pathophysiology of non-alcoholic fatty liver disease, has been added. In Chapter 10 (ischemic heart disease), detailed discussion on atherosclerosis had been added. In Chapter 11 (congestive heart failure), detailed discussion on regulation of cardiac output and pathophysiology of congestive heart failure has been added. Chapters "hypertension" (12) and "circulatory shock" (13) have been entirely rewritten. In Chapter 14 (obstructive and restrictive lung diseases) topics of bronchial asthma, and chronic obstructive pulmonary disease have been rewritten. Chapters 15 (ventilatory disorders), 16 (respiratory failure), 19 (disorders of motor control) and 20 (cerebrovascular accidents) have been entirely rewritten. In Chapter 21 (disorders of consciousness), pathophysiology of syncope, orthostatic hypotension and postural tachycardia syndrome has been discussed in detail. The pathophysiology of pain has been discussed in detail in Chapter 22. In Chapter 23 (pituitary gland) discussion on pathophysiology of growth disorders has been expanded. Acute renal failure and chronic kidney failure have been discussed in great detail in Chapters 28 and 29.

In view of changes detailed above, 2nd edition of *Pathophysiology* shall prove to be an ideal companion to both undergraduate and postgraduate students in clinical medicine. The new edition maintains its relevance to BPharm students also.

The author would like to thank Mr SK Jain, Managing Director, CBS Publishers & Distributors for his support and cooperation in the publication of this book. The contribution of Mr YN Arjuna, Senior vice-President—Publishing, Editorial and Promotion, in publication of the book is thankfully acknowledged.

RK Marya

Preface to the First Edition

The true aim of medical education is not merely remembering the list of facts about a disease but also to really understand the whole mechanism of the disease process. With such a knowledge, when a clinician is faced with a new situation, he can rationalize the given symptoms and signs and reach the correct diagnosis. Therefore, in recent years, it is being increasingly realized that understanding of the pathophysiology of diseases is of fundamental importance in the practice of clinical medicine. With comprehension of pathophysiology of a disorder, one can transform the symptoms, physical findings and diagnostics into a coherent model of the disease. The diagnosis and treatment of a disorder thus becomes logical and rational, rather than empirical. In this book the fabric of physiology and pathophysiology has been interwoven in such a fashion that a sound basis is created for understanding the clinical features of various medical disorders from a textbook of medicine.

The book is expected to be a useful aid to the study of medical disorders, from a textbook of medicine both at undergraduate as well as post-graduate levels. It is also meant to be used as a textbook of pathophysiology by BPharm students.

I am highly grateful to Professor RK Keswani, former Professor of Surgery and Director, Medical College, Rohtak, who originally suggested to me the idea of writing this book. Professor Keswani, after retirement from government service, is currently engaged in private surgical practice. He expressed the necessity of a book giving a brief account of modern concepts of physiology and pathophysiology for use of senior medical and surgical specialists engaged in private practice. I hope this group of readers would also be benefited by perusal of this book.

Grateful thanks are also due to may wife Mrs Veena Marya for her generous help in the preparation of this book.

I would like to thank Mr SK Jain, Managing Director and Mr VK Jain, Production Director of M/S CBS Publishers & Distributors, New Delhi for cooperation in the publication of this book. I would also like to thank Mr Satish Kalra for skillfully composing the book.

Any suggestions for improvement of this book are most welcome.

RK Marya

Contents

Preface to the Second Edition v
Preface to the First Edition vii

1. **Anemias** 1
   Erythropoiesis 1
   Hemoglobin 2
   Iron Metabolism 3
   Parameters of Iron Status of the Body 5
   Iron Overload 6
   Folic Acid Metabolism 9
   Vitamin B_{12} (Cyanocobalamin) 9
   Pathophysiology of Anemias 10
   Red Cell Indices 10
   Laboratory Diagnosis of Anemia 11
   Hemolytic Anemia 15
   Acute Post-hemorrhagic Anemia 19
   Some Special Types of Anemia 21

2. **Inflammation and Repair** 24
   Acute Inflammation 28
   Cardinal Signs 28
   Acute Inflammatory Response 28
   Allergic Inflammation 35
   Chronic Inflammation 36
   General Features of Chronic Inflammation 36

3. **Disorders of Hemostasis** 38
   Formation of Platelet Plug (Primary Hemostasis) 38
   Coagulation of Blood (Secondary Hemostasis) 39
   Mechanism of Coagulation 39
   The Extrinsic Pathway 40
   The Intrinsic Pathway 40
   Natural Anticlotting Mechanisms 41
   Fibrinolytic System 42
   Physiological Basis of Tests of Hemostasis 43
   Activated Partial Thromboplastin Time (aPTT) 43
   Prothrombin Time (PT) 43
   Specific Coagulant Factors 44
   Thrombin Time (TT) 44
   Fibrin Degradation Products (FDPs) Assay, D-dimer Assay 45

Bleeding Disorders	45
Purpura	46
Disorders of Coagulation	47
Thrombosis	48
Arterial Thrombosis	48
Deep Venous Thrombosis (DVT)	49
Venous Stasis	50
Vascular Injury	50
Hypercoagulability	51
Outcomes of Thrombosis	51
Disseminated Intravascular Coagulation (DIC)	52
Causes of DIC	52
Pathophysiology of DIC	54
Clinical Manifestations of DIC	55
Summary of Clinical Manifestations of DIC	56
Blood Indices in DIC	56

4. Disorders of Esophagus — 58

Physiological Considerations	58
Functions	59
Deglutition	59
The Oral Stage	60
The Pharyngeal Stage	60
Esophageal Stage	60
Dysphagia	62
Etiology	62
Achalasia	63
Esophageal Manometry	65
Diaphragmatic (Hiatal) Hernia	65
Gastroesophageal Reflux Disease (GERD)	68
Pathophysiology	68

5. Disorders of Stomach — 73

Functional Anatomy and Physiology	73
Innervation	74
Secretory Functions of Stomach	74
Gastric Acid Secretion	74
Blockers of Acid Secretion	76
Motor Functions of Stomach	76
Estimation of Gastric Acid Output	76
Maximum Acid Output (MAO)	77
Pathophysiology of Peptic Ulcer	77
Role of *Helicobacter pylori*	78
Role of Stress	80
Complications of Peptic Ulcers	80
Gastric Outlet Obstruction	81
Infantile Hypertrophic Pyloric Stenosis	82
Pathophysiology	82

6. Disorders of Intestines — 84
- Small Intestine — 84
- Defense Mechanisms of the Small Intestine — 85
- Malabsorption Syndrome — 87
- Lactose Intolerance — 87
- Tropical Sprue — 89
- Small Bowel Syndrome — 90
- Bacterial Overgrowth Syndrome — 90
- Postgastrectomy Malabsorption Syndrome — 91
- Diabetic Steatorrhea — 91
- Colon — 91
- Diarrhea — 92
- Irritable Bowel Syndrome — 94
- Inflammatory Bowel Disease — 94
- Cancer Risk — 96
- Hirschsprung's Disease — 96

7. Disorders of Pancreas — 98
- Acute Pancreatitis — 98
- Alcoholic Pancreatitis — 99
- Potential Complications of Acute Pancreatitis — 100
- Biliary Pancreatitis — 100
- Chronic Pancreatitis — 100

8. Disorders of Liver — 103
- Functional Anatomy — 103
- Functions of the Liver — 104
- Carbohydrate Metabolism — 105
- Protein Metabolism — 106
- Ammonia Metabolism — 106
- Lipid Metabolism — 107
- Detoxification/Inactivation Function — 108
- Pathophysiology of Jaundice — 109
- Bilirubin Metabolism — 109
- Hepatic Uptake — 110
- Conjugation Reactions — 110
- Excretion into Bile — 110
- Liver Function Tests — 111
- Summary — 116
- Alcohol liver Disease — 116
- Alcoholic Hepatitis — 117
- Alcoholic Cirrhosis — 118
- Nonalcoholic Fatty Liver Disease — 120
- Liver Cirrhosis — 121
- Portal Hypertension and its Complication — 123
- Causes of Portal Hypertension — 123
- Consequences of Portal Hypertension — 124
- Pathophysiology of Ascites — 124

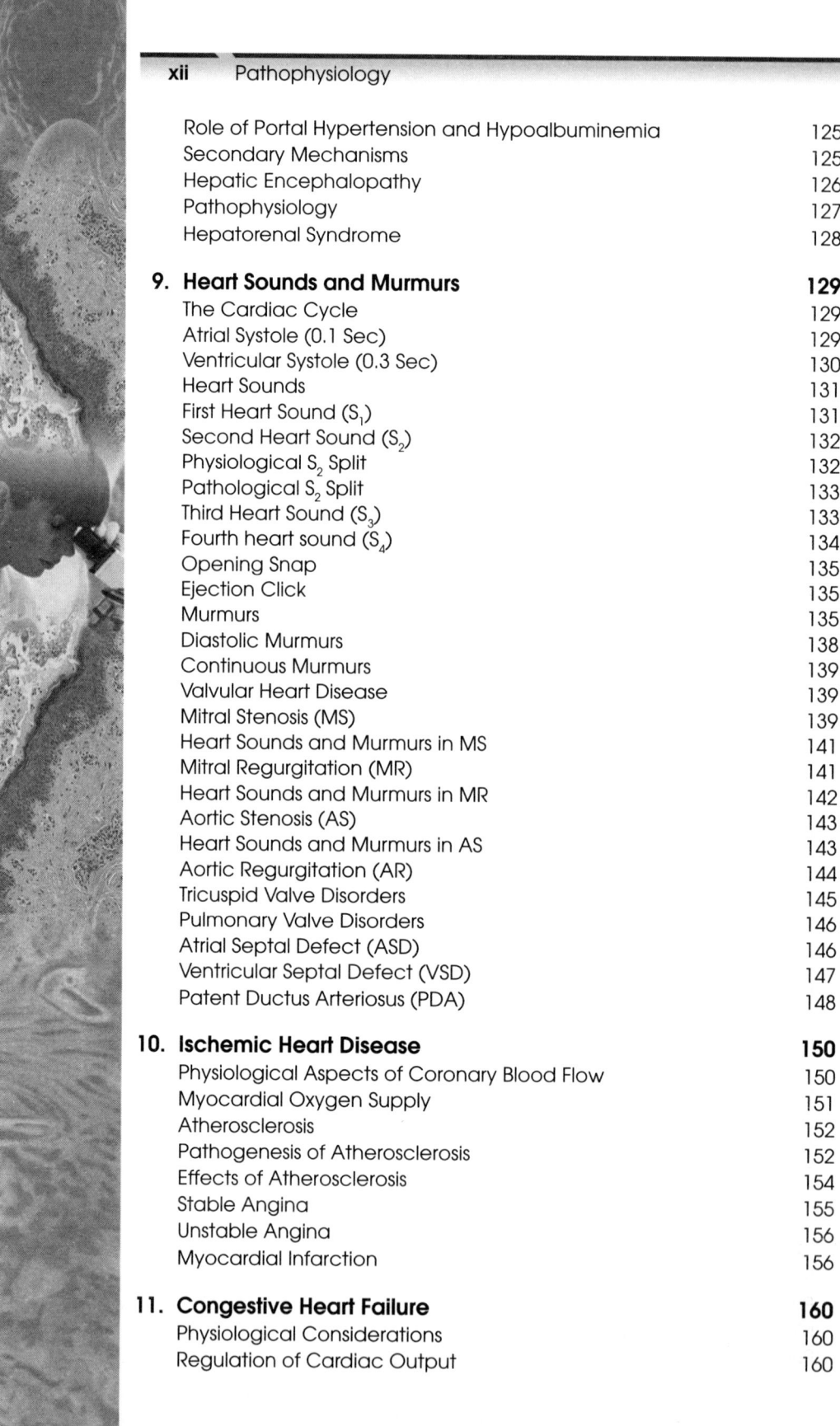

xii Pathophysiology

Role of Portal Hypertension and Hypoalbuminemia	125
Secondary Mechanisms	125
Hepatic Encephalopathy	126
Pathophysiology	127
Hepatorenal Syndrome	128

9. Heart Sounds and Murmurs — 129

The Cardiac Cycle	129
Atrial Systole (0.1 Sec)	129
Ventricular Systole (0.3 Sec)	130
Heart Sounds	131
First Heart Sound (S_1)	131
Second Heart Sound (S_2)	132
Physiological S_2 Split	132
Pathological S_2 Split	133
Third Heart Sound (S_3)	133
Fourth heart sound (S_4)	134
Opening Snap	135
Ejection Click	135
Murmurs	135
Diastolic Murmurs	138
Continuous Murmurs	139
Valvular Heart Disease	139
Mitral Stenosis (MS)	139
Heart Sounds and Murmurs in MS	141
Mitral Regurgitation (MR)	141
Heart Sounds and Murmurs in MR	142
Aortic Stenosis (AS)	143
Heart Sounds and Murmurs in AS	143
Aortic Regurgitation (AR)	144
Tricuspid Valve Disorders	145
Pulmonary Valve Disorders	146
Atrial Septal Defect (ASD)	146
Ventricular Septal Defect (VSD)	147
Patent Ductus Arteriosus (PDA)	148

10. Ischemic Heart Disease — 150

Physiological Aspects of Coronary Blood Flow	150
Myocardial Oxygen Supply	151
Atherosclerosis	152
Pathogenesis of Atherosclerosis	152
Effects of Atherosclerosis	154
Stable Angina	155
Unstable Angina	156
Myocardial Infarction	156

11. Congestive Heart Failure — 160

Physiological Considerations	160
Regulation of Cardiac Output	160

Extrinsic Regulation of Cardiac Output	162
Congestive Heart Failure	162
Systolic versus Diastolic Failure	163
High Output versus Low Output Heart Failure	164
Right Sided versus Left Sided Heart Failure	164
Compensatory Mechanisms in CHF	164
Frank-Starling Mechanism	164
Increased Adrenergic Discharge	165
Redistribution of Cardiac Output	166
Hormonal Mechanisms	166
Decompensated Congestive Heart Failure	167
Pathophysiological Basis of Various Symptoms and Signs of CHF	167
Physiological Principals of Therapeutics in CHF	168
Role of Salt Restriction and Diuretics	168
Vasodilators (ACE Inhibitors)	168
Sympathomimetics	169
Digitalis	169

12. Hypertension — 171

Determinants of Arterial Blood Pressure	171
Regulation of Arterial Blood Pressure	173
Neural Regulatory Mechanisms	173
Long-term Arterial Blood Pressure Regulation	174
What is Hypertension?	175
Pathogenesis of Essential Hypertension	176
Complications of Untreated Essential Hypertension	178
Physiological Basis of Treatment of Essential Hypertension	181
Pharmacological Measures	181

13. Circulatory Shock — 182

Classification of Shock	182
Hypovolemic Shock	182
Cardiogenic Shock	182
Distributive Shock	183
Obstructive Shock	183
Endocrine Shock	183
Hypovolemic Shock	184
Compensatory Mechanisms	184
Symptoms of Hypovolemic Shock in Relation to the Stages of Shock	186
Cardiogenic Shock	188
Septic Shock	188
Multiple Organ Dysfunction Syndromes (MODs)	191

14. Obstructive and Restrictive Lung Diseases — 196

Normal Defense Mechanisms of Lungs	196
Physical and Anatomic Factors	196
Mucociliary Clearance	196
Phagocytic and Inflammatory Cells	197

Immune Responses	198
Airway Resistance	198
Lower Airway Resistance	200
Bronchomotor Muscle Tone	200
Radial Traction by Lung Parenchyma	200
Transmural Pressure	201
Mucus in Airways	201
Obstructive Lung Disease	202
Bronchial Asthma	203
Chronic Obstructive Pulmonary Disease (COPD); Chronic Obstructive Lung Disease (COLD)	205
Cigarette Smoke	206
Genetic Factors	206
COPD with Predominant Bronchitis	206
COPD with Prominent Emphysema	208
Restrictive Lung Disease	209
Reduced Lung Volumes	210
Decreased Lung Compliance	211
Hypoxia	211
Pulmonary Hypertension	211

15. Ventilatory Disorders — 212

Neural Control of Respiration	212
Brain Stem Respiratory Centers	212
Chemical Control	213
Anatomic and Physiologic Dead Space	214
Alveolar Ventilation versus Pulmonary Ventilation	215
Hypoventilatory Syndromes	215
Sleep Apnea Syndrome	217
Hyperventilation	218

16. Respiratory Failure — 220

Physiological Aspects of Diffusion of Gases	220
The Respiratory Parenchyma	220
Diffusion Capacity of Lungs	221
Effect of Ventilation–Perfusion Ratio on Pulmonary Gas Exchange	221
Respiratory Failure	222
Hypoxemic Type	223
Hypercapnic Type	223
Adult Respiratory Distress Syndrome (ARDS)	224
Causes of ARDS	224
Effects on Gas Exchange	225
Effect on Work of Breathing	226
Pulmonary Hypertension	226
Infant Respiratory Distress Syndrome (IRDS)	226

17. Physiological Principles of Oxygen Therapy — 228

Oxygen Transport in Blood	228
Effects of Inhalation of Pure Oxygen	229

Role of Oxygen Therapy in Hypoxia	229
Hazards of Oxygen Therapy	230
Oxygen Toxicity	231
Retinopathy of Prematurity (Retrolental Hyperplasia)	231

18. Pulmonary Function Tests — 233
Tests of Lung Volume	233
Measurement of Functional Residual Capacity	234
Interpretation	235
Spirometric Response to Inhaled Bronchodilators	236
Diffusion Capacity (Transfer Factor)	236
Flow Volume Loops	237
Arterial Blood Gases	238
Oxygenation Status	238
Exercise Testing	239

19. Disorders of Motor Control — 240
General Considerations	240
Role of Sensory Information in Motor Activity	241
Upper and Lower Motor Neurons	242
Regulation of Muscle Tone	243
The Muscle Spindles	243
Stretch Reflex	244
Inverse Stretch Reflex	245
Withdrawal (Flexor) Reflex	245
Clinical Testing of Reflexes	245
Babinski Sign	246
Regulation of Muscle Tone	247
Disorders of Muscle Tone	248
Tremor	248
Resting Tremor	248
Physiologic Tremor	249
Upper Motor Neuron Paralysis	250
Lower Motor Neuron Paralysis	251

20. Cerebrovascular Accidents — 253
General Considerations	253
Cerebral Blood Flow	255
Tissue Level Effects of Cerebral Ischemia	256
Effects of Global Cerebral Ischemia	256
Acute Ischemic Stroke	257
Intracerebral Hemorrhage	258
Pathophysiology	259

21. Disorders of Consciousness — 261
Reticular Activating System	261
Functions of RAS	262
Disorders of Consciousness	263

Coma	263
Syncope	264
Orthostatic Hypotension	266
Postural Tachycardia Syndrome (POTS)	267

22. Pain — 269

Nociceptive Pain	269
Pain Receptors	270
Chemical Mediators of Pain	270
Transmission of Pain Signals: Fast and Slow Pain	271
Site of Pain Perception	271
Visceral Pain	272
Characteristics of Visceral Pain	273
Effect of Age on Visceral Pain Perception	274
Referred Pain	274
Mechanism of Referred Pain	274
Hyperalgesia	276
Endogenous Pain Modulation	276
Implications in Management of Pain	278
Neuropathic Pain	278
Causes of Neuropathic Pain	280
Pathophysiology	281
Chronic Pain Syndrome	282
Effects of Pain	282
Chronic Pain Responses	282
Implications in Pain Management	284

23. Pituitary Gland — 286

Functional Anatomy	286
Anterior Pituitary Gland (Adenohypophysis)	288
Hypothalamic Control of Anterior Pituitary Gland	288
Hypophysiotropic Hypothalamic Hormones	288
Growth Hormone (GH)	289
Insulin-like Growth Factors (IGFs)	289
Effect of Age on GH Secretion	290
Prolactin	290
Adrenocorticotropic Hormone (ACTH)	292
Thyroid Stimulating Hormone (TSH)	293
Gonadotropins	293
Syndromes of Anterior Pituitary Hypersecretion	294
Hyperprolactinemia	294
Acromegaly and Giantism	294
Syndromes of ACTH Excess (Cushing Disease and Nelson's Syndrome)	295
Anterior Pituitary Deficiency Syndromes	296
Posterior Pituitary Gland (Neurohypophysis)	296
Antidiuretic Hormone	296
Syndrome of Inappropriate Antidiuretic Hormone Secretion (SIADH)	298

Growth Disorders	299
Physiology of Growth	299
Short Stature	302
Tall Stature	302

24. Thyroid Gland — 304

Functional Anatomy	304
Biosynthesis and Release of Thyroid Hormones	304
Mode of Action of Antithyroid Agents	306
Transport of Thyroid Hormones	307
Actions of Thyroid Hormones	307
Regulation of Secretion	308
Hyperthyroidism	309
Graves' Disease	309
Thyroid Storm (Hyperthyroid Crisis)	310
Hypothyroidism	310
Iodine Deficiency Hypothyroidism	311
Adult Hypothyroidism	312
Skin	312
Voice	312
Cardiovascular System	313
Respiratory System	313
Gastrointestinal System	313
Hematological System	313
Nervous System	313
Metabolism	314
Biochemical Profile	314
Myxedema Coma (Myxedema Crisis)	314

25. Adrenal Gland — 315

Biosynthesis of Adrenal Corticosteroids	316
Fetal Steroid Biosynthesis	316
Regulation of Adrenal Steroidogenesis	317
Regulation of Glucocorticoid Secretion	317
Regulation of Mineralocorticoid Secretion	317
Regulation of Adrenal Androgen Secretion	318
Transport in Blood	319
Actions of Glucocorticoids	319
Actions of Mineralocorticoids	321
Escape Phenomenon	321
Hyperfunction of Adrenal Cortex	322
Cushing Syndrome	322
Primary Aldosteronism (Conn's Syndrome)	322
Secondary Hyperaldosteronism	323
Syndromes of Adrenal Androgen Excess (Congenital Adrenal Hyperplasia)	324
Adrenocortical Insufficiency	325
Adrenal Medulla	325

xviii Pathophysiology

Effects of Adrenergic Receptor Stimulation	326
Sympathoadrenal Response in Some Pathophysiologic States	326
Pheochromocytoma	328

26. Endocrine Pancreas — 329

Physiological Considerations	329
Insulin	329
Actions of Insulin	330
In Liver	330
In Skeletal Muscle	330
In Adipose Tissue	330
Glucagon	330
Actions	331
Blood Glucose Homeostasis	331
Postprandial State	331
Postabsorptive State	332
Pathophysiology of Diabetes Mellitus	333
Hyperglycemia and its Consequences	333
Ketosis and its Consequences	337
Increased Protein Catabolism and its Consequences	338
Hypoglycemia	339
Hypoglycemia Unawareness	340

27. Metabolic Bone Disease — 341

Functional Anatomy	341
Compact Bone	341
Remodeling of Bone	343
Bone Formation	343
Bone Resorption	343
Role of Parathyroid Hormone in Bone Metabolism	344
Role of Vitamin D in Bone Metabolism	345
Role of Osteocytes in Bone Metabolism	345
Metabolic Bone Disease	345
Osteoporosis	345
Senile/Postmenopausal Osteoporosis	346
Osteomalacia and Rickets	349
Pathophysiology of Vitamin D Deficiency States	350
Paget's Disease	351
Osteitis Fibrosa Cystica	352

28. Acute Renal Failure — 355

Physiological Considerations	355
Urine Formation	355
Glomerular Filtration	356
Tubular Mechanisms	356
Acute Renal Injury/Acute Renal Failure	357
Prerenal ARI	357
Relation between GFR and Plasma Levels of Creatinine and Urea	359

Renal ATI (Renal (Intrinsic) Azotemia)	359
Acute Tubular Necrosis (ATN)	360
Initiation Phase	361
Maintenance Phase	361
Recovery Phase	362
Biochemical Abnormalities in ARI	363
Postrenal ARI	364
RIFLE Criteria in ARI	365

29. Chronic Kidney Failure — 366

Renal Handling of Different Solutes in Chronic Kidney Disease	366
Pathophysiology of Uremia	367
General Cellular Dysfunction	368
Hypothermia	369
Anemia and Immune Dysfunction	369
Renal Osteodystrophy	370
Acidosis	370
Hyperkalemia	371
Cardiovascular Dysfunction	371
Fluid and Electrolyte Imbalance	371
Uremic Neuropathy	372
Uremic Encephalopathy	372
Malnutrition	372
Endocrine Abnormalities	373
Skin	374

30. Acid-Base Disorders — 375

The Concept of pH	375
Acid-base Buffers	375
Regulation of Hydrogen Ion Balance	377
Role of Respiration	378
Role of Kidneys	378
Anion Gap Concept	379
Acid-base Disorders in Clinical Practice	380
Primary Acid-base Disorders	380
High Anion Gap MA	380
Normal Anion Gap (Hyperchloremic) MA	381
Acid-base Analysis	384
Mixed Acid-base Disorders	384

Index — *387*

1

Anemias

ERYTHROPOIESIS

All the blood cells arise from a pool of pluripotent stem cells (progenitor cells) present in the bone marrow. A process of self-renewal without differentiation maintains stem cell population. Some of them migrate to other areas and produce lymphocytes. A process of commitment converts others into erythroid line of cells, myeloid line of cells or platelet forming cells. Certain humoral substances like erythropoietin, colony stimulating factors or thrombopoietin push the stem cells into the respective line of development. From the bone marrow stem cells, a separate line of development leads to production of various types of lymphocytes in lymphoid tissues (Fig. 1.1)

Every day, about 1% of total circulating erythrocytes are released into blood circulation from the bone marrow. An equal number are destroyed every day by the tissue macrophages located in the liver, spleen and bone marrow. Erythropoiesis is regulated by a glycoprotein, erythropoietin, secreted by the endothelial cells of peritubular capillaries in the renal cortex. Hypoxia is the most important stimulus for the release of erythropoietin. Erythropoietin exerts its chief effect on the stem cells,

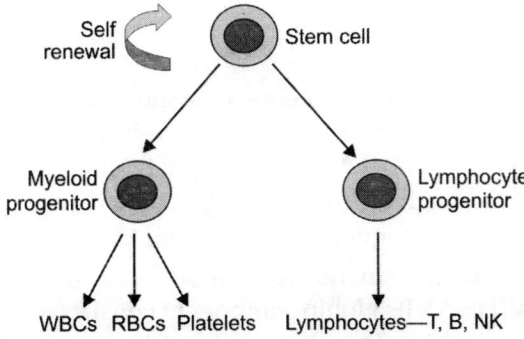

Fig. 1.1: Hemopoiesis (diagrammatic).

2 Pathophysiology

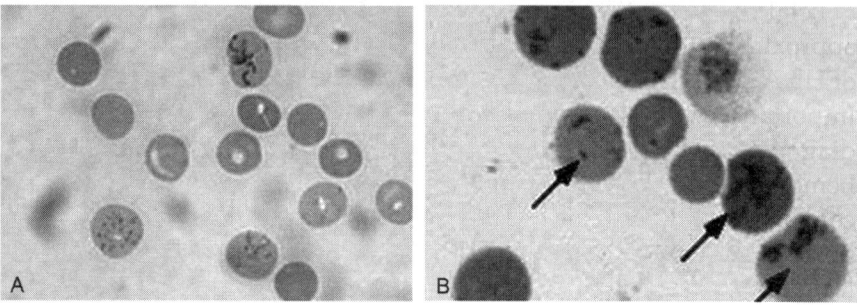

Fig. 1.2: Reticulocytosis in a patient of hemolytic anemia (A) and a patient of pernicious anemia after administration of vitamin B_{12} (B).

causing them to differentiate into erythroid line of development. It seems to be necessary for normal hemoglobin synthesis in the maturing erythroblasts. Erythropoiesis is an extravascular process. Red cell enters the circulation (bone marrow sinusoids) at the stage of reticulocyte. A reticulocyte is named after the fact that with a special stain, a network of basophilic material (remnants of ribosomes) can be demonstrated in its cytoplasm. Within 24–48 hours in circulation, the basophilic material finally disappears and cell is now called a young erythrocyte. Normal erythropoiesis depends on the presence of adequate nutrients such as iron, amino acids, vitamins (notably folic acid and vitamin B_{12}) and certain hormones (notably thyroxine, and cortisol).

Normal peripheral blood contains 0.5–2.5% of total red cells as reticulocytes. Reticulocyte count is used as a marker of the rate of red cell production. In aplastic anemia, reticulocyte count is extremely low. Reticulocyte count is also low in iron deficiency anemia or vitamin B_{12} deficiency anemia and liver cirrhosis. An elevated reticulocyte count is a characteristic feature of hemolytic anemia. In pernicious anemia, administration of a large parenteral dose of vitamin B_{12} may increase the reticulocyte count as high as 50%, indicating an explosive increase in red cell maturation in the bone marrow (Fig. 1.2).

HEMOGLOBIN

Hemoglobin is a conjugated protein with a molecular weight of 64,400. It consists of four subunits of heme, each containing an iron atom in ferrous (Fe^{++}) state and a protein, globin, constituted by four polypeptide chains. Polypeptide chains of globin (α, β, γ and δ chains) vary in the total number of amino acids and the sequence of amino acids.

Hemoglobin present in the red blood cells of an adult is called Hemoglobin A (Hb A). Its globin component consists of two alpha chains (141 amino acids each) and two beta chains (146 amino acids). Thus, Hb A is said to have $\alpha_2 \beta_2$ pattern of globin component.

Fetal hemoglobin has $\alpha_2\gamma_2$ chains (Hb F = $\alpha_2\gamma_2$). In normal adults, approximately 2.5% of hemoglobin is present as Hb A_2 ($\alpha_2\delta_2$). Presence of Hb A_2 in such a small concentration has no physiological significance. Importance of Hb A_2 estimation lies in the fact that its elevated level is diagnostic of the existence of β thalassemia trait. In another type of hemoglobinopathy, called Sickle cell anemia, the red cells of the patient contain hemoglobin S (Hb S). Hb S has $\alpha_2\beta_2$ pattern, but in the β chain, at position 6, amino acid valine is present instead of normal glutamic acid. Mutation of one amino acid drastically alters the physical property of Hb S, resulting in the disorder known as sickle cell anemia. Various types of hemoglobins can be differentiated by high-performance liquid chromatography (HPLC).

Hemoglobinopathies mentioned above result from a genetic defect in the globin component of hemoglobin. The disorder persists throughout life. Hemoglobinopathies are characterized by shortened life span of the red cells resulting in hemolytic anemia. The heme component of hemoglobin may be altered in some acquired and potentially reversible defects. Methemoglobin and carboxy-hemoglobin are examples of such variants of Hb A. Methemoglobin results from intake of certain drugs which oxidize iron component of heme from ferrous (Fe^{++}) to ferric (Fe^{+++}) state. Ferric iron is incapable of oxygen transport resulting in hypoxia. Similarly, attachment of CO to iron atom (carboxy-hemoglobin) also renders it useless for oxygen transport. The resulting acute hypoxia in either case can be fatal.

IRON METABOLISM

Iron is one of the most abundant metal present in the body. It serves numerous vital functions. As a component of hemoglobin and myoglobin, iron is involved in the transport of oxygen to the tissues. Iron is present in most of the cells as a component of vital cytochromes enzymes involved in oxidative and energy transfer reactions.

Average dietary content of iron is about 10 mg per day. Of this, approximately 10% can be absorbed, mostly in duodenum and jejunum. Dietary iron from food of animal sources called heme-iron. It is present in meat, fish, liver, etc. The intestine can absorb 10–20% of dietary heme-iron as compared to 0–10% absorption of non-heme or inorganic iron salts present in vegetarian food (green leafy vegetables, dried beans, cereals and eggs, etc.).

Absorption of non-heme iron is decreased by high-fiber diet, tea or coffee if taken with food, high calcium content of food and oxalates. Spinach is rich in iron, but since it contains a large amount of oxalates as well, the bioavailability of iron is poor from this source. Absorption of non-heme iron is favored by the presence of ascorbic acid (citrus fruit,

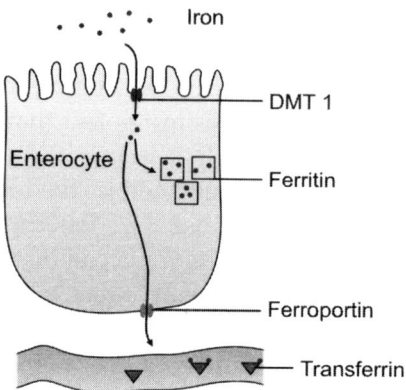

Fig. 1.3: Mechanism of iron absorption in the small intestinal enterocyte.

tomatoes etc). In the vegetables, iron is mostly present as ferric form (Fe^{+++}) whereas only ferrous (Fe^{++}) can be absorbed in the intestines. Gastric acid and a reducing agent (e.g. ascorbic acid) help in conversion of ferric to ferrous form of iron.

In the intestinal epithelial cells, there is a regulatory control over absorption of iron. In Fe^{++} state, iron crosses the luminal border with the help of divalent metal transporter-1 (DMT-1). In the cytosol of the intestinal epithelial cell, Fe^{++} can take one of the two possible routes:

1. It may cross the baso-lateral border of the epithelial cell into the blood stream. The efflux of iron across the basolateral membrane and into the circulation is mediated by the iron transport protein ferroportin. In addition to ferroportin, the basolateral efflux of iron from enterocytes requires another transport protein called hephaestin. Although the exact role of this protein has not been defined, its ability to oxidize ferrous to ferric iron is predicted to be important for its function (Fig. 1.3)

2. Some cytosolic Fe^{++} is converted to Fe^{+++} and combines with a storage protein called apoferritin to constitute ferritin. Ferritin cannot cross the baso-lateral border of the enterocytes. Within a few days, this form of iron is lost from the body along with the desquamated intestinal epithelial cells.

The fraction of absorbed iron that crosses the basolateral border of the enterocytes and that becomes ferritin varies with the status of iron stores of the body. When the body iron stores are saturated, most of the absorbed iron becomes ferritin in the enterocytes and does not enter the body. In iron deficiency states, a larger percentage of absorbed iron enters blood circulation and only small amount becomes ferritin and lost from the body. This regulatory control over intestinal absorption (*mucosal block hypothesis*) is critically important for prevention of iron overload, since once iron enters the body, it cannot be excreted.

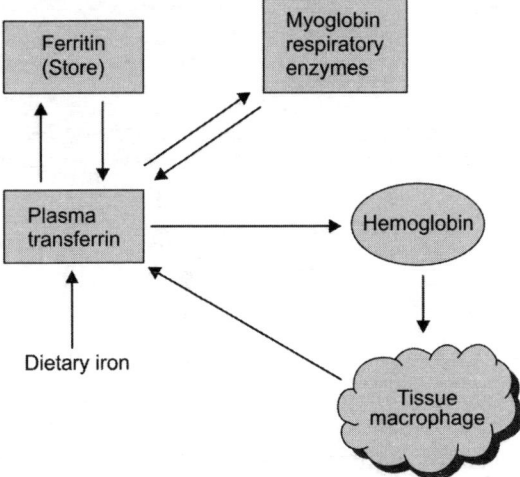

Fig. 1.4: Iron metabolism.

Iron is transported in plasma in combination with a transport protein called transferrin. Iron is stored mainly in the parenchymal cells and macrophages of liver, and in macrophages of bone marrow, and spleen. In these tissues, iron, in ferric state, combines with a storage protein called apoferritin to form ferritin. However, small amount of ferritin is present practically in the all the tissue cells. Under steady state conditions, the serum ferritin level correlates with total body iron stores. From the iron stores, iron is released into plasma and utilized for formation of hemoglobin, myoglobin and respiratory enzymes, etc. (Fig. 1.4).

Excessive ferritin accumulation within cells results in formation of large aggregates of ferritin called hemosiderin. Iron in ferritin or hemosiderin state can be released from the storage tissues, although it is less readily available from hemosiderin. Under light microscope, hemosiderin can be seen in the cytoplasm as yellow to brown granules. Ferritin can be identified only under electron microscope.

There is practically no physiological mechanism of iron excretion from the body (Fig. 1.4). That is why in iron deficiency states, parenteral administration of iron should be undertaken with outmost care and only when absolutely necessary.

Parameters of Iron Status of the Body

1. **Serum iron:** Normal range 80–180 µg/dl
2. **Total iron binding capacity (TIBC):** Normal—250–450 µg/dl. TIBC level is increased in iron deficiency.
3. **Transferrin saturation**

$$\frac{\text{Serum iron concentration} \times 100}{\text{TIBC}}$$

6 Pathophysiology

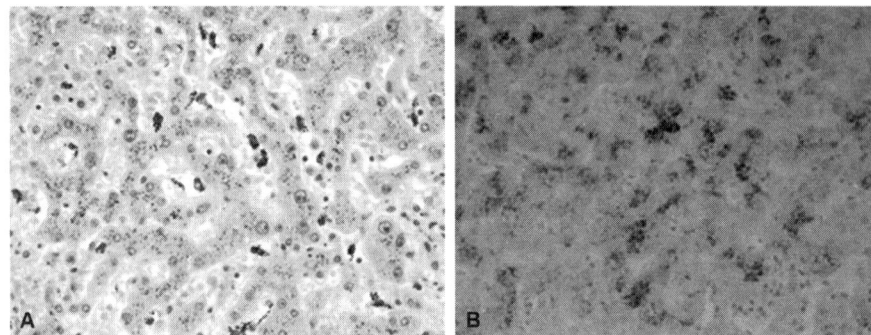

Fig.1.5: Hepatic iron. Normal (A) and iron overload (B).

Normal range: TIBC saturation values <15% indicate iron deficiency whereas values >60% are indicative of iron overload.

4. **Serum ferritin:** Ferritin is normally present only in the tissues as stored iron, from where a small amount leaks into plasma. Estimation of serum ferritin is a sensitive index of status of body iron stores. Normal range: 18–250 ng/ml in males 12–160 ng/ml in females.
5. **Bone marrow iron:** Presence of iron stored in the bone marrow can be visualized by examination of a bone marrow smear stained with Prussian blue stain. Bone marrow biopsy for assessing the status of body iron status is often considered a gold standard, but seldom done to confirm iron deficiency since it is an invasive procedure and other tests mentioned above are quite reliable. For diagnosis of iron overload, liver biopsy is more useful (Fig. 1.5B).

Iron Overload

Iron deficiency states are very common all over the world populations and have been discussed later in this chapter. Iron overload may occur in two forms:
1. Primary hemochromatosis
2. Transfusional hemosiderosis

1. *Primary (Hereditary) Hemochromatosis*

Hereditary hemochromatosis is characterized by an accelerated rate of intestinal iron absorption and progressive iron deposition in various tissues. Actually, iron absorption is only slightly increased (2–4 mg/day as compared to normal 1–2 mg/day). By the age of 40–50 years, when the disease manifests, body contains 20–40 g of iron (Fig. 1.6). Hemosiderin deposited in various organs results in widespread tissue damage. The most affected organ is liver, where excessive iron is found to be deposited in hepatocytes (Fig. 1.7A), that leads to cirrhosis. In addition

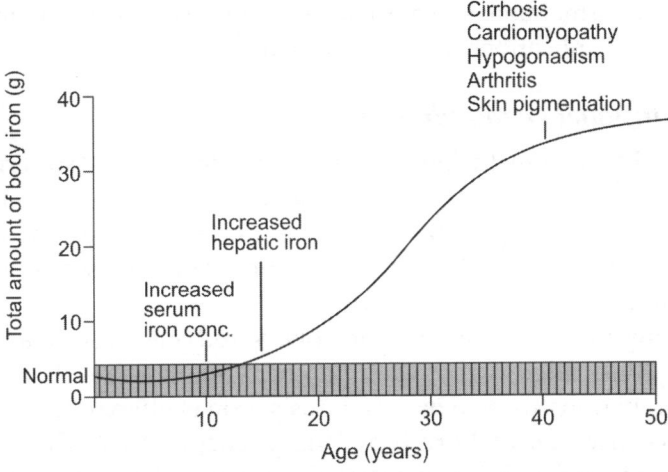

Fig 1.6: Typical total body iron in a case of hereditary hemochromatosis.

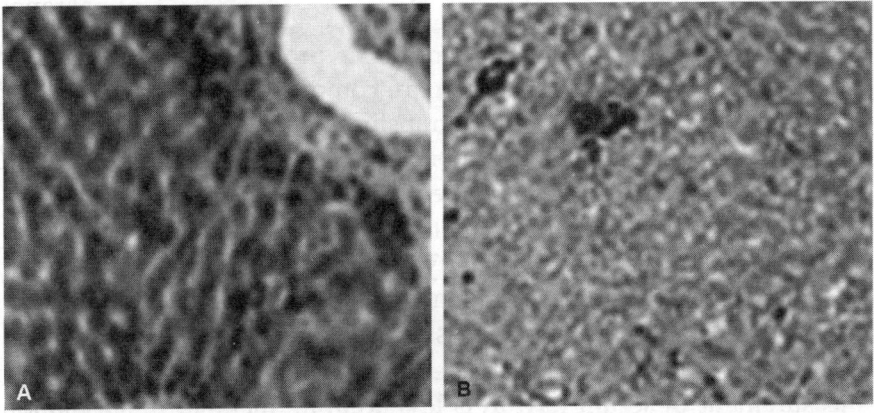

Fig 1.7: Iron deposit in hepatic parenchymal cells (A) and in Kupffer cells (B).

hypopituitarism, hypogonadism, cardiomyopathy, diabetes, arthritis, or hyperpigmentation of skin may occur. Because of the severe sequelae of this disease if left untreated, early diagnosis, i.e. before symptoms or signs appear is important.

Hemochromatosis is the most common genetically carried disease (13% of all persons in the US are said to carry the gene) and about 1 in 200–400 persons has hemochromatosis. Most of the patients are of European origin. Men are affected with hemochromatosis nearly 2–3 times as often as women because the latter have inbuilt system of iron loss throughout their reproductive life through menstruation, pregnancy, and lactation. That is why the disorder manifests around 40 years of age in men compared to 50 years in women. Early diagnosis and therapeutic phlebotomy to maintain low normal body stores is crucial and can prevent all known complications of hemochromatosis.

2. *Transfusional Hemosiderosis*

Repeated blood transfusions are lifesaving in patients suffering from thalassemia and other cases of hereditary hemoglobinopathies. Repeated transfusion leads to rapid iron loading, because each unit of blood contains 200 to 250 mg of iron and can cause an iron overload disorder known as transfusional hemosiderosis (Fig. 1.8).

Since this iron is derived from hemolysed red cells, tissue macrophages become iron-loaded earlier than parenchymal tissue cells (Fig. 1.7B). However, in transfusional hemosiderosis, iron is ultimately deposited in the same sites as in hereditary hemochromatosis (hepatocytes, myocardium, and endocrine tissues). Cardiomyopathy is more prominent in patients with transfusional iron overload than in those with hemochromatosis, probably because of rapid iron loading.

Liver involvement is common. Early cirrhotic changes can be observed as early as 7 years of age in some children with thalassemia. Cardiac involvement is a major determinant of the prognosis in iron-overload states. Hypertrophy and dilatation are common. The average time for the development of heart failure in transfused, unchelated patients is said to be 10 years. Cardiomyopathy alone accounts for more than 70% of the causes of death of thalassemia patients

Endocrine dysfunction affects virtually all glands. Pituitary involvement causes delayed puberty in more than 50% of patients. Up to 15% may develop insulin-dependent diabetes mellitus (IDDM). Thyroid, parathyroid, and exocrine pancreas are also affected.

The body iron burden is best determined by quantitative liver biopsy; measurement of serum ferritin is less accurate method. In such cases, iron overload has to be treated by chelation therapy.

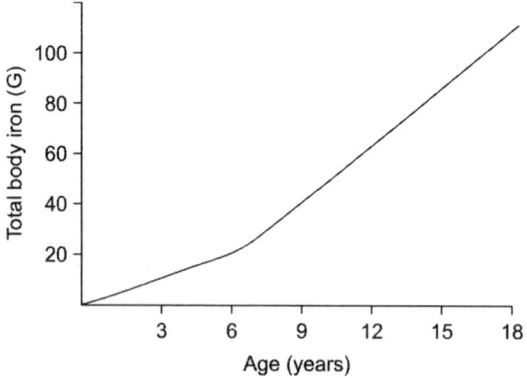

Fig. 1.8: Transfusional hemosiderosis. Projected total body iron in a child who received repeated blood transfusion without chelation therapy.

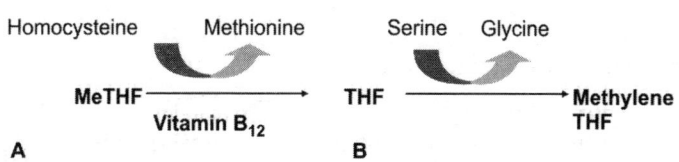

Fig. 1.9: Folic acid metabolism. THF = tetrahydrofolate; MeTHF = methyltetrahydrofolate.

Folic Acid Metabolism

Folic acid (pteroylglutamic acid) is present in many fruits and vegetables. Body stores of folic acid are adequate for a few weeks only. Therefore, folic acid deficiency can arise rapidly in cases with malnutrition or malabsorption syndrome. It can also arise due to increased demand by rapid cellular proliferation (pregnancy, hemolytic anemia, psoriasis, etc.). In developing countries, more than 50% of pregnant women may develop folic acid deficiency anemia unless folic acid supplements are routinely given. Certain drugs (such as methotrexate, anticonvulsants, alcohol) interfere with metabolism of folic acid and therefore tend to produce folic acid deficiency disorders. Folic acid deficiency may lead to glossitis, diarrhea, depression, confusion, anemia, and fetal neural tube defects and brain defects (during pregnancy). Folic acid deficiency is accelerated by alcohol consumption.

Folic acid, present in the food as pteroylpolyglutamate, is absorbed mostly in the jejunum. In the intestinal lumen and enterocytes, polyglutamate is broken down to monoglutamate, reduced to tetrahydrofolate and methylated. Thus, folic acid appears in the plasma as methyltetrahydrofolate (MeTHF).

Further metabolism of MeTHF is shown in Fig. 1.9. The final product, methylene THF is required in the synthesis of thymidine, an important component of DNA. The vitamin B_{12}-mediated reaction (Fig. 1.9A) generates amino acid methionine that is essential for myelin synthesis in the nervous tissue. As seen from Fig. 1.9, normal generation of methylene THF depends on adequate supply of both folic acid and vitamin B_{12}. Deficiency of either vitamin can result in defect in all the tissues with rapid rate of cellular proliferation, e.g. bone marrow and gastrointestinal tract.

Vitamin B_{12} (Cyanocobalamin)

Meat (especially liver), milk and milk products are the only dietary sources of vitamin B_{12}. The vitamin is absorbed in the ileum. A specific cobalamin-binding protein, more commonly known as intrinsic factor of Castle (IF) is essential for its intestinal absorption. The IF is a glycoprotein secreted by the acid-producing oxyntic cells of the gastric glands. Vitamin B_{12} is stored in the liver. Hepatic stores of vitamin B_{12} are large. Symptoms of vitamin B_{12} deficiency usually appear 3–6 years after total gastrectomy. Such large storage of a water soluble vitamin is unique.

Dietary deficiency of vitamin B_{12} is rare. More common causes of vitamin B_{12} deficiency are partial or total gastrectomy or intestinal malabsorption syndrome. The name Addisonian type of pernicious anemia is given to the deficiency disorder caused by an autoimmune gastric atrophy leading to complete cessation of secretion of hydrochloric acid, IF and pepsinogen by the stomach.

PATHOPHYSIOLOGY OF ANEMIAS

Anemia is defined as a reduction in red cell mass below the normal range, for the age and sex of the individual. It is also reflected in hemoglobin concentration. In adults, hematocrit below 40% (or Hb below 13 g/dL) in males and below 35% (or Hb below 12 g/dL in females) is cutoff level for diagnosis of anemia. The normal range of hematocrit, hemoglobin and other hematological parameters is shown in Table 1.1.

Estimation of hemoglobin level is usually adequate for the diagnosis of anemia except in conditions with expanded plasma volumes such as pregnancy or congestive heart failure. In such patients, estimation of hemoglobin gives falsely low values (dilutional anemia). On the other hand, an acute reduction in plasma volume (severe dehydration due to heat stress, diuretics or severe burns) may give falsely high values of hemoglobin or RBC count due to hemoconcentration.

RED CELL INDICES

From the RBC count, hemoglobin concentration and hematocrit (PCV) value, certain indices (or absolute values) of the red cells of the person

Table 1.1: Important normal values in hematology

	Men	Women
Hemoglobin, g/dL	13–18	12–16
Hematocrit, %	40–52	35–47
Red cell count, millions/mL	4.4–5.9	3.8–5.2
White cell count, thousands/mL	4–11	4–11
Mean corpuscular volume (MCV), μ^3	80–100	80–100
Mean corpuscular hemoglobin (MCH), pg	26–34	26–34
Mean corpuscular hemoglobin concentration (MCHC)%	32–36	32–36
Platelet count, thousand//mL	150–440	150–440
Reticulocyte count, %	0.5–1.5	0.5–2.5
Erythrocyte sedimentation rate, mm 1st hr	0–10	0–20

can be calculated. These absolute values are used in the laboratory diagnosis of anemia. The method of calculation and normal range of various red cell indices are shown in Table 1.2.

Laboratory Diagnosis of Anemia

Figure 1.10 summarizes the steps in the laboratory diagnosis of anemia.

1. *Hypochromic Microcytic Anemia*

i. *Iron deficiency anemia*

Iron deficiency is the commonest cause of hypochromic microcytic anemia. It is the most prevalent single deficiency state on a worldwide basis. It is important economically because it diminishes the capability of individuals

Table 1.2: Calculation and normal range of red cell indices

Absolute value	Normal range	Calculation
Mean corpuscular volume (MCV)	80–100 µ³	$\dfrac{PCV (\%) \times 10}{RBC\ count\ (millions/\mu l)}$
Mean corpuscular hemoglobin (MCH)	26–34 pg	$\dfrac{Hb\ (g/dL) \times 10}{RBC\ count\ (millions/\mu l)}$
Mean corpuscular hemoglobin concentration (%)	32–38%	$\dfrac{Hb\ (g/dL) \times 100}{PCV\ (\%)}$

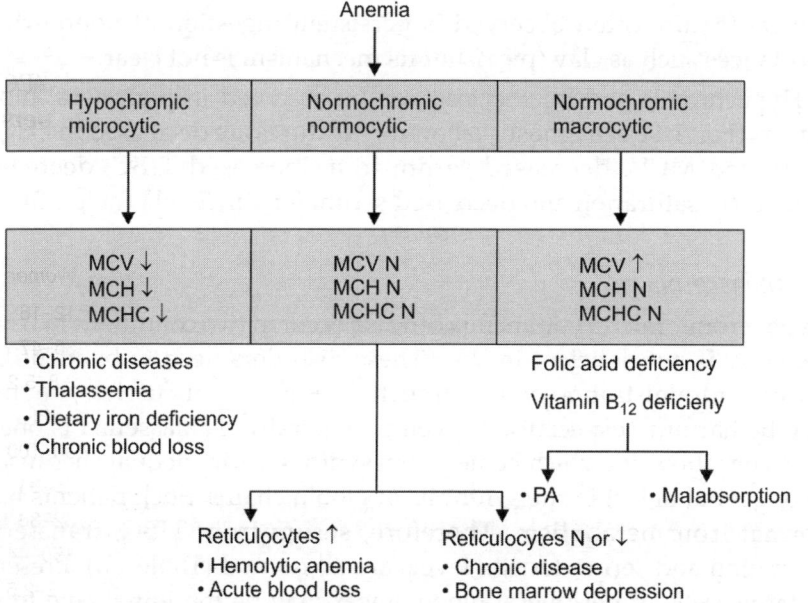

Fig. 1.10: Diagnosis of anemia on the basis of laboratory indices.

who are affected to perform physical labor, and it diminishes both growth and learning in children. Such patients seem to be more prone to infections.

Iron deficiency anemia is usually the end result of a long period of negative iron balance. The daily requirement of iron in males is very little. Except malnourished individuals, males are not prone to develop iron deficiency anemia. Therefore, in a male patient with such type of anemia, causes such as gastrointestinal blood loss, malabsorption or hookworm infestation should be looked for.

Females in the reproductive age group are prone to develop iron deficiency because of loss of iron in menstruation, pregnancy and lactation. Excessive menstrual losses or repeated pregnancies are the usual causes of iron deficiency anemia in women. Gastric surgery and achlorhydria are other causes of iron deficiency anemia which may occur both in males and females. Achlorhydria may be the result rather than the cause of iron deficiency.

Most cells require iron for growth and proliferation due to its presence in proteins involved in hemoglobin synthesis, DNA synthesis and mitochondrial respiration. Cellular iron deficiency causes cell cycle arrest and reduces cell proliferation. Thus defective structure and function can be demonstrated in many tissues with high rate of cellular proliferation other than bone marrow, especially in epithelia. Decreased lymphocyte proliferation may account for defective immune function resulting in more frequent infections. Besides anemia, other characteristic features of iron deficiency include spoon-shaped nails, atrophy of lingual papillae, glossitis, dysphagia and atrophic gastritis with achlorhydria. Another clinical feature often observed is persistent ingestion of nonnutritive substances such as clay (pica), but its mechanism is not clear.

Hypochromia and microcytosis can be observed in peripheral blood smears (Fig. 1.11). Diagnostic laboratory features are decreased MCHC%, decreased MCV, decreased serum iron, increased TIBC, decreased transferrin saturation and decreased serum ferritin level (Table 1.3).

ii. *Thalassemia*

Hypochromic microcytic anemia can also occur in two conditions in which the body is not deficient in iron. These disorders need to be identified because administration of iron in such cases is not only useless, but may also be harmful, especially if given parenterally. Thalassemia is one of such conditions, in which hemoglobin synthesis is inadequate because of a congenital defect in the synthesis of globin chains. Such patients have normal iron metabolism. Therefore, serum iron, TIBC, transferrin saturation and serum ferritin levels are all normal (Table 1.3). Presence of target cells in peripheral blood smear may be the initial clue to the disorder. Estimation of Hb A2 is diagnostic.

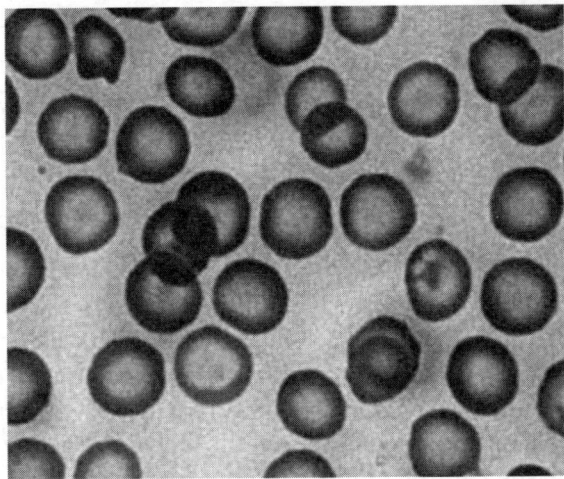

Fig 1.11: Hypochromic microcytosis. Central pallor in the red blood cells is enlarged.

Table 1.3: Differential diagnosis of hypochromic microcytic anemia

Laboratory test	Range of normal values	Iron deficiency anemia	Anemia of chronic disease	Thalassemia
Serum iron, µg per dL	60 to 100	<60	<60	N
Total iron-binding capacity, µg per dL	250 to 400	>400	<250	N
Transferrin saturation, %	20 to 60	<16	<20	N
Serum ferritin, ng per mL	100 to 300	<100	>300	N

N = within normal range

iii. Anemia of chronic diseases

This term refers to the anemia commonly observed in patients with a variety of infective, inflammatory or neoplastic diseases that persist one to two months or more. Such anemia is especially common in elderly hospitalized population. Anemia of chronic disorders may be normochromic normocytic but more often, it is hypochromic microcytic type. The latter type of anemia is characterized by low serum iron; low TIBC, low transferrin saturation and elevated serum ferritin level (Table 1.3). Typically, iron stores are within normal limits or elevated. The chronic illness produces complex cytokine-mediated disturbances, which include impaired bone marrow proliferation and impaired erythropoietin production. Most important effect is the shift of iron metabolism from transferrin-bound iron-available state to ferritin incorporated storage state. Poor availability of iron results in a picture of iron deficiency anemia.

Over the last few years, many investigators have come to feel that hepcidin is the central factor in producing anemia of chronic inflammation.

Hepcidin, a peptide hormone produced by the liver, is now said to be the principal regulator of systemic iron homeostasis. Hepcidin controls plasma iron concentration and tissue distribution of iron by inhibiting intestinal iron absorption, iron recycling by macrophages, and iron mobilization from hepatic stores. Hepcidin acts by inhibiting cellular iron efflux through binding to and inducing the degradation of ferroportin, the sole known cellular iron exporter. Synthesis of hepcidin is homeostatically increased by iron loading and decreased by anemia and hypoxia. Hepcidin synthesis is also elevated during infections and inflammation, causing a decrease in serum iron levels and contributing to the development of anemia of inflammation, probably as a host defense mechanism to limit the availability of iron to invading micro-organisms. Regardless of the fundamental defect, the fact is that many patients with chronic diseases cannot mobilize and utilize iron that is present in sufficient amounts in the iron stores of the body.

2. *Macrocytic Normochromic Anemia*

Deficiency of folic acid or vitamin B_{12} produces macrocytic normochromic type of anemia (MCV : ↑ : MCHC : N). As explained earlier, an interaction of both the vitamins results in production of methylenetetrahydrofolate, which is involved in the synthesis of DNA (Fig. 1.9). Deficiency of either of the two vitamins impairs DNA synthesis and thereby cell division. RNA synthesis is unaffected. Therefore, the cytoplasmic components of the cells are synthesized in excessive amounts during the delay between cell divisions. The tissues with rapid rate of cellular proliferation are most affected, e.g. bone marrow and epithelial cells of the alimentary canal.

In the bone marrow of individuals with macrocytic anemia, the developing red cells are larger than normal at each stage of development and have a characteristic non-condensed chromatin pattern. Such cells are called **megaloblasts** (cf. normoblasts). A large percentage of megaloblastic cells are destroyed before their release in to circulation. Due to this ineffective erythropoiesis, macrocytic anemia tends to be more severe than other types of deficiency anemia. Abnormalities in the development of leukocytes (giant metamyelocytes) and platelets may also be noticed. Massive destruction of immature red cells in the bone marrow liberates large amounts of the enzyme LDH.

In the peripheral blood, besides increase in mean corpuscular diameter, the red cells tend to have a large variation in size (anisocytosis) and shape (poikilocytosis). Hypersegmentation of neutrophils (10–12 lobes) may also be observed (Fig. 1.12). Total leukocyte count and platelet count are subnormal.

Impaired cell division in the epithelial tissue produces atrophy of buccal, gastric and intestinal mucosa. Consequently, glossitis, loss of appetite and diarrhea are common.

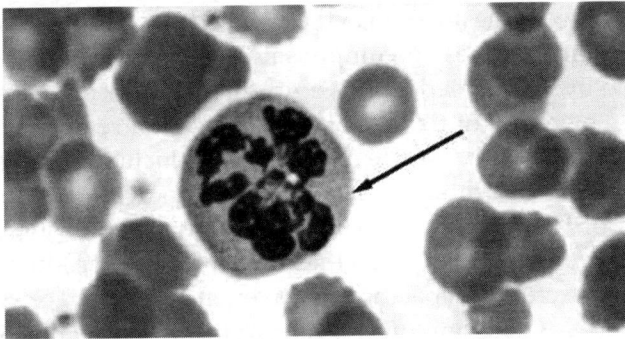

Fig. 1.12: Normochromic macrocytosis and a hypersegmented neutrophil.

The *nervous system* involvement is a characteristic feature of vitamin B_{12} deficiency. It is related to the independent role of vitamin B_{12} in the synthesis of methionine (Fig. 1.9) an essential component of myelin. The neurological damage chiefly involves white matter of dorsal and lateral columns of spinal cord, the cerebrum and peripheral nerves. These abnormalities account for paresthesias, weakness, unsteady gait and positive Romberg sign. In more severe vitamin B_{12} deficiency, spasticity, hyperreflexia, clonus and positive Babinski sign may be observed.

Addisonian pernicious anemia, because of autoimmune destruction of gastric mucosa, mostly occurs in the Western world. In tropical countries, vitamin B_{12} deficiency is usually due to intestinal malabsorption syndrome or gastric resection. On the other hand, folic acid deficiency is fairly common all over the world, especially in pregnant women. Poor people, whose diet lacks animal proteins and fresh green vegetables, are more prone to develop folic acid deficiency. Tropical sprue and gluten-induced enteropathy are other causes of folic acid deficiency. Macrocytic anemia may also develop because of interference of folic acid metabolism by alcohol, anticonvulsants or methotrexate.

3a. *Normochromic Normocytic Anemia with High Reticulocyte Count*

High reticulocyte count indicates rapid red blood cell regeneration. Two important causes are:
- Hemolytic anemia
- Acute post-hemorrhagic anemia

Hemolytic Anemia

Hemolytic type of anemia should be suspected if anemia is associated with unconjugated hyperbilirubinemia.

The life span of normal red blood cells is approximately 120 days. Due to various intracorpuscular (hereditary or congenital) or extracorpuscular (acquired) defects, the life span of the red cells may be markedly reduced. The bone marrow tries to compensate for increased rate of red cell destruction by accelerated rate of erythropoiesis. Increased reticulocyte count is an evidence of this fact. When the rate of red cell regeneration cannot keep pace with the rate of red cell destruction, anemia develops. Moreover, increased rate of red cell destruction overloads the excretory pathways of hemoglobin degradation products (bilirubin). Jaundice (hemolytic type) develops when the rate of bilirubin production exceeds the bilirubin excretory capacity of the liver. Increased red cell destruction results in increased serum LDH level, but the levels are not as high as in megaloblastic anemia. Hemolytic anemia is initially normocytic normochromic. Macrocytosis may develop if folic acid stores are exhausted by increased rate of erythropoiesis.

In patients with hemolytic anemia, decreased red cell survival can be demonstrated by radioactive chromium technique but such measurement is seldom necessary for the confirming the diagnosis of hemolytic anemia. More important task is to find out the cause of excessive rate of hemolysis. Study of red cell morphology in a peripheral blood smear often gives a clue to the cause of hemolysis. Spherocytosis is a relatively common abnormality (Fig. 1.13). Besides hereditary spherocytosis, spherocytes are commonly seen in patients with autoimmune hemolytic anemia.

Target cells with deficient hemoglobin are hallmark of thalassemia (Fig. 1.14A). Target cells well filled with hemoglobin are seen in patients with Hb C. Sickled crescent-shaped cells are hallmark of sickle cell anemia (Fig. 1.14B).

i. *Congenital (hereditary) spherocytosis*

This disorder is caused by a congenital defect in the skeleton of red cell membrane. Two important proteins, namely, spectrin and ankyrin,

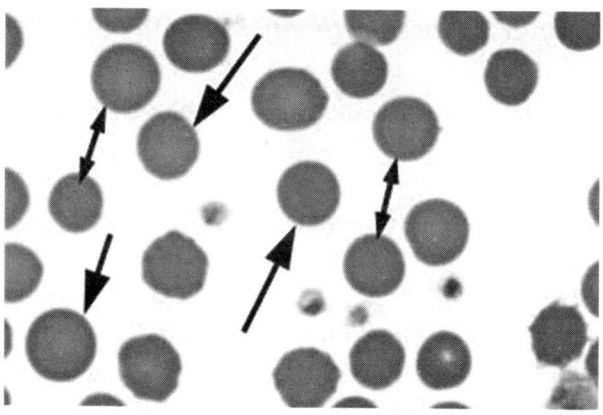

Fig. 1.13: Spherocytes—absence of normal central pallor in the red blood cells.

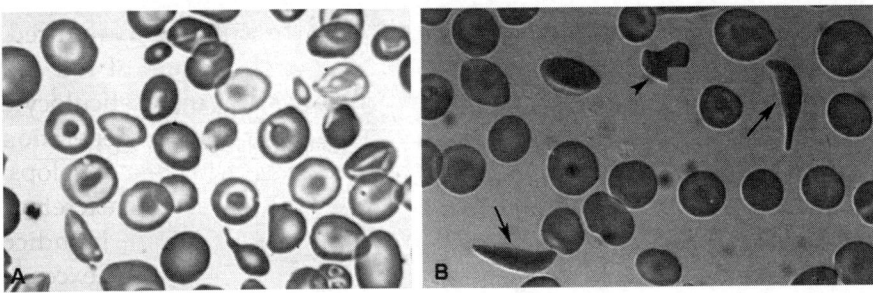

Fig. 1.14: (A) Target cells in a patient with thalassemia and (B) sickled cells (marked with arrows).

maintain the normal shape of red blood cells. A genetic defect in the synthesis of either of the two proteins results in reduced surface area to volume ratio of the red cells. The cells tend to attain a shape with smallest surface area for a given volume, i.e. a sphere. Spherical shape makes the red cells less flexible. Spherocytes cannot bend or twist during passage through narrow capillaries and hence are damaged. The spleen seems to possess a special ability to detect and trap even mildly damaged red cells. Thus, besides hemolytic anemia, splenomegaly is an important clinical feature of this disorder. The defect is inherited as an autosomal dominant trait. An important diagnostic laboratory feature is increased osmotic fragility (at 0.6–0.8% saline rather than 0.45% saline).

ii. *Glucose-6-phosphate dehydrogenase (G6PD) deficiency*

The red blood cells derive most of energy through HMP shunt mechanism of glycolysis. The shunt generates a large amount of a reducing compound called NADPH, which maintains red cell glutathione in reduced state. The reduced glutathione is essential for maintaining iron atoms of hemoglobin in ferrous (Fe^{++}) state. Glucose-6-phosphate dehydrogenase (G6PD) is the critical enzyme which pushes glucose-6-phosphate into shunt pathway (Fig. 1.15).

Most patients with G6PD deficiency do not ordinarily suffer from excessive hemolysis or anemia. However, the red cells are poorly protected against oxidants. Any exposure to oxidants results in the formation of methemoglobin (Fe^{+++}), destruction of red cell membrane and hemolysis. Such episodes of hemolysis occur during certain infections or after intake of drugs such as antimalarials (chloroquine, primaquine), sulphonamides, analgesics (aspirin) or even ingestion of certain beans.

Although the hemolysis is predominantly extravascular, intravascular hemolysis may also occur, leading to hemoglobinemia and hemoglobinuria during the hemolytic episode. G6PD deficiency is the most common human enzyme defect. The disorder is inherited as X-chromosome linked recessive trait, and hence occurs only in males. Estimation of G6PD activity in the red cells is diagnostic.

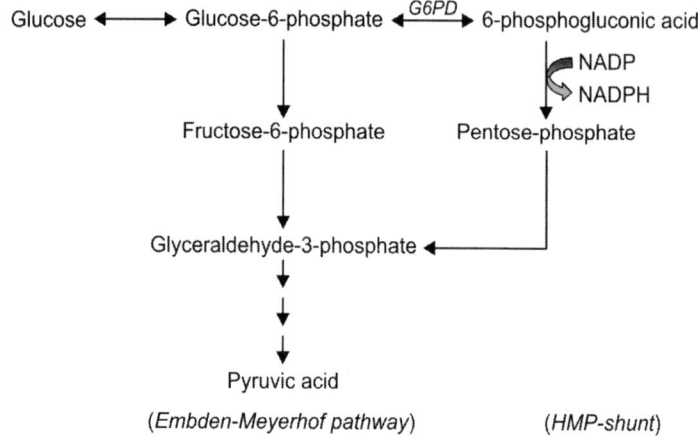

Fig. 1.15: Hexose-mono-phosphate (HMP) shunt pathway in Embden-Meyerhof pathway of glycolysis. (G6PD = Glucose-6-phosphate dehydrogenase enzyme)

iii. *Congenital disorders of hemoglobin*

There are a number of congenital defects in which the globin chains of hemoglobin are abnormal. These defects can mainly be divided into:
a. The hemoglobinopathies when there is an alteration in the amino acid sequences of a polypeptide chain of hemoglobin, e.g. Hb S, Hb C, Hb D.
b. The thalassemia in which the amino acid sequence is not disturbed but synthesis of one of the two types of chains (α or β) is impaired.

In the hemoglobinopathies, the altered amino acid sequence results in an abnormality in the solubility of hemoglobin. Consequently, there is a striking abnormality in red cell morphology, which renders the red cell more prone to hemolysis, especially in the spleen.

In thalassemia, suppression of either α or β chains results in deficient hemoglobin synthesis leading to profound hypochromia. Moreover, absence of one type of polypeptide chain results in excessive production of the other type. This results in a disturbance in hemoglobin solubility and hence excessive hemolysis.

Sickle cell anemia

This hemoglobinopathy is caused by the presence of amino acid valine instead of glutamic acid at position 6 of the β chains of hemoglobin. This variant is known as hemoglobin S (Hb S), because when deoxygenated, it polymerizes and distorts the red cell membrane in to a sickle shape or a crescent shape (Fig. 1.14B). Hb S is highly prevalent in the black population of Africa, but may be found in other countries also. Sickle cell anemia occurs in those individuals who are homozygous for Hb S gene. In such patients the entire hemoglobin is Hb S type. In individuals who are heterozygous for Hb S gene, the red cells contain Hb S (50%) as well as normal Hb A (50%). Such individuals are said to have sickle cell trait. They act as carriers for the abnormal gene but do not suffer from hemolytic anemia. Individuals with sickle cell trait are highly resistant to falciparum type of malaria.

The sickle cells are not only abnormal in shape but also less elastic than normal biconcave red cells. The abnormal morphology makes the sickle cells more prone to hemolysis as well as gives a tendency to block the capillaries. The resultant tissue hypoxia causes further sickling. The vicious cycle results in amplification of microscopic obstruction to large areas of infarction in different organs. The hypertonic and acidic environment of renal medulla is particularly prone to sickling and infarction.

In view of the pathophysiology discussed above, it would be easy to understand that sickle cell anemia is characterized by recurrent attacks of vaso-occlusive phenomenon called 'painful crises" in various parts of the body.

The thalassemia

The type of thalassemia (α or β) usually carries the name of the under-produced chain or chains. In either case, the condition may be homozygous (thalassemia major) or heterozygous (thalassemia minor). Beta-thalassemia is common in Mediterranean region, where as α thalassemia is seen in Southeast Asia. Anemia is mild in patients with thalassemia minor, but very severe in those with thalassemia major. The severe anemia becomes apparent by 4 months of age when β chains replace γ chains of fetal hemoglobin. In the deficiency of one type of polypeptide chain, the red cells develop the tetramers of the other type, making hemoglobin unfit for oxygen transport.

iv. *Acquired hemolytic anemia*
Acquired hemolytic anemia may be broadly classified into two types:
a. Immunological
b. Non-immunological

In immunological hemolytic anemia, auto-antibodies are formed against red cell membrane antigens causing inappropriate destruction of red cells. The presence of "cold antibodies" or "warm antibodies" can be detected by Combs' test.

Causes of non-immune hemolytic anemia include mechanical trauma (incompetent cardiac valves), thermal injury (burns) and infections (*Plasmodium falciparum*).

Acute Post-Hemorrhagic Anemia

When the blood loss occurs in small amounts over a prolonged period, anemia develops only when iron stores of the body are exhausted. This type of chronic blood loss produces hypochromic microcytic type of anemia. On the other hand, a large acute blood loss, whether external or internal, results in anemia which is normochromic normocytic type with high reticulocyte count. The anemia is primarily dilutional. Due to increased erythropoietic response such an anemia disappears in 6–8 weeks.

3b. Normochromic Normocytic Anemia with Normal or Low Reticulocyte Count

The anemia of chronic diseases is usually hypochromic microcytic type, but may be normochromic normocytic type. The latter type of anemia is commonly seen in patients with uremia, chronic liver disease or hypothyroidism. The anemia does not respond to hematinics but improves with improvement in the underlying disease.

4. Aplastic Anemia

It is rare but most serious type of anemia. Primarily, there is hypoplasia of bone marrow leading to pancytopenia. The diagnosis is confirmed by histologic examination of bone marrow (Fig. 1.16). Aplastic anemia may be idiopathic or secondary to drugs or radiation. However, except cytotoxic drugs, the reported association between aplastic anemia and most of the drugs (chloramphenicol, carba mazepine, phenytoin, quinine, and phenylbutazone, etc.) is based mainly on case reports but at a very low probability. As an example, chloramphenicol treatment is said to be followed by marrow aplasia in less than 1 in 40,000 treatment courses.

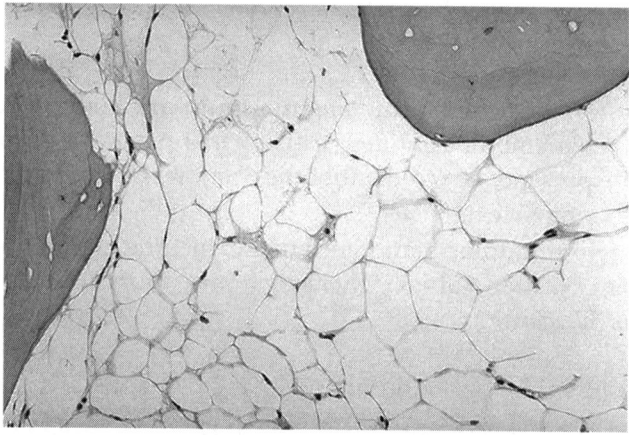

Fig. 1.16: Aplastic bone marrow

Some Special Types of Anemia
a. *Anemia in the Elderly Population*

Anemia has several consequences in the elderly. It has been associated with increased mortality, a higher incidence and more severe cardiovascular disease, cognitive impairment, decreased physical function, and an increased risk of falls and fractures. These adverse effects may be seen even in patients with mild anemia.

Contrary to a common impression, aging by itself is unlikely to lead to anemia. Cross-sectional and longitudinal studies of *healthy older individuals* have shown that the average hemoglobin levels remain stable between ages 60 and 90 years, but the incidence and prevalence of anemia increase with age. These paradoxical observations suggest that anemia in older individuals is probably due to the increased prevalence of comorbidity in this population.

Causes of anemia in the population over age 65 years are relatively few. According to an analysis of one survey 33% of anemia in older adults was due to folic acid, B_{12}, or iron deficiency alone or in combination. In another 33% cases the anemia could be attributed to chronic diseases including renal insufficiency. In the remaining 34% cases there was no apparent cause (unexplained anemia, UA).

Iron deficiency is frequently seen in the elderly and usually is a result of acute or chronic blood loss through the gastrointestinal tract. Therefore, diagnosis of iron deficiency anemia in the elderly must be followed by evaluation of the gastrointestinal tract as a possible source of bleeding. In 20 to 40 percent of patients, the source is in the upper gastrointestinal tract from peptic ulcer disease, gastritis, esophagitis or gastric cancer. The blood loss in the colon is the cause of anemia in 15 to 30 percent of cases, most often caused by colon cancer, polyps or colitis. Chronic blood loss from genitourinary tract cancer, chronic hemoptysis and bleeding disorders may result in iron deficiency but are much less common causes. Older persons may also become iron deficient because of inadequate intake or inadequate absorption of iron. Without blood loss, anemia takes several years to develop.

b. *Unexplained Anemia*

In approximately one-third cases of anemia, occurring in the elderly males or females, cannot be attributed to nutritional deficiency, inflammatory disease, or renal insufficiency. The term "unexplained anemia" (UA) is used to identify this group.

These cases seem to represent a wide array of situations including inadequate diagnostic investigations, early cases of myelodysplasia, and unrecognized renal insufficiency. Some of these cases may represent an early exhaustion of erythropoietic progenitors and inadequate erythropoietin production. The production of erythropoietin in response to anemia seems to be compromised in individuals over age 70. It is likely that an age-associated decline in androgen contributes to some extent to a decline in erythroid mass and may thus be a contributing factor to unexplained anemia.

Myelodysplasia occurs most often in older age groups. Anemia is a common feature, and early in the disease may be difficult to classify. The red blood cells are typically macrocytic and examination of the peripheral blood smear may indicate qualitative or quantitative abnormalities in white blood cells or platelets. However, bone marrow examination would be required for accurate diagnosis. At an early stage of the disorder, such cases are often labeled as UA, but in the majority of such patients, the anemia will become more severe and ultimately there will be evidence of myelodysplasia.

UA is most commonly mild, with hemoglobin levels only approximately 1 g/dL lower than the WHO standard. The red blood cells are typically of normal size and examination of the peripheral smear reveals no evidence for intravascular destruction or morphological features suggestive of myelodysplasia. Because UA is typically mild, it is likely to be overlooked. In fact, in one population-based cohort that included elderly patients with even more significant anemia, the medical records of affected individuals did not mention anemia as a problem in 75% of the cases. This casual acceptance in older populations may not be advisable. Not only can a decline in important functional measures be related to mild anemia, but longitudinal studies have demonstrated increased mortality among individuals with even mild anemia. Thus, although in younger individuals mild anemia may be well tolerated, in many older individuals, it is associated with important negative consequences.

c. Anemia of Renal Insufficiency

A progressive decline in glomerular filtration rate is the most common age-related physiologic change. In persons with comorbidities such as diabetes mellitus or hypertension, the decline may be more pronounced. It accounts for large part for the anemia associated with kidney failure. Thus, it would not be surprising if a number of older individuals experience a reduction in their ability to produce erythropoietin and developed anemia of chronic renal insufficiency.

Under normal circumstances, erythropoietin levels increase with advancing age. It may be a compensatory response to sub-clinical blood loss or increased erythropoietin resistance of red cell precursors. However, for subjects with a history of diabetes mellitus and/or hypertension, the age-associated rise in erythropoietin is either significantly less, or not existent. In fact, erythropoietin levels have been shown to be less than expected in the larger group of elderly individuals who meet criteria for UA, and this occurs even in the absence of clinically evident renal insufficiency. Reduced red blood cell survival may also occur and aggravate anemia. Anemia of renal insufficiency is normocytic and normochromic type.

Further Reading

Artz AS, Fergusson D, Drinka PJ, et al. **Mechanisms of unexplained anemia in the nursing home.** *J Am Geriatr Soc.* 2004; 52:423–7.

Batts, KP. **Iron overload syndromes and the liver.** *Modern Pathology* 2007; 20:S31–S39.

Guralnik JM, Eisenstaedt RS, et al. **Prevalence of anemia in persons 65 years and older in the United States: evidence for a high rate of unexplained anemia.** *Blood* 2004; 104:2263–68

Joosten E, Pelemans W, Hiele M, et al. **Prevalence and causes of anemia in a geriatric hospitalized population.** *Gerontology.* 1992; 38 : 111–7.

Weiss G, Goodnough LT. **Anemia of chronic disease.** *N Engl J Med.* 2005; 352:1011–23.

2
Inflammation and Repair

In unstained state, in contrast to the red blood cells, white blood cells (leukocytes) and platelets are colorless (Fig. 2.1). The generic function of leukocytes is to participate in the defense of the body against bacteria and viruses and constitute a part of the immune system. Leukocytes constitute a large group of cells; some circulating in the blood, others fixed to the tissues; some contain granules in their cytoplasm (granulocytes) others being non-granulocytes (lymphocytes, monocytes). Most of them are phagocytic (granulocytes, monocyte-macrophages, fixed tissue-macrophages,) other perform their function by releasing bactericidal globulins (B-lymphocytes).

Polymorphonuclear neutrophils are the most numerous white blood cells(50–70%, Table 2.1). Neutrophils perform their function in the tissue spaces outside the blood vessels. The average lifespan of a neutrophil in circulation is approximately 12 hours. All the time, some neutrophils are squeezing out of blood capillaries and wander around in the tissue spaces

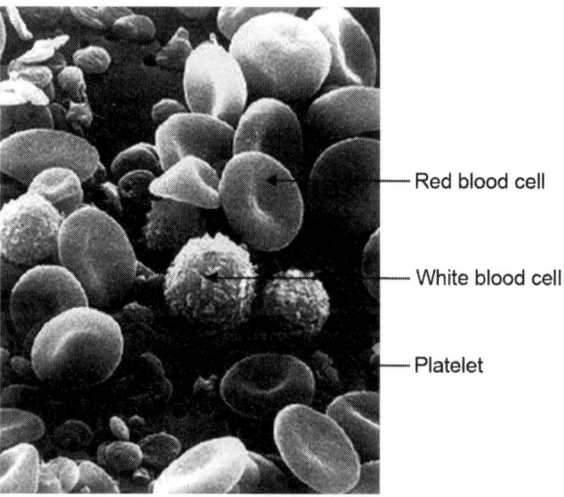

Fig. 2.1: Blood cells.

Table 2.1:	Normal values of various leukocytes		
Cell	Cell/μl (average)	Cell/μl (normla range)	% of total WBCs
Total WBCs	9000	4000–11000	—
Neutrophils	5400	3000–6000	50–70
Eosinophils	275	150–300	1–4
Basophils	35	0–100	0–1
Lymphocytes	2750	150–4000	20–40
Monocytes	540	300–600	2–8

looking for any bacterium or a foreign matter. They survive in the tissue spaces for a few days and die. Neutrophils constitute the first line of defense of tissues against foreign organisms. Within a few hours of the onset of an acute infection, the number of neutrophils in circulation increases 4–5 folds. This increase is due to mobilization of young neutrophils (band form) from storage pool of neutrophils, i.e. neutrophils already formed and stored in the bone marrow. A number of chemicals released from the area of inflammation are collectively called granulocyte-releasing factors reach the bone marrow causing release of neutrophils from the storage pool. The rate of production of granulocytes is simultaneously increased by another group of chemicals collectively called colony stimulation factors released into circulation from inflamed tissues.

Neutrophils are the primary white blood cells that respond to a bacterial infection; so the most common cause of neutrophilia is a bacterial infection, especially pyogenic infections. However, neutrophils are also increased in any acute inflammation, so their blood count will be raised after a heart attack, other infarct or burns. As neutrophil ages, its nuclear lobes increase progressively ... from band form to five lobes. During acute inflammation, the young neutrophils (band form) enter the circulation in large numbers. This is called "shift to the left" (Fig. 2.2).

Eosinophils normally present in circulation are rather a few (1–4%). However, skin and submucosa of respiratory, gastrointestinal and

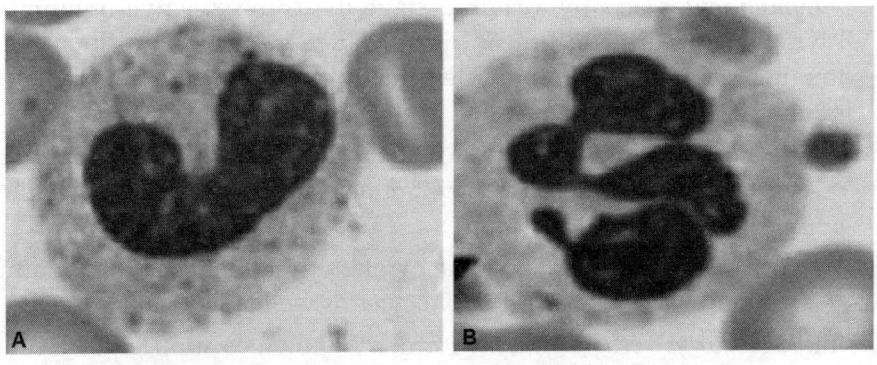

Fig. 2.2: Neutrophils—(A) young (band form); (B) mature.

genitourinary tracts contain large number of neutrophils. In these tissues, during allergic reactions, the number of eosinophils and mast cells is markedly increased and their degranulation results in tissue injury and other features of inflammatory response. In spite of intense research during the last many decades, the function of eosinophils in allergic states remains obscure. Eosinophils do not have any role in ordinary bacterial infections. Eosinophils' antiparasitic activity (on intestinal worms) is believed to be related to the presence an extremely potent toxin called major basic protein (MBP).

Basophils constitute only 0–1% of circulating leukocytes. Their exact function is not clear. Mast cells, which histologically resemble the blood basophils, are present in large numbers out side the blood capillaries in many tissues. Mast cells play an important role in allergic reactions. Immunoglobulin IgE attaches itself to the mast cells. Subsequent exposure to the specific antigen results in antigen-IgE reaction on the surface of mast cells. Degranulation of mast cells releases histamine, bradykinin, serotonin and heparin. These agents produce local manifestations of allergy.

Monocyte: Macrophages constitute the second line of defense in acute inflammatory conditions. At the site of an acute inflammation, neutrophils appear first. Macrophages appear 24–48 hours later. The monocytes circulating in the blood (10–18 μ) migrate to the tissues and undergo further differentiation. Their size may increase up to 80 μ and are then called macrophages. A macrophage contains large number of lysosomal granules and mitochondria. It shows a larger phagocytic power than a neutrophil. Some of these tissue macrophages get attached to tissue cells and remain viable for several months. Tissue macrophage system includes macrophages lining the sinusoids of liver (Kupffer's cells), spleen, lymph nodes and bone marrow. They are also present in the lungs (alveolar macrophages), bone (osteoclasts), brain (microglia) and skin (Langerhans' cells).

Lymphocytes occupy a central stage in acquired active immunity. B-lymphocytes are concerned with production of humoral immunity (immunoglobulins). T-lymphocytes, chiefly concerned with cell-mediated immunity, are of three types:

i. *Cytotoxic T-cells (T_C cells)* act as killer cells and attack cells containing viruses or mutant cells. They are also involved in the process of incompatible graft rejection.

ii. *Helper T-cells (T_H cells)* secrete cytokines that enhance the immune response of activated B-lymphocytes as well as activated T_C cells.

iii. *Regulatory T cells (T_{reg} cells)* formerly known as suppressor T cells, are crucial for the maintenance of immunological tolerance. Their major role is to shut down T cell-mediated immunity toward the end of an immune reaction.

Inflammation is the complex biological response of vascular tissues to harmful stimuli, such as pathogens, damaged cells, or irritants. Avascular tissues such as cornea, articular cartilage, intervertebral disc, etc. do not show inflammatory response. Inflammatory response is a protective attempt by the organism to remove the injurious stimuli as well as initiate the healing process. Inflammation is not a synonym for infection. Even in cases where inflammation is caused by infection, the two are not synonymous: infection is caused by an exogenous pathogen, while inflammation is the response of the organism to the pathogen.

Inflammation can be classified as either acute or chronic. *Acute inflammation* is the initial response of the body to harmful stimuli and is achieved by the increased movement of plasma and leukocytes (initially neutrophils) from the blood into the injured tissues. A cascade of biochemical events propagates and matures the inflammatory response, involving the local vascular system, the immune system, and various cells within the injured tissue. It comes to an end with in a few hours or days. Prolonged inflammation persisting for weeks or months is known as *chronic inflammation*. Whereas, neutrophil accumulation in the lesion is a hallmark of acute inflammation, chronic inflammatory lesion is characterized by the presence of lymphocytes, monocytes, macrophages and plasma cells. Another hallmark of chronic inflammation is simultaneous processes of tissue destruction and healing resulting in the formation of scar tissue. Inflammation may result from two sets of causes; exogenous and endogenous:

A. *Exogenous factors*

- *Mechanical injury* (traumatic injury)
- *Physical injury* (extremely low or high temperature, ionizing irradiation, microwaves)
- *Chemical injury* (caustic agents, poisons, venoms, etc.)
- *Biological injury* (viruses, microorganisms, protozoan and metazoan parasites)
- *Ischemic injury*

B. *Endogenous factors*

- The immunopathological responses such as *allergic* inflammations and *autoimmune* inflammatory disorders
- Endogenous products of tissue metabolism such as gout.

ACUTE INFLAMMATION

Cardinal Signs

Acute inflammation is a short-term process, usually appearing in a few minutes or hours and ceasing once the injurious stimulus has been removed. It is characterized by five cardinal signs:
- Redness
- Warmth
- Swelling
- Pain
- Loss of function

The first four (classical signs) were described by Celsus about 2000 years ago, while *loss of function* was added to the list later by Virchow in 1870. Redness and warmth are due to increased blood flow at body core temperature to the areas such as skin, which normally are at a lower temperature; swelling is caused by accumulation of fluid and plasma proteins in the extravascular spaces; pain is due to release of chemicals that stimulate pain nerve endings or sensitize them to other stimuli. Loss of function has multiple causes, chiefly pain and local edema.

These five signs appear when acute inflammation occurs on the body's surface. In case of acute inflammation of internal organs all the five signs may not be apparent.

ACUTE INFLAMMATORY RESPONSE

The acute inflammatory response may be discussed under two headings: (1) The vascular response and (2) the cellular response.

1. The Vascular Response

Alterations in the microvasculature (arterioles, capillaries and venules) of the injured tissue are the earliest response to the injury. It consists of: (a) hemodynamic changes and (b) changes in vascular permeability.

a. *Hemodynamic Changes*

i. Transient vasoconstriction of the arterioles and reduced blood flow is the immediate response irrespective of the type of injury. It usually lasts only a few seconds but may be prolonged up to five minutes if the injury is very severe. It is followed by:

ii. Persistent and progressive vasodilatation, which begins in the arterioles and spreads to the capillaries and venules as well. This change becomes prominent within an hour of injury. Vasodilatation results in increased blood flow to the microvasculature and accounts for the clinical signs of redness and warmth. Vasodilatation is brought about by the release of vasodilator mediators by the injured tissue cells as well by the blood cells attracted by the injury.

iii. Transudation of fluid into the extra-cellular space (edema) is another consequence of vasodilatation. Starling forces, chiefly capillary hydrostatic pressure and plasma protein oncotic pressure, govern the tissue fluid exchange across the capillary wall. It involves tissue fluid formation at the proximal segment of the capillary followed by reabsorption in the distal segment. Vasodilatation, by increasing the capillary hydrostatic pressure shifts the balance of the Starling forces in favor of greater exudation and decreased reabsorption. Thus, local edema results.

iv. Stasis. Loss of fluid from the capillaries leads to increased viscosity of blood flowing through the capillaries, with resultant *stasis* due to the increase in the concentration of the cells within blood. Stasis allows leukocytes to marginate along the endothelium, a process critical to their recruitment into the tissues. Normal flowing blood prevents this, as the shearing force along the periphery of the vessels moves blood cells into the middle of the vessel. Nutritional supply to the tissue may be so compromised that it may become ischemic, even necrotic.

b. *Increased Vascular Permeability*

All the blood vessels are lined by a continuous layer of endothelial cells, which provide a passive diffusion barrier. It permits free diffusion of water and solutes but restricts the movement of larger molecules such as plasma proteins and cellular components of blood. The endothelial cells are joined together by tight junctions. In inflammatory conditions, the excessive fluid transferred into extracellular space consists not only of usual water and solutes (called *transudate*), but also contains a high concentration of plasma proteins. Such a fluid is called an *exudate*. The exudate is formed because of markedly increased vascular permeability. The causes of increased vascular permeability include the following:

1. Opening of endothelial intercellular tight junctions, particularly in the post-capillary venules due to contraction of endothelial cells. It is mediated by release of histamine, bradykinin and other chemical mediators of inflammation. This response begins immediately after injury usually lasts for a short duration (15–30 minutes).

2. Direct injury to endothelial cells results in necrosis and appearance of physical gaps at the site of detached endothelial cells. This type of increased permeability lasts for hours or even days.

3. Endothelial injury is also mediated by leukocytes. Margination followed by leukocyte adhesion may result in activation of leukocytes.

The activated leucocytes release proteolytic enzymes and toxic free radicals which cause endothelial injury and increased vascular leakiness.

4. The capillaries, newly formed during the process of repair, are excessively leaky.

Mediators of Increased Vascular Permeability

The primary source of vasoactive mediators of increased permeability during an inflammatory process are derived from injured tissue cells as well as plasma (Fig. 2.3)

2. The Cellular Response

Inflammatory response, which lasts more than a few hours, is characterized by accumulation of white blood cells within the area of injury. In bacterial infections, physical or thermal injury, polymorphonuclear neutrophils are first to arrive ("first line of defense"). Twenty-four to forty-eight hours later, large number of macrophages can be seen in the inflamed area. In allergic inflammation, eosinophils and mast cells predominate. In viral infections, lymphocytes are first to arrive.

A. *Polymorphonuclear Neutrophils and Monocyte Macrophages*

The accumulation of neutrophils and monocytes macrophages at the site of inflammation is due to the presence of locally generated chemical mediators called chemotactic factors.

i. *Chemotaxis:* The chemotactic-mediated transmigration of leukocytes involves initial crossing of several barriers (endothelial basement

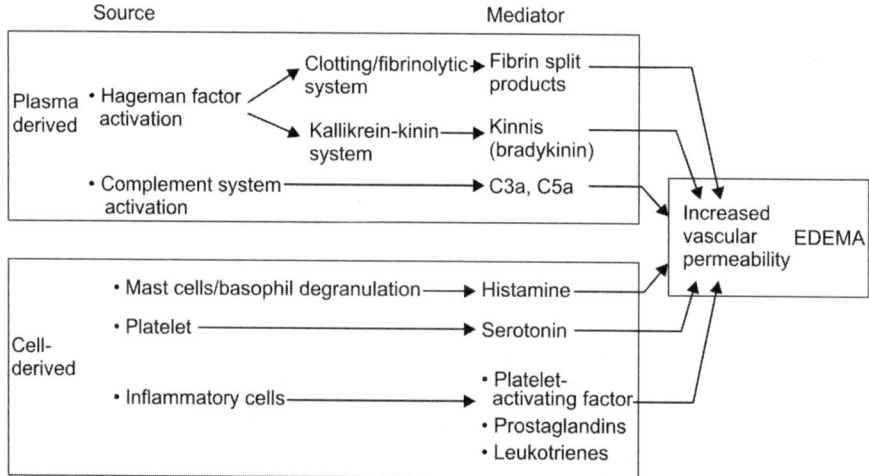

Fig. 2.3: Vasoactive mediators of increased vascular permeability during inflammation.

membrane and matrix), followed by transport in the interstitial fluid to the inflamed area. The process is called chemotaxis. The chemical agents which act as potent chemotactic agents include leukotrienes, platelet factor, components of complement system (C5a in particular), cytokines (IL–8 in particular), soluble bacterial products, monocyte chemo-attractant protein and eotaxin factor (for eosinophils). There is an increasing concentration gradient of chemotactic agents between an adjacent blood capillary the site of inflammation and leukocyte migration follows the gradient (Fig. 2.4).

ii. *Margination:* This is the first step towards transmigration of leukocytes out of the blood capillaries. Normal blood flow is characterized by an axial stream of red cells, leukocytes and platelets and a peripheral cell-free layer of plasma close to the vessel wall. Due to slowing of blood flow and stasis, the central stream of cells widens and blood cells including leukocytes come closer to the vessel wall. This phenomenon is known as margination.

iii. *Adhesion:* Marginated leukocytes tend to stick briefly to the endothelial cells or roll over them. Injury leads to neutralization of the normal charge on the leukocytes and endothelial cells, resulting in a loose transient adhesion of leukocytes to the endothelial cells.

iv. *Emigration (diapedesis):* During chemotactic response, there is a characteristic change in the morphological orientation of the leukocyte (neutrophil or monocyte). It loses its classical rounded appearance and becomes wedge-shaped. At first, the leading edge passes into the space between two adjacent endothelial cells, damaging the basement membrane and passes out of the vessel wall. By amoeboid movements, rear part of the cell containing lysosomal granules and lastly the nucleus leaves the blood vessel.

v. *Phagocytosis:* Neutrophils and macrophages have an inherent capacity to recognize and engulf foreign particles. Coating of the bacteria by plasma proteins containing IgG and/or complement (opsonization) renders them more liable to phagocytosis. When a neutrophil or a macrophage becomes bound to a bacterium (or a foreign particle), there is a localized contraction of the cell under the point of contact, resulting in the formation of a cup-shaped invagination. Through the pseudopodia thrown out at the margins of the cups, the bacterium, enclosed in a vacuole, is internalized into

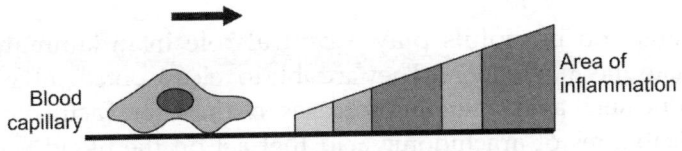

Fig. 2.4: Chemotaxis.

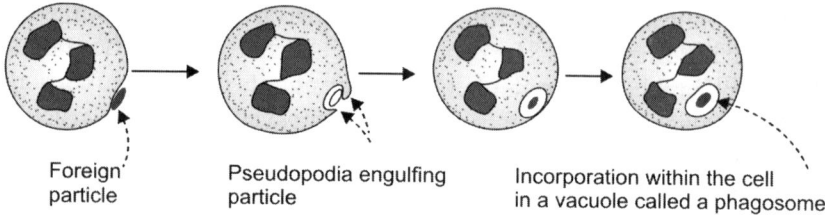

Fig. 2.5: The process of phagocytosis.

the phagocyte and called a **phagosome** (Fig. 2.5). Movement of the phagosome towards the granule-rich areas of the cytoplasm results in fusion of phagosome to an adjacent lysosome. Next, the lysosomal granules are discharged into the phagosome. This phenomenon is known as *degranulation*. The lysosomal membrane is incorporated into the vacuole membrane. The resulting structure is called a **phagolysosome**. Generally, the release of lysosomal granules is restricted to the phagolysosome. However, when the phagosome formation occurs in a granule-rich area or the phagocyte attempts to engulf too large a particle, lysosomal granules may be discharged into extracellular space causing damage to the host tissue cells in the vicinity.

vi. *Bacterial killing and digestion:* This is the ultimate objective of phagocytosis. Anti-microbial agents act by the following two mechanisms:

Oxygen-dependent bactericidal mechanisms: Degranulation is accompanied by activation of two enzymes present in the leukocyte granules, namely NADPH-oxidase and myeloperoxidase. Activation of NADPH-oxidase is associated with a sharp increase in oxygen consumption in the leukocyte (the respiratory burst) leading to generation of highly toxic superoxide (O_2^-) and hydrogen peroxide (H_2O_2). Myeloperoxidase catalyzes the formation of highly toxic hypochlorous acid (HClO).

Oxygen-independent bactericidal mechanisms: Lysosomal granules contain a number of agents which do not require oxygen for their bactericidal activity. These agents include lysosomal hydrolases, permeability increasing factor, defensins, lysozyme and cationic protein.

B. *Mast Cells/Basophils*

Mast cells and basophils play a central role in inflammatory and immediate allergic reactions. They are able to release potent inflammatory mediators, such as histamine, proteases, chemotactic factors, cytokines and metabolites of arachidonic acid that act on the blood capillaries, smooth muscle, connective tissue, mucous glands and inflammatory cells.

Both mast cells and basophils contain special *cytoplasmic granules* which store mediators of inflammation. The extracellular release of the mediators from the mast cells (*degranulation*) may be induced by:

a. Physical destruction, such as high temperature, mechanical trauma, ionizing irradiation, etc.
b. Chemical substances, such as toxins, venoms, proteases
c. Endogenous mediators, including tissue proteases, cationic proteins derived from eosinophils and neutrophils
d. Immune mechanisms which may be IgE-dependent or IgE-independent

The increase in the number of mast cells and basophils, and the enhanced secretion at sites of inflammation, can accelerate the elimination of the cause of tissue injury or, paradoxically, may lead to a chronic inflammatory response. Thus, manipulating mast-cell and basophil adhesion may be an important strategy for controlling the outcome of allergic and inflammatory responses.

C. Eosinophils

Eosinophil is a leukocyte that resides predominantly in submucosal tissue and is recruited to sites of specific immune reactions, including allergic diseases. **The large specific granules** contain four distinct cationic proteins which exert a range of biological effects on host cells and microbial targets: *major basic protein* (MBP), *eosinophil cationic protein* (ECP), *eosinophil derived neurotoxin* (EDN), and *eosinophil peroxidase* (EPO). In addition, histaminase and a variety of hydrolytic lysosomal enzymes are also present in the large specific granules. These proteins have major effects not only on the potential role of eosinophils in host defense against helminthic parasites, but also in contributing to tissue dysfunction and damage in eosinophil related inflammatory and allergic diseases. Compared to neutrophils, eosinophils have limited phagocytic activity which is mainly aimed at killing multicellular parasites. Another possible beneficial function of eosinophils is the *inactivation* of mediators of anaphylaxis.

Systemic Effects of Acute Inflammation

1. **Fever** is due to release of interleukin 1 (a cytokine), prostaglandins or tumor necrosis factor from the inflammatory tissues, either of which can disturb the hypothalamic temperature regulating center. Fever may also be induced by certain constituents in the cell wall of dead bacteria called pyrogens
2. **Leukocytosis** is a feature of infections or even non-infectious inflammations. Typically, the total leukocyte count is between 15,000 and 20,000/µL. Usually, in bacterial infections, leukocytosis is due to neutrophilia; in viral infections due to lymphocytosis; and in allergic conditions due to eosinophilia. Some infections, e.g. typhoid fever,

however, are associated with leucopenia (neutropenia with relative lymphocytosis).

3. *Lymhangitis-lymphadenitis* in the lymph vessels and lymph nodes draining the area of inflammation is commonly seen. These responses represent either a non-specific reaction to chemical mediators released into the inflamed tissues or an immunological response to foreign antigen.

4. *Acute phase proteins.* Acute inflammation is commonly accompanied by increased concentrations of several plasma proteins such as C-reactive protein, alpha-2 macroglobulin, and fibrinogen (collectively called **acute phase proteins**). Precise function of these proteins in inflammation is largely unclear. However, when measured in the laboratory, they can serve as useful markers of inflammation. These proteins also increase the **erythrocyte sedimentation rate (ESR)**, a *nonspecific* indicator of inflammation. Finally, prolonged or widespread inflammation can deplete complement leading to decreased levels of certain components of complement in the serum.

5. *Other symptoms* such as decreased appetite, lactacidosis, negative nitrogen balance and increased slow-wave sleep are commonly seen in acute infections. Most of these seem to be produced interleukin 1.

6. *Shock* may develop in severe acute inflammatory conditions. Tumor necrosis factor (TNF α), a cytokine, is one of the mediators of acute inflammation. Bacteremia/septicemia may result in the release of a massive amount of TNF α leading to wide-spread vasodilatation and increased vascular permeability. These changes lead to intravascular volume loss, hypotension and circulatory shock. Microthrombi may be formed throughout the body which may lead to disseminated intravascular coagulation (DIC), bleeding and death.

Outcomes of acute inflammation: The acute inflammatory response may have one of the following four outcomes depending on whether or not injury results in significant tissue loss or the inflammatory stimulus is rapidly removed: (1) resolution, (2) healing, (3) suppuration, or 4) chronic inflammation.

1. *Resolution:* Such an outcome follows complete removal of the agent or micro-organism that triggered the inflammatory response. The process includes the removal of any injured (necrotic) host cells. This is the ideal outcome for acute inflammation. It is more likely if cellular damage has been minimal, e.g. resolution of lobar pneumonia.

2. *Healing may involve two processes:*
   i. **Regeneration:** The replacement of damaged or lost tissue by normal tissue of a similar type. It occurs only in tissues that contain cells

capable of dividing (e.g. epithelial tissues such as the epidermis of the skin).

ii. **Repair:** *Scar formation, fibrosis.* It involves replacement of damaged or lost tissue by collagen fibers (scar tissue). This is the healing mechanism for those tissues that cannot regenerate (dermis, nerve, muscle, etc.).

3. **Suppuration and abscess formation:** If there has been a large amount of cellular necrosis, or if there is a great deal of bacterial contamination, exudates and dead leukocytes (pus) can accumulate forming an abscess. In time, connective tissue walls off the abscess and limits its spread. Resolution and healing cannot take place until adequate drainage of the abscess has been provided.

4. **Chronic inflammation:** Normally, the acute inflammatory response to cellular injury has subsided by the time tissue healing begins. If tissue destruction is prolonged, inflammation and attempts at healing occur at the same time. This produces the picture of chronic inflammation.

Mechanism of Final Resolution of Acute Inflammation

Acute inflammation normally resolves by mechanisms that have remained somewhat elusive. Emerging evidence now suggests that an active, coordinated program of resolution is initiated in the first few hours after an inflammatory response begins. After entering tissues, granulocytes promote the switch of arachidonic acid-derived prostaglandins and leukotrienes to lipoxins, which initiate the termination sequence. Neutrophil recruitment thus ceases and programmed death by apoptosis is engaged. Consequently, apoptotic neutrophils undergo phagocytosis by macrophages, leading to neutrophil clearance and release of anti-inflammatory and reparative cytokines such as transforming growth factor-β_1. The anti-inflammatory program ends with the departure of macrophages through the lymphatics.

Allergic Inflammation

An allergic reaction is the result of an inappropriate immune response triggering inflammation. A common example is hay fever, which is caused by a hypersensitive response by skin mast cells to allergens. Presensitized mast cells respond by degranulation, releasing vasoactive chemicals such as histamine. These chemicals propagate an excessive inflammatory response characterized by blood vessel dilation, production of proinflammatory molecules, cytokine release, and recruitment of leukocytes. Severe inflammatory response may mature into a systemic response known as anaphylaxis.

CHRONIC INFLAMMATION

Chronic inflammation occurs when the damaging stimulus persists and the process of *continuing tissue necrosis, organization, and repair all occur concurrently*. In addition to acute inflammation, the specific defenses of the immune system are activated around the area of damage, and tissues are infiltrated by activated lymphoid cells.

The chronic inflammatory tissue shows:
- Necrotic cell debris
- Acute inflammatory exudate
- Vascular and fibrous granulation tissue
- Lymphoid cells
- Macrophages
- Collagenous scar

Chronic inflammation may be caused by one of the following three mechanisms:

i. *Chronic inflammation following an acute inflammation:* When tissue destruction is extensive or bacteria survive and persist at the site of inflammation, e.g. osteomyelitis or pneumonia leading to a lung abscess.

ii. *Recurrent attacks of acute inflammation:* Repeated attacks of acute inflammation may culminate in chronicity of the disease process, e.g. pyelonephritis resulting from recurrent attacks of urinary tract infection, or repeated attacks of acute cholecystitis culminating in chronic cholecystitis

iii. *Chronic inflammation starting de novo:* In such cases, the inflammatory agent produces a chronic inflammatory response to begin with.

General Features of Chronic Inflammation

Ordinarily, agents that produce an acute inflammatory response are removed by the neutrophils and macrophages by phagocytosis and digestion. However, certain agents cannot be removed by acute inflammatory response, e.g. *Mycobacterium tuberculosis*, fungus or a suture. The mechanism of dealing with such indigestible agents is termed chronic or granulomatous inflammation. Chronic inflammation response primarily serves to contain the pathological process, as well as, to remove the offending agent, if possible. Though, chronic inflammatory responses may somewhat differ in detail, depending on the offending agent, the following features are common to all chronic inflammations: (A) mononuclear cell infiltration, (B) tissue destruction and necrosis, and (C) proliferative changes.

A. Mononuclear Cell Infiltration

i. *Macrophages:* The macrophages comprise the most important cells in chronic inflammation. These cells are recruited by chemotactic migration from the circulation as well as by local proliferation. Activated macrophages release several biologically active substances such as neutral and acid proteases, oxygen-derived reactive metabolites and cytokines. These agents bring about tissue destruction, neovascularization and fibrosis. Chronic inflammatory lesions usually show some other chronic inflammatory cells:

ii. *Lymphocytes:* These cells are a prominent feature of chronic inflammatory lesion. They perform vital functions both in cell-mediated and humoral immune responses. The T-lymphocytes function not only as cytotoxic killer cells but also regulate macrophage recruitment and activation through secretion of lymphokines (cytokines) and modulate antibody production.

iii. *Plasma cells:* These cells are also usually present in a chronic inflammatory lesion. Plasma cells are immune-activated B-lymphocytes rich in cytoplasmic reticulum. These cells are the primary source of antibodies specific to the antigen present at the site of chronic lesion.

B. Tissue Destruction

It is one of the important features of most of the chronic inflammatory responses. As mentioned above, it is brought about by several biologically active substances released by activated macrophages.

C. Proliferative Changes

Summary of differences between acute inflammation and chronic inflammation	
Acute inflammation	Chronic inflammation
Abrupt injury	Persistent injury
Onset is well-defined	Vague onset
Prominent symptoms	Symptoms often subdued, and /or insidious
Prominent vascular effects and exudate	Mild tissue effects
Exudate rich in neutrophils	Exudate rich in lymphocytes and macrophages
Connective tissue proliferation occurs after inflammation subsides	Connective tissue proliferation is concurrent with on-going inflammation

As a result of necrosis, proliferation of small blood vessels is stimulated. Eventually, collagen is laid down and healing by fibrosis occurs.

Further Reading

Kumar V, et al. **Robbins and Cotran Pathologic Basis of Disease:** Elsevier Health Sciences 2009.

Ryan GB, Majno G. **Acute inflammation. A review.** Am J Pathol. 1977 ; 86:183–276.

3
Disorders of Hemostasis

HEMOSTASIS

When a blood vessel is injured, a number of mechanisms operate to minimize and ultimately arrest bleeding. Hemostatic events may be summarized as the following five overlapping steps:

1. Initial constriction of injured blood vessel
2. Formation of a platelet plug
3. Humoral facilitation of vasoconstriction
4. Coagulation of blood
5. Ultimate fibrous tissue growth into the blood clot permanently sealing the breach in the vessel wall

The clot is finally removed by proteolytic enzymes (fibrinolysis).

Formation of Platelet Plug (Primary Hemostasis)

When the platelets come in contact with the damaged endothelial lining of the blood vessel and particularly with the collagen fibers exposed in the blood vessel wall, a series of changes occur in the platelets. The platelets begin to swell up and assume an irregular shape. A number of processes protrude from their surface and become very sticky. Consequently the platelets stick to the collagen fibers and secrete large quantities of ADP and a prostaglandin, thromboxane-A, which activates other platelets in the blood, making them sticky as well. The activated sticky platelets tend to aggregate and form a platelet plug which may close the opening in the vascular wall. In day-to-day life, numerous small leaks tend to occur in the capillaries but are immediately dealt with by the platelet plugs. Because the platelet plug is basically soft, it is not able to stop bleeding from a large leak in the blood vessels. In that case also, activated platelets play an equally important role in the process of coagulation of blood and clot retraction.

Coagulation of Blood (Secondary Hemostasis)

In this process, a soluble plasma protein fibrinogen is converted into a gel like insoluble protein fibrin. Fibrin is laid down as highly adhesive long threads in the form of a network. These fibrin threads not only stick to one another but also to the adjacent vascular wall forming an efficient plug in the vascular opening. Erythrocytes, leukocytes and platelets are also entrapped in the fibrin threads. Within minutes, the clot contracts, making the clot a very firm bung which stops bleeding from the injured vessel permanently.

MECHANISM OF COAGULATION (Fig. 3.1)

Step 1: Generation of prothrombin activator

In spite of the presence of all the clotting factors in the blood, the blood does not clot spontaneously, unless a vessel wall has been injured. This is due to the fact that normally all the factors are present in an inactive form and therefore, prothrombin activator is absent from the blood. Moreover, the blood contains small amounts of naturally occurring anticoagulants.

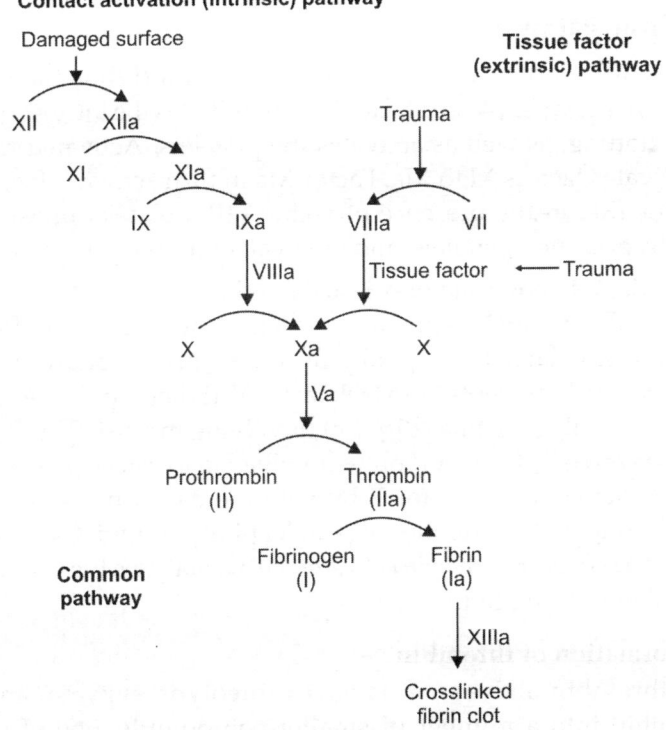

Fig. 3.1: Steps of coagulation

In short, clotting occurs only when the blood contains prothrombin activator.

Prothrombin activator is formed by a cascade of reactions in which activation of one factor leads to activation of the next clotting factor. This sequence of changes can occur in two pathways, the extrinsic pathway, and the intrinsic pathway, each ultimately leading to the generation of prothrombin activator (Fig. 3.1). Both pathways begin when a blood vessel is injured and bleeding has occurred. The reactions of extrinsic system are initiated by a factor called tissue-thromboplastin *released by the injured tissues around the vessel wall*. The intrinsic system is initiated by activation of a factor (XII), *present in the plasma itself*, by the vascular injury.

The Extrinsic Pathway

In the extrinsic pathway, the injured tissue releases several substances which are together known as tissue thromboplastin (or tissue factor or factor III). They include phospholipids from the cell membrane and a glycoprotein. The tissue factor combines with factor VII. Next, tissue factor—factor VII complex, in the presence of Ca^{++} activates factor X to factor Xa. The steps subsequent to the activation of factor X are common to extrinsic and intrinsic pathways.

The Intrinsic Pathway

Exposure of blood to the collagen fibers underlying the vascular endothelium activates plasma factor XII and initiates the intrinsic pathway of blood clotting, as well as activates the platelets. Activated factor XII [XIIa] activates factors XI to XIa. Factor XIa in turn activates factors IX to IXa. Factor IXa, in the presence of factor VIIIa, platelet-phospholipids released by activated platelets, and ionic calcium, convert factors X to Xa.

As mentioned above, factor X is activated by tissue factor—factor VII complex in the extrinsic pathway, as well as by factor IXa along with factor VIIIa and platelet phospholipids in the intrinsic pathway. Serious bleeding occurs in patients who lack factor VIII (hemophilia-A) or factor IX (hemophilia-B, Christmas disease) (involving intrinsic pathway) only or in those who lack factor VII only (involved in extrinsic pathway). This shows that activation of factor X by both the pathways is essential for normal clotting. In the presence of platelet phospholipid, Ca^{2+} and factor Va, *factor Xa acts as prothrombin activator,* i.e. it catalyzes the conversion of prothrombin to thrombin.

Step 2: **Formation of thrombin**
The prothrombin activator acts as a proteolytic enzyme, and splits prothrombin into a number of smaller compounds, one of which is thrombin.

$$\text{Prothrombin} \xrightarrow[\text{Ca}^{++}]{\text{Prothrombin activator}} \text{Thrombin}$$

Step 3: **Formation of fibrin threads**

$$\text{Fibrinogen} \xrightarrow{\text{Thrombin}} \text{Fibrin monomers} \xrightarrow[\text{Polymerization}]{\text{XIIIa, Ca}^{++}} \text{Fibrin threads}$$

Thrombin, acting as a proteolytic enzyme removes four low molecular weight peptides from each molecule of fibrinogen to form a fibrin monomer. Fibrin monomers tend to polymerize spontaneously. But the process is catalyzed by another plasma factor called fibrin stabilizing factor (activated factor XIII). Thrombin activates factor XIII also. In the presence of Ca^{++}, factor XIIIa causes formation of covalent cross-linkages between fibrin threads. Thus, a dense meshwork of fibrin threads is formed, which traps the remaining components of plasma as well as the blood cells to form a solid mass called the blood clot. The blood clot becomes adherent to the injured vascular walls, plugging it permanently.

Natural Anticlotting Mechanisms

Normally, the flowing blood does not clot in the blood vessels. Even after injury to a blood vessel, the clot is limited to the area of bleeding and does not extend inside the vessel. Obviously, some mechanisms operate in the circulation which prevent intravascular clotting. Some of the known anticlotting mechanisms are as follows:

1. **Smoothness of normal intact endothelial linings** is one of the most important factors. The intrinsic or extrinsic clotting pathways cannot be initiated as long as the endothelium is not injured.
2. **Heparin** is a powerful anticoagulant but its concentration in the normal circulation is so low that its independent physiological role is doubtful. However, the circulating heparin may supplement the activity of antithrombin-III.
3. **Antithrombin-III** is probably the most important anticoagulant in the normal circulation. It is an α-globulin. It inhibits thrombin, factor Xa and IXa. Its activity is markedly enhanced by combination with heparin.
4. **Protein C** is another natural anticoagulant present in the plasma. As such, it is inactive. It is activated by exposure to thrombin formed during clotting. Thrombin interacts with an endothelial modulator to activate protein C. Activated protein C inhibits factors Va and VIIa.

$$\text{Endothelial cells} \longrightarrow \text{Thrombomodulin} \searrow \xrightarrow{\text{Thrombin}}$$
$$\text{Protein C} \longrightarrow \text{Activated protein C}$$

5. Some of the activated intermediates of the process of coagulation enter the circulation but are quickly removed by the **macrophages** in the liver and elsewhere.
6. The **fast velocity of blood flow** in larger blood vessels in itself prevents coagulation. Slowing of blood flow is one of the important contributory factors in genesis of intravascular blood clotting (thrombosis).

Fibrinolytic System

$$\text{Plasminogen} \xrightarrow[\text{Plasminogen activator}]{\text{Thrombin}} \text{Plasmin}$$

$$\text{Fibrin} \xrightarrow{\text{Plasmin}} \text{Fibrin degradation products (FDPs)}$$

Following a vascular injury and clot formation, the discontinuity of the vessel wall is gradually repaired by proliferation of adjacent fibroblasts, smooth muscle cells and endothelial cells. The clot, no more required, is gradually dissolved by degradation of fibrin into small soluble fragments called fibrin-degradation products (FDPs). The phenomenon, called *fibrinolysis*, is a normal secondary response in hemostasis. The dissolution of clot occurs by the action of a proteolytic enzyme, plasmin, activated in the clot. Normal plasma contains a protein plasminogen (mol.wt. 92,000) synthesized in the liver. Cleavage of a single peptide bond converts plasminogen into an active proteolytic enzyme called plasmin. The cleavage of plasminogen into plasmin can occur under the effect of (i) thrombin, or (ii) plasminogen activator.

When a clot is formed, plasminogen is also incorporated in it. Thrombin formed during the process of clotting slowly begins to convert plasminogen into plasmin. Moreover, the deposition of fibrin within the vessel wall gives rise to stimuli which trigger the release of plasminogen activator from the endothelial cells. Plasmin system plays a role not only in (i) dissolution of a blood clot but also in (ii) tissue remodeling in inflammation, (iii) ovulation and (iv) mechanisms by which tumor cells invade a tissue.

Fibrin degradation product (FDPs), also known as fibrin split products, are components of the blood produced by clot degradation. These are produced by the action of plasmin on deposited fibrin. The most notable subtype of fibrin degradation products is D-dimer (Fig. 3.2). The levels of FDPs rise after any thrombotic event. Estimation of plasma D-dimer concentration is used as a laboratory test in the diagnosis of disseminated intravascular coagulation.

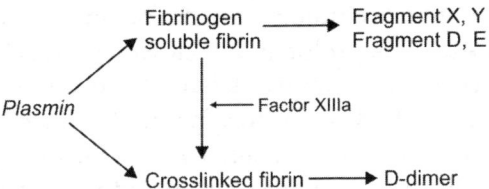

Fig. 3.2: Actions of plasmin.

Physiological Basis of Tests of Hemostasis

1. Tests of Primary Hemostasis

Bleeding time

Prolonged bleeding time is a characteristic feature of a defect in primary hemostasis (purpura). The result of this test is highly operator-dependent. Bleeding time extimation is performed by measuring the duration required for bleeding to stop from a fresh superficial cut (1 mm deep, 1 cm long) made on the volar surface of the forearm. The cessation of bleeding results from the formation of a primary hemostatic plug. Bleeding time is prolonged with platelet counts below 75,000/µL, although that finding provides no insight into reason the count is low.

Platelet Count

Platelet count helps to differentiate the thrombocytopenic and non-thrombocytopenic types of purpura. Platelet count is also low in cases with disseminated intravascular coagulation.

2. Tests of Secondary Hemostasis

Estimation of clotting time is an undependable test of secondary hemostasis. Instead, a battery of laboratory tests is used to evaluate different aspects of secondary hemostasis.

Activated Partial Thromboplastin Time (aPTT)

This is a simple test of intrinsic pathway of coagulation. To the citrated plasma of the patient is added a mixture of kaolin (which activates factor XII), Ca^{++}, and a phospholipid. Clot formation occurs at normal rate if all the factors of the *intrinsic* pathway and the *common pathway* (Fig. 3.1) are present in normal concentrations. This test is more sensitive to deficiency of factor VIII and factor IX.

Prothrombin Time (PT)

This is a test for the extrinsic system of coagulation. In this test, tissue thromboplastin derived from the brain (tissue factor, Factor III) and Ca^{++}

are added to the patient's citrated plasma. The time taken for the mixture to clot is estimated. PT is prolonged in cases with a defect in any of the factors involved in the extrinsic system and common pathway of coagulation (Factors VII, X, V, prothrombin, and fibrinogen) (Fig. 3.1). If both aPTT and PT are prolonged, deficiency of factors X, V or II exists. If aPTT is prolonged, but PT is normal, bleeding can be attributed to deficiency of factor VIII or IX. If aPTT is normal, but PT is prolonged, congenital deficiency of factor VII exists. Patients on oral anticoagulant therapy also show normal aPTT and prolonged PT.

Specific Coagulant Factors

After initial screening by aPTT and PT, concentration of a specific coagulant factor can be investigated by bioassay.

Thrombin Time (TT)

This is a test for final conversion of fibrinogen to fibrin. This test bypasses both the intrinsic and extrinsic pathways, because thrombin is added to the patient's citrated plasma. TT is prolonged in cases with

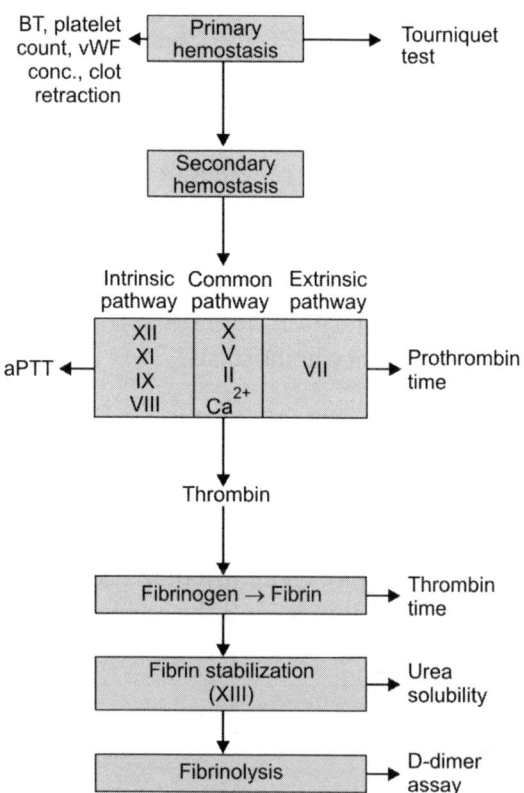

Fig. 3.3: Physiological basis of various tests of hemostasis.

hypofibrinogenemia or those suffering from disseminated intravascular coagulation (DIC).

Fibrin Degradation Products (FDPs) Assay, D-dimer Assay

Assay of both FDPs and D-dimer help to evaluate the status of the fibrinolytic system. FDPs assay is a measurement of all of the fragments of clot dissolution, while D-dimer is a more specific measurement for one of the crosslinked, breakdown fragments. This a diagnostic investigation in of DIC. The D-dimer assay has replaced measurement of FDPs as the preferred assay owing to the greater specificity of D-dimer assays for detecting fibrinolysis versus fibrinogenolysis (Fig. 3.2). In addition, the detection of circulating D-dimer has greater sensitivity for the diagnosis of DIC. A positive D-dimer result indicates the presence of an abnormally high level of fibrin degradation products. It shows that there may be significant thrombus formation and break down. It may be due to, for example, a venous thromboembolism (VTE) or DIC. Typically, the D-dimer level is markedly elevated in DIC. When used to monitor DIC treatment, decreasing levels indicate good prognosis.

BLEEDING DISORDERS

Bleeding disorders can be broadly classified into two categories:
i. Bleeding disorders caused by a defect in the **primary hemostasis**: Such disorders are collectively called purpura. In purpura, bleeding occurs in the skin or mucous membranes of nose, gastrointestinal tract or genitourinary tract either spontaneously or immediately after a relatively minor trauma. Characteristic physical examination findings are petechiae, purpura or ecchymoses. Petechiae are pinpoint hemorrhages (< 2 mm) in the skin, and purpura (0.2–1 cm) and ecchymoses are larger hemorrhages. Primary hemostatic disorders are characterized by prolonged bleeding time (Fig. 3.4).

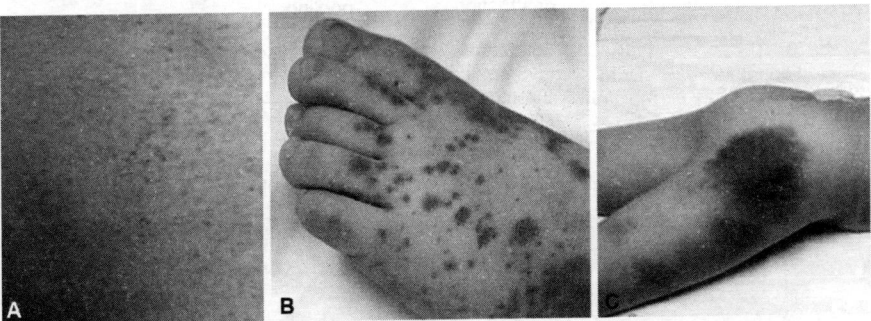

Fig. 3.4: Disorders of primary hemostasis: (A) Petechiae; (B) purpura; (C) ecchymoses.

ii. Bleeding disorders caused by a defect in **secondary hemostasis** (defect in process of coagulation). In this case bleeding occurs several hours or even days after an injury, when the effect of (normal) primary hemostatic mechanisms wanes. Such bleeding mostly occurs in deep tissues like muscles, joints. Characteristic clinical findings are hemarthroses and muscle hematomas.

Purpura

Basically purpura may result from a deficiency of platelets in the blood (thrombocytopenic purpura) or some other causes (nonthrombocytopenicic purpura). **This classification helps in differential diagnosis of purpura** (Fig. 3.5).

1. Immune Thrombocytopenic Purpura

Idiopathic thrombocytopenic purpura (ITP), also known as primary immune thrombocytopenic purpura and autoimmune thrombocytopenic purpura, is defined as isolated thrombocytopenia with normal bone marrow and the absence of other causes of thrombocytopenia. Two distinct clinical syndromes manifest as an acute condition in children and a chronic condition in adults. *ITP is primarily a disease of increased peripheral platelet destruction,* with most patients having antibodies to specific platelet membrane glycoproteins. The resulting splenic sequestration and phagocytosis by mononuclear macrophages causes thrombocytopenia. Relative marrow failure may contribute to this condition, since studies show that most patients have either normal or diminished platelet production.

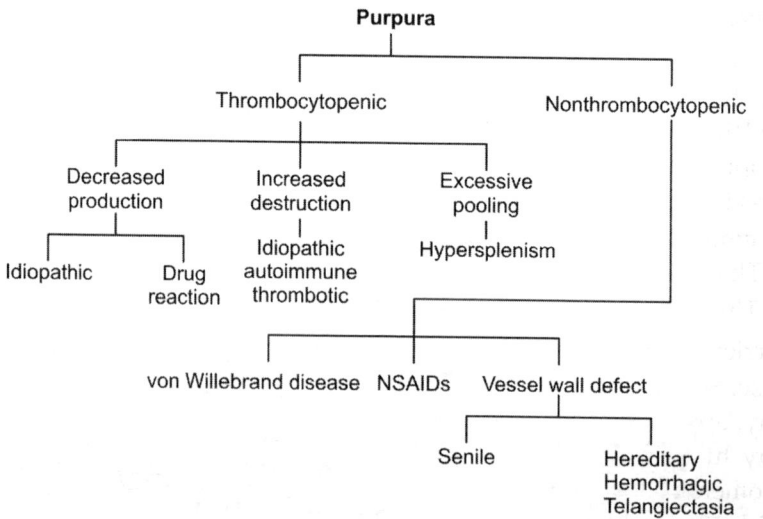

Fig. 3.5: Various pathophysiological mechanisms of purpura.

Acute ITP often follows an acute infection in children and has a spontaneous resolution within 2 months. Chronic ITP occurs mostly in adults and persists longer than 6 months without a specific cause. With platelet counts from 20,000/μL to 50,000/μL, petechiae and ecchymoses are observed following mild trauma. With platelet counts less than 10,000/μL, generalized petechiae, ecchymoses, and mucosal bleeding occur.

2. *von Willebrand Disease*

von Willebrand disease (vWD) is the most common inherited bleeding disorder. Its prevalence is estimated to be as high as 1 case per 1000 population. This disease is caused by deficiency of von Willebrand factor (vWF). The synthesis of vWF is coded by a gene on chromosome 12. It is transmitted as an incompletely dominant autosomal trait. vWF is required for platelet adhesion to endothelial cells during primary hemostasis. vWF also acts as a carrier for factor VIII in plasma. Absence of vWF results in a hybrid hemostatic defect. In mild forms, the clinical picture is dominated by cutaneous and mucosal bleeding resembling purpura. In severe form, low plasma factor VIII level produces a clinical picture resembling hemophilia. In classic hemophilia A, the factor VIII activity level is low because of a defect in the synthesis of factor VIII itself, whereas in von Willebrand disease, the factor VIII activity level is low because of a deficiency in its carrier protein.

Disorders of Coagulation

Clotting disorders result from a congenital or an acquired defect in one or more factors involved in coagulation of blood.

1. *Congenital Clotting Disorders*

Congenital disorders usually result from deficiency of only one clotting factor. In 80–90% of such cases, the defect is a congenital deficiency of factor VIII synthesis (hemophilia A). In 10–20% cases, factor IX is deficient (hemophilia B). Deficiencies of other factors (II, V, VII, XI, and XIII) account for less than 1% of such cases.

Hemophilia A is caused by a congenital deficiency of coagulation factor VIII. The disorder is transmitted as an X-chromosome linked recessive trait. Therefore in successive generations, females with $\overset{\bullet\bullet}{XX}$ pattern act as carriers whereas males with $\overset{\bullet}{XY}$ pattern show manifestations of the disease. Spontaneous mutations may occur during embryogenesis. That is why, approximately one-third of all cases of hemophilia do not have family history. The deficiency of factor VIII is not an all or none phenomenon. Severe reduction (< 40 percent of normal) or absence of the factor leads to a bleeding disorder. Mild deficiency of factor VIII may go unnoticed till late childhood.

The clinical hallmarks of hemophilia A are joint and muscle hemorrhages, easy bruising, and prolonged and potentially fatal hemorrhage after trauma or surgery. However, excessive bleeding does not occur after minor cuts or abrasions since primary hemostatic mechanisms are normal. Hemarthroses are often first noted when the child begins to walk. Untreated, joint hemorrhage will usually lead to severe limitation of movement at the joints. The pathologic processes continue after the bleeding has stopped, with inflammation causing damage to the blood-filled joints. This is a vicious circle, since the inflammation that follows bleeding into a joint leads to synovitis, which in turn increases the likelihood of more frequent hemarthroses; ultimately leading to a permanent disability.

Hemophilia B (Christmas disease) is caused by congenital deficiency of clotting factor IX. Gene for this factor is also located on X chromosome, but its locus is away from the gene for the synthesis of factor VIII. Clinically, hemophilia B resembles hemophilia A. The two types can be differentiated by laboratory tests for factor VIII and factor IX. Acquired clotting disoders are far more common, e.g. clotting defects in liver disease, vitamin K deficiency in the newborn and DIC (described below).

THROMBOSIS

Over 150 years ago, Virchow first postulated that a triad of conditions predisposes to thrombus formation:
  i. Abnormalities in the vessel wall
 ii. Alterations in blood flow
iii. Hypercoagulability of blood.

The first two components of Rudolf Virchow's triad were based on his necropsy observations; the third reflects Virchow's hypothesis that is only now being substantiated. Virchow was primarily referring to venous thrombosis; the same mechanisms are held responsible for arterial thrombosis. Currently, factor (i) seems to be of paramount importance in arterial thrombosis since arterial thrombosis is rare in the absence of this abnormality. All the three factors seem to contribute to venous thrombosis. That the pathophysiology of arterial thrombosis differs from that of venous thrombosis is reflected by the different ways in which they are treated. In broad terms, arterial thrombosis is treated with drugs that target platelets, and venous thrombosis is treated with drugs that target proteins of the coagulation cascade.

Arterial Thrombosis

High blood flow rate is considered one of the factors that maintain fluidity of blood. However, this statement is more applicable to venous thrombosis. The arterial thrombosis develops despite normal high blood flow rate (high shear stress). Arterial thrombosis generally develops as a result of underlying vascular abnormalities, typically atherosclerotic vascular disease. Atherosclerosis affects medium and large sized arteries and is rarely found in arteries smaller than 500 microns in diameter. The aorta and other large arteries, such as femoral, coronary, carotid, cerebral, and renal, are typically affected.

Any damage to the endothelial lining of a blood vessel acts as a nidus for platelet adhesion and aggregation. The primary trigger of arterial thrombosis is rupture of an atherosclerotic plaque which attracts circulating platelets. The thrombus initially resembles a platelet plug, that is, tightly adherent mass of platelets, a small amount of fibrin and a few red and white blood cells. Activated platelets then release the contents of granules, which further promote platelet recruitment, adhesion, aggregation and activation. The clots formed in arterial thrombosis are called "white clots" due to their composition of fibrin and platelets. (In contrast, whole blood tends to clot in venous thrombosis. The rich red cell content of a venous clot gives it the name "red thrombus.)

Hypertension, turbulent blood flow, excessive viscosity of blood (polycythemia, leukemia) can act only as contributory factors but an atherosclerotic trigger seems essential in arterial thrombosis. The ultimate effect of arterial thrombosis is partial or complete obstruction to the blood flow in the affected artery resulting in ischemia or infarction in the concerned organ.

DEEP VENOUS THROMBOSIS (DVT)

The origin of venous thrombosis is frequently multifactorial, with all the three components of the Virchow's triad of variable importance in individual patients. The formation, propagation, and dissolution of venous thrombi represent a balance between thrombogenesis and the body's protective mechanisms, specifically the circulating inhibitors of coagulation and the fibrinolytic system. *In practical terms, the development of venous thrombosis is best understood as the activation of coagulation in areas of reduced blood flow. This explains why the most successful prophylactic regimens are anticoagulation and minimization of venous stasis.*

Studies have shown that low flow sites, such as, behind venous valve pockets, and at venous confluences are at most risk for the development of venous thrombi. However, stasis alone is not enough to facilitate the development of venous thrombosis. Although, patients that are immobilized for long periods of time seem to be at high risk for the development of DVT, an additional stimulus is also required (Table 3.1).

Table 3.1: Virchow's triad in deep vein thrombosis

1. Stasis:
- Immobilization
- Limb paralysis (stroke, plaster cast, spinal cord injury)
- Heart failure
- Varicose vein or chronic venous insufficiency
- Pregnancy

2. Intimal injury:
- Direct vessel injury
- Surgery
- Central venous catheter
- Trauma
- Chemotherapy
- Vasculitis
- Sepsis

3. Hypercoagulable state:
- Pregnancy
- Hormone replacement therapy
- Malignancy
- Nephrotic syndrome

Venous Stasis

Venous return from the legs is enhanced by contraction of the calf muscles, which propels blood upward from the extremities. It is helped by venous valves, which prevents blood from pooling in the lower extremities. Venous stasis may contribute to thrombogenesis by allowing stagnation of the blood with associated local hypoxia and endothelial cell release of an activator of factor X.

Immobility occurs in many conditions such as spinal cord injury, stroke, orthopedic surgery. In each case, immobility is an independent risk factor contributing to development of lower-extremity venous thrombosis. Increased venous pressure as a result of varicosed veins or damaged valves is often an additional contributory factor.

Vascular Injury

The vascular endothelium can be damaged by direct trauma; exposure to endotoxin; inflammatory cytokines, such as interleukin-1 and tumor necrosis factor; thrombin; or low oxygen tension. Injured endothelial cells synthesize tissue factor and plasminogen activator inhibitor-1, which promote thrombogenesis. Damaged endothelial cells also produce less tissue plasminogen activator, the principal activator of fibrinolysis, which further tips the balance toward thrombosis. Common examples of direct venous injury in an elderly population include patients undergoing hip or knee surgery, prostatectomy, hysterectomy, or an extremity fracture.

Hypercoagulability

Patients with hypercoagulable states are at great risk for developing a thrombotic event. However, not all persons with a well-defined hypercoagulable state will develop an overt thrombosis since at least one other factor of the triad must be present. Moreover, not all persons with thrombosis have an identifiable hypercoagulable state. Hypercoagulability may result from an increase in concentration of coagulant factor(s) or activation of coagulant factors.

Elevated levels of various coagulation factors particularly fibrinogen, factors V, VII, VIII and X have been observed in pregnant women or women on oral contraceptives or hormone replacement therapy. Fibrinogen and factors V and VII are acute phase reactants. Their plasma levels may be elevated in almost any disorder associated with tissue damage or inflammation.

Many cases of venous thrombosis can be attributed to an inappropriate low grade activation of coagulation rather than increased concentration of coagulant factors. Tissue factor, responsible for extrinsic system of coagulation, seems to be released during parturition, or conditions such as minimal trauma or presence of interleukin 1 or endotoxins, etc. Stasis of blood results in deficient wash out of tissue factor. Deficient hepatic clearance of activated coagulation factors may represent an important contributory factor in patients with liver disease.

The vast majority of calf vein thrombi dissolve completely without therapy. Approximately 20% propagate proximally. Propagation usually occurs before embolization. The process of adherence and organization of a venous thrombus does not begin until 5–10 days after thrombus formation. Until this process has been established fully, the non-adherent disorganized thrombus may propagate and/or embolize.

Outcomes of Thrombosis

Thrombus formation can have one of the following outcomes: embolization, dissolution, and organization.

1. Embolization occurs when the thrombus breaks free from the vascular wall and becomes mobile. Venous emboli (most likely from deep venous thrombosis in the lower extremities) will travel through the systemic circulation, reach the right side of the heart, and travel through the pulmonary artery resulting in a pulmonary embolism. On the other hand, arterial thrombosis resulting from hypertension or atherosclerosis can become mobile and the resulting emboli can occlude any artery or arteriole downstream of the thrombus formation. This means that cerebral stroke, myocardial infarction, or any other organ can be affected.

2. Dissolution occurs when fibrinolytic mechanisms break up the thrombus and blood flow is restored to the vessel. This may be aided by drugs (for example, after occlusion of a coronary artery). The best response to fibrinolytic drugs is within a couple of hours, before the fibrin mesh-work of the thrombus has been fully developed.
3. Organization and recanalization involves the ingrowth of smooth muscle cells, fibroblasts and endothelium into the fibrin-rich thrombus. If recanalization proceeds it provides capillary-sized channels through the thrombus for continuity of blood flow through the entire thrombus but may not restore sufficient blood flow for the metabolic needs of the downstream tissue.

DISSEMINATED INTRAVASCULAR COAGULATION (DIC)

Disseminated intravascular coagulation is a process that involves enhanced coagulation followed by enhanced anticoagulation activity. Both stages of the disorder contribute to morbidity and mortality. Its etiology can be quite diverse. The coagulation process is initiated by the excessive production of *prothrombin activator* via either the extrinsic or intrinsic pathway of coagulation, more often the former pathway. Under normal circumstances, the coagulation activity remains localized because of simultaneous activation of inhibitory mechanisms. In DIC, the inhibitory mechanisms that normally localize coagulation are overwhelmed by the massive systemic activation of the coagulation process. The result is widespread thrombosis, with end-organ ischemia and dysfunction causing the prominent symptoms. Thrombosis may be overshadowed by generalized bleeding. Hemorrhage is caused by the combination of consumption of coagulation factors, reduced fibrinogen levels, thrombocytopenia and circulation of *fibrin degradation products* (FDPs) acting as anticoagulants. Excessive fibrinolytic mechanisms are also activated in response to the widespread formation of thrombi. This disorder is sometimes referred to as consumption coagulopathy. However, since pathophysiology is multifactorial, and consumption of coagulation factors is only one of them, DIC seems a more appropriate term.

Causes of DIC

The common etiological factor in the causation of DIC is the systemic release of tissue factors that initiate extrinsic pathway of coagulation. Disseminated intravascular coagulation is always secondary to an underlying disorder (e.g. massive trauma especially cerebral trauma, cancer, infection, or obstetric catastrophe) that is usually obvious. A common and serious error in managing DIC is to waste time trying to correct abnormal laboratory values by giving blood product infusions.

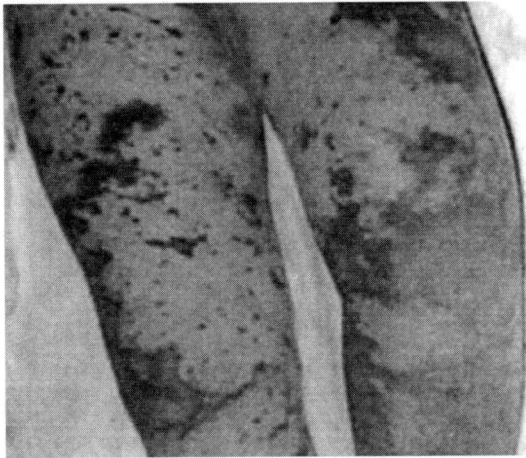

Fig. 3.6: Purpura fulminans.

More effective therapy would be to treat the underling etiological factor that initiated the process.

1. Septicemia

Infection is a common cause of acute, severe DIC. DIC can be caused by nearly any type of microorganism. Components of these microorganisms activate cytokines (chiefly tumor necrosis factor and interleukin-6), inducing an inflammatory response and triggering coagulation. Anything that enhances the spread of the infection (immunosuppression, hepatic insufficiency) can lead to the development of DIC. Sepsis-associated DIC is particularly instrumental in infarctive necrosis of the microcirculation of the skin, i.e. purpura fulminans (Fig. 3.6).

2. Severe Trauma

Severe trauma, particularly involving brain tissue, is associated with DIC. The release of tissue factor from damaged tissue into the systemic circulation leads to coagulation activation. The DIC seen in trauma is greatly enhanced by concurrent shock. With impaired perfusion of blood containing the monocyte macrophages, activated coagulation factors can accumulate in the blood, further enhancing DIC.

3. Malignancy

Solid tumors (particularly metastatic adenocarcinomas) and hematological malignancies may be complicated by DIC. Tissue factor expressed on the surface of tumor cells has been implicated in the development of DIC. Slow, ongoing tumor-initiated DIC is often more thrombotic than hemorrhagic in presentation. On the other hand, DIC in cancer may present as brisk hemorrhage, especially following rapid cell death after effective therapy resulting in tumor lysis syndrome.

4. Obstetric Catastrophes

Several obstetric complications can result in DIC. Amniotic fluid embolism, placenta previa, and abruptio placentae can cause acute activation of the coagulation systems. More than 50% of cases of DIC are caused by obstetrical complications. Tissue factor from a retained dead fetus or abruptio placentae gradually enters the maternal systemic circulation and initiates DIC. Although DIC can be explosive in these patients, it can be short-lived if the obstetric catastrophe is corrected. These patients are generally otherwise healthy and the intact monocyte-macrophage system rapidly clears the circulation of activated products of coagulation.

Pathophysiology of DIC

Major sequence of events in DIC includes the following (Fig. 3.7):
- Exposure of blood to procoagulant substances
- Fibrin deposition in the microvasculature
- Organ damage and failure
- Depletion of coagulation factors and platelets (consumptive coagulopathy)
- Bleeding

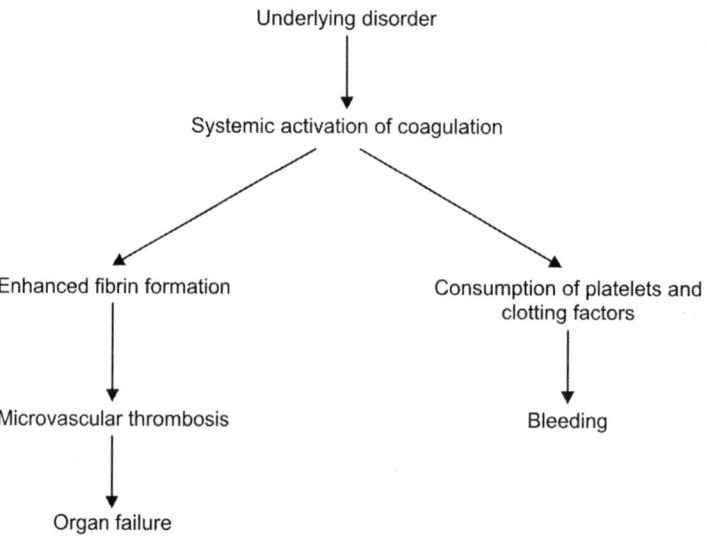

Fig. 3.7: Mechanism of DIC and its consequences.

A. Thrombotic Phase

DIC is due to excessive activation of coagulation. In addition, there is an inability to neutralize circulating activated procoagulants as physiologic inhibitors are over-whelmed. Potent thrombogenic stimuli cause uncontrolled, continued, and excessive generation of circulating thrombin. The consequence is pathologic fibrin deposition throughout the microvasculature.

Excessive thrombin generation is detectable at 3–5 hours after the occurrence of bacteremia or endotoxemia. *Ample evidence exists for a pivotal role of the tissue factor/factor VIIa system in the initiation of thrombin generation.* Hence, activation of coagulation in disseminated intravascular coagulation is tissue factor-driven; the intrinsic pathway of coagulation does not seem to play an important role.

Microvascular thrombosis causes tissue ischemia, contributing to the development of multiorgan dysfunction syndrome. Circulating red blood cells are sheared by the mechanical stress caused by intravascular fibrin strands. A microangiopathic hemolytic anemia may develop secondary to sepsis-induced DIC.

B. Bleeding Phase

Excess thrombin and subsequent widespread deposition of fibrin enhance platelet aggregation and consumption of coagulation factors. In addition, excessive circulating plasmin produced in response to widespread intravascular microthrombi acts to degrade fibrinogen, fibrin, and other coagulation factors. The consumption of these factors, as well as fibrinolysis, enhances hemorrhage.

C. Impaired Coagulation Inhibitor Systems

An impaired function of various natural regulating pathways of coagulation activation may amplify the further thrombin generation and contribute to fibrin formation. Plasma levels of the most important inhibitor of thrombin, antithrombin III, are usually markedly reduced in patients with disseminated intravascular coagulation. This reduction is caused by an increased consumption, due to ongoing thrombin generation. In addition to the decrease in antithrombin III, a significant depression of the protein C system may occur. Consequently, procoagulant state is enhanced.

Clinical Manifestations of DIC

The diagnosis of DIC is clinical. Clinical manifestations of DIC are bleeding and thrombosis, alone or in combination, with ensuing progressive organ dysfunction, supported by evidence of perturbations in selected laboratory data. At the microcirculatory level, both thrombosis and hemorrhage into an organ result in ischemia, tissue damage, and progressive organ failure. Additionally, hypotension with resultant impaired organ perfusion exacerbates organ dysfunction.

Bleeding is typically acute and from multiple sites. Intravenous and intra-arterial line sites, previously dry for days, may begin to ooze. Epistaxis and gum bleeding are common as are petechiae and purpura, which can progress to purpura fulminans, especially in cases due to septicemia. Blood, hemoglobin, or both may appear in the urine. Less commonly, there may be evidence of thrombosis with acrocyanosis and pregangrenous changes of the digits, genitalia, and nose. Metabolic derangements are frequently observed in patients with acute severe DIC.

Summary of Clinical Manifestations of DIC

- Extensive skin and mucous membrane bleeding
- Hemorrhage from surgical incisions, wound sites, catheter or venipuncture sites
- Thrombosis
- Purpura fulminans
- Peripheral acrocyanosis
- Pregangrenous changes in digits, genitalia and nose.

Possible consequences of DIC: Signs of multiple organ dysfunctions —
- Liver function may deteriorate and jaundice may develop.
- Cardiac abnormalities may be demonstrated by elevation in serum cardiac enzymes, cardiac rhythm disturbances, or both.
- Renal function declines, as evidenced by oliguria and rising serum creatinine levels or blood urea nitrogen values, or both.
- Pulmonary insult leads to diffuse alveolar hemorrhage and adult respiratory distress syndrome.
- Central nervous system abnormalities include altered mental status, seizures, and focal neurological deficits.
- Gastrointestinal injury manifests mainly through mucosal ulcerations with consequent bleeding.
- Adrenal insufficiency may result from adrenal gland infarction with subsequent hemorrhagic necrosis.
- Skin manifestations include petechiae and purpura fulminans from hemorrhagic skin necrosis.

Blood Indices in DIC

No single laboratory test is sensitive or specific enough to definitively diagnose DIC. Rather, laboratory tests serve to confirm one's clinical suspicion. A combination of simple and readily available laboratory tests confirms the clinical diagnosis of DIC. These tests include the platelet count, prothrombin time, activated partial thromboplastin time, thrombin time, fibrin degradation product assay, D-dimer assay, and peripheral blood smear. Should these tests be normal, a cause other than DIC should be sought to explain the patient's situation.

Further Reading

Bick, RL. **Disseminated intravascular coagulation. Current concepts of etiology, pathophysiology, diagnosis, and treatment.** *HematolOncolClin N Am* 2003, **17**:149–76.

Hoyer, LW. **Hemophilia A.** N Engl J Med 1994; 330:38–47.

Levi, M. **Disseminated intravascular coagulation: what's new?** *Crit Care Clin* 2005, **21**:449–67.

Mackman, N. **Triggers, targets and treatments for thrombosis.** Nature 2008, 451: 914–18.

4
Disorders of Esophagus

PHYSIOLOGICAL CONSIDERATIONS

The esophagus connects the pharynx to the stomach. It is a flattened muscular tube of 18 to 26 cm length from the upper sphincter to the lower sphincter. Beginning in the neck at the pharyngoesophageal junction the esophagus descends anteriorly to the vertebral column through the superior and posterior mediastinum. After traversing the diaphragm at the diaphragmatic hiatus, the esophagus extends through the gastroesophageal junction to end at the orifice of the cardia of the stomach.

Topographically, there are three distinct regions: cervical, thoracic, and abdominal. The cervical esophagus extends from the pharyngoesophageal junction to the suprasternal notch and is about 4 to 5 cm long. The thoracic esophagus extends from the suprasternal notch to the diaphragmatic hiatus. The abdominal esophagus extends from the diaphragmatic hiatus to the orifice of the cardia of the stomach. Structurally, the esophageal wall is composed of four layers: innermost mucosa, submucosa, muscularis propria, and adventitia. Unlike the remainder of the GI tract, the esophagus has no serosa.

Between swallows, the esophagus is collapsed. During swallowing, the lumen can distend up to approximately 2 cm in the anterior–posterior dimension and up to 3 cm laterally to accommodate a swallowed bolus. The *mucous membrane is lined by* a nonkeratinized stratified squamous epithelium. It covers the entire inner surface of the esophagus, except the LES, where both squamous and columnar epithelium may coexist. The *submucosa* contains connective tissue as well as lymphocytes, plasma cells, neurons (Meissner's plexus), and mucous glands. The esophageal glands are small racemose glands of mucous type. Their secretion is important in esophageal clearance and tissue resistance to acid.

The gastroesophageal junction is located at the level of the diaphragm. On *histological examination;* the gastroesophageal junction can be identified by an abrupt transition from the stratified squamous epithelium of the esophagus to the simple columnar epithelium of the gastric mucosa. On

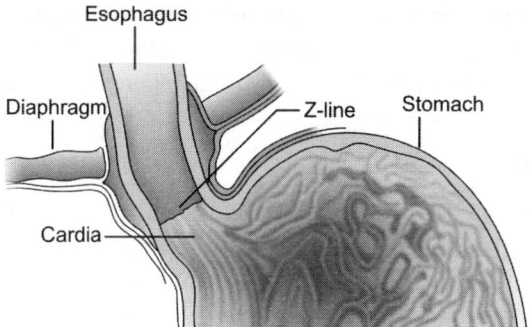

Fig. 4.1: Gastroesophageal junction.

endoscopy; the esophageal lumen appears as a smooth, pale pink tube with visible submucosal blood vessels. The transition from esophageal to gastric mucosa is known as the Z-line and consists of an irregular circumferential line between two areas of different colored mucosa. The gastric mucosa is darker than the pale pink esophageal mucosa. Peristaltic waves can be seen during endoscopic examination. The upper margin of the longitudinal folds of the stomach can also be used as an appropriate endoscopic definition of the gastroesophageal junction (Fig. 4.1).

The esophageal secretions are mostly mucoid in nature. The mucus helps in the propulsion of food during deglutition. The mucosa of the lower end of the esophagus contains many large compound mucous glands. The secretion of these glands protects the esophagus from digestion by strong gastric acid which often regurgitates into the lower end of the esophagus.

The muscular coat of the esophagus consists of two anatomically and physiologically distinct regions, namely a proximal striated muscle portion (cervical esophagus) and a distal smooth muscle portion (thoracic and abdominal esophagus). The extrinsic innervation of the esophagus is by vagus nerve. The vagal fibers that innervate the striated muscle arise from the nucleus ambiguus (NA, the somatic component), whereas the smooth muscle is innervated by vagal fibers arising from the dorsal motor nucleus (DMN, the autonomic component) of the vagal nucleus.

Functions

The esophagus serves two chief functions:
- Transport of food from the oral cavity to the stomach (deglutition).
- Prevention of retrograde flow of gastric contents (gastroesophageal reflux).

Deglutition

Deglutition or swallowing is a three stage process that transfers the chewed food from the mouth to the stomach. The first or the oral stage is voluntary. The next two stages, namely, the pharyngeal stage and the esophageal stage are reflex in nature. The reflex activity is coordinated by a *swallowing center located in the medulla oblongata and lower pons.*

The Oral Stage

When the chewed food is ready for swallowing, it is voluntarily rolled back into the pharynx by the backward and upward pressure of the tongue against the palate. This initiates the involuntary or the reflex mechanisms of swallowing.

The Pharyngeal Stage

Oral opening of the pharynx, specially the *tonsillar pillars, soft palate* and epiglottis contain sensory receptors for the swallowing reflex. *The afferent fibers* pass via V and IX cranial nerves to the tractus solitarius in the brain stem. The *swallowing center* consists of a group of neurons located in the reticular formation of the medulla and lower pons. This center brings about coordinated and sequential contraction of a number of striated and smooth muscles in the pharynx and esophagus. *The efferent fibers* involved in this reflex are carried by V, IX, X and XII cranial nerves constituting a pharyngeal plexus.

In the pharyngeal stage of swallowing:

i. The soft palate is elevated, sealing the nasopharynx and preventing the food from entering it
ii. The larynx is elevated and thus the epiglottis closes the superior opening of the larynx
iii. The vocal cords are approximated and the breathing is temporarily stopped (*deglutition apnea*).

The multiple responses mentioned above leave no chance for the food to enter the respiratory passages. At the same time, upper 3–4 cm of the esophagus (normally under tonic contraction constituting the upper esophageal sphincter) relaxes. A rapid peristaltic wave starting in the pharyngeal muscles passes into the esophagus; thereby propelling food into the upper part of esophagus. Once the bolus of food has passed in to the esophagus, normal breathing is resumed and the upper esophagus goes into tonic contraction once again. This stage is completed in 1–2 seconds.

Esophageal Stage

The peristaltic wave, which begins in the pharynx, travels down the esophagus up to its lower end, pushing the bolus of food ahead of it. The lower 2–5 cm of esophagus normally remains tonically contracted constituting the lower esophageal sphincter. As the peristaltic wave approaches this segment, the sphincter relaxes and the bolus of food enters the stomach without encountering any resistance. This stage is completed in 5–10 seconds.

In the upright position, the liquids and semisolid foods, under the effect of gravity, reach the lower end of esophagus ahead of the primary peristaltic wave described above. The primary peristaltic wave always starts from the pharynx as a part of the swallowing reflex. It may not be able to push a bolus of solid food all the way down the esophagus. In that case, the secondary peristaltic waves are initiated by the distension of esophagus by the bolus of food. The secondary peristaltic waves can originate in any part of esophagus depending on the position of the residual bolus of food. One or more secondary peristaltic waves may be required to transfer the bolus into the stomach.

Upper and Lower Esophageal Sphincters

At the upper and the lower ends of the esophagus, the tonic contraction of its muscle converts these regions into *physiological sphincters*. These regions are normally closed and open only during deglutition, when the peristaltic waves pass over them. However, histologically, no difference can be detected between the region of sphincteric action and the rest of esophagus.

The upper esophageal sphincter (UES) refers to an intraluminal high pressure zone, 2–4 cm in length that exists at the upper end of the body of the esophagus. It does not correlate with any anatomically defined sphincter. The high pressure zone is created by tonic contraction of (striated) inferior pharyngeal constrictor and cricopharyngeal muscles due to a continuous neural discharge. The upper esophageal sphincter serves to prevent the entry of air into the esophagus during normal respiration as well as prevents esophageal contents from refluxing into the pharynx and respiratory tree. During swallowing, the tonic neural discharge to the two muscles mentioned above transiently ceases as a component of swallowing reflex activity. The UES abruptly but briefly relaxes to allow the passage of bolus of food from the pharynx to the upper esophagus and goes into tonic contraction again.

The *lower esophageal sphincter (LES)* refers to an intraluminal high pressure zone that exists between the esophageal body and stomach. Any well defined thickening of smooth muscle (i.e. an anatomical sphincter) cannot be demonstrated in this zone also. When a bolus of food reaches this zone, LES briefly relaxes to allow its passage into the stomach. In the remaining period, LES remains closed and thus prevents any reflux of gastric contents (food, gastric juice, air) into the esophagus. *The tonic contraction of LES is due to a unique intrinsic property of smooth muscle of that zone.* The resting tone of LES can be modulated by neural, hormonal, myogenic and mechanical influences. LES tone is increased by gastrin (e.g. high protein meal), but decreased by orally ingested fats, chocolates, ethanol, nicotine, caffeine. The tone is decreased by some gastrointestinal hormones such as VIP, CCK, as well as estrogens and progesterone (e.g. during pregnancy). Pharmacological agents such as dopamine, nitroglycerin, anti-cholinergics and beta-adrenergic agonists also decrease LES tone.

An increased intragastric pressure results in simultaneous increase in LES tone. This mechanism prevents gastroesophageal reflux during activities that briefly increase intra-abdominal pressure such as sneezing, coughing, straining, etc. The reflex relaxation of LES during deglutition is mediated by the action of vagal fibers on the intrinsic neurons of myenteric plexus which release an inhibitory neurotransmitter (VIP) on the smooth muscle of the sphincter.

DYSPHAGIA

Dysphagia is the term used to describe the subjective sensation of food being obstructed as it passes from the oral cavity to the stomach. Dysphagia should be differentiated from odynophagia, a condition in which the patient feels pain during swallowing, but no sensation of obstruction. Odynophagia is usually caused by acute inflammatory conditions of the esophagus.

As mentioned earlier, the esophagus consists of two anatomically and physiologically distinct regions, namely a proximal striated muscle portion (cervical esophagus) and a distal smooth muscle portion (thoracic and abdominal esophagus). Diseases that affect these two regions are quite different

Diseases that affect the cervical esophagus (striated muscle) are essentially neuromuscular disorders that also affect the oropharynx. These diseases do not generally affect smooth muscle of the thoracic esophagus. By themselves, the motility disorders of the striated muscle segment are not of great diagnostic problem as their clinical presentation is overwhelmed by the symptoms caused by involvement of striated muscle of the oral cavity and pharynx.

Etiology

Dysphagia is classified as *oropharyngeal* or *esophageal* depending on where it occurs.

Oropharyngeal dysphagia: Oropharyngeal dysphagia is difficulty emptying material from the oropharynx into the esophagus. *It results from an abnormal function proximal to the esophagus.* Patients complain of difficulty in initiating swallowing, nasal regurgitation, and tracheal aspiration followed by coughing. Most often, oropharyngeal dysphagia occurs in patients with neurological conditions or muscular disorders that affect skeletal muscles.

Neurological Conditions

- Stroke
- Parkinson's disease
- Multiple sclerosis
- Some motor neuron disorders (amyotrophic lateral sclerosis, progressive bulbar palsy, pseudobulbar palsy)
- Bulbar poliomyelitis

Muscular Conditions

- Myasthenia gravis
- Dermatomyositis
- Muscular dystrophy
- Cricopharyngeal incoordination

Esophageal dysphagia: Esophageal dysphagia is difficulty in passing food down the esophagus. It results from either a motility disorder or a mechanical obstruction of the esophagus.

Motility Disorder

- Achalasia
- Diffuse esophageal spasm
- Systemic sclerosis

Mechanical Obstruction

- Peptic stricture
- Esophageal cancer
- Lower esophageal rings
- Extrinsic compression
- Caustic ingestion

Achalasia

Functionally, the intramural motor neurons of the Auerbach's plexus are of two types: inhibitory and excitatory. The inhibitory motor neurons relax esophageal smooth muscle by releasing nitric oxide (NO) and vasoactive intestinal peptide (VIP). The excitatory motor neurons produce contraction of esophageal smooth muscle by releasing acetylcholine and substance P. Achalasia is characterized by failure of the lower esophageal sphincter to relax during swallowing. The fundamental defect lies in the degeneration of Auerbach's plexus especially of VIP and/or NO- secreting

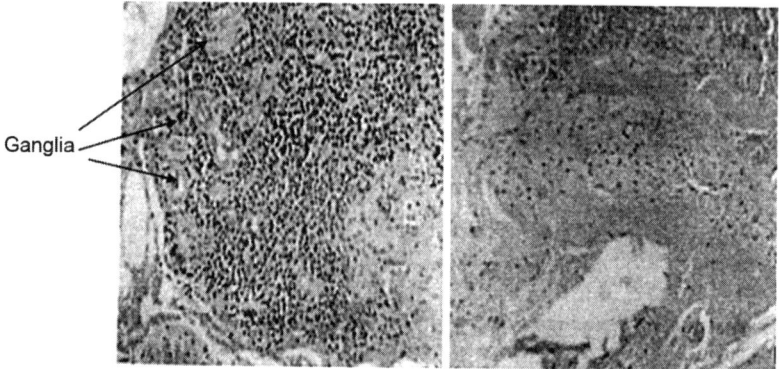

Fig. 4.2: Histology of distal esophagus. Left: normal, showing numerous ganglion cells. Right: from a patient of achalasia, showing inflammatory cells and almost complete absence of ganglia.

neurons in the lower esophagus (Fig. 4.2). This results in impaired LES relaxation and loss of peristaltic sequencing of the esophageal contractions, producing symptoms of dysphagia, chest pain, and regurgitation. During each meal, food tends to collect in the esophagus, from where it slowly passes into the stomach. Ultimately; marked dilatation of esophagus results. Achalasia can occur at any age, but is more common in adults over 25. The chief symptom of the disorder is difficulty in swallowing. Patients typically describe food sticking in the chest after it is swallowed. In a patient with achalasia, dysphagia occurs with both solid and liquid food. Moreover, the dysphagia is consistent, meaning that it occurs during virtually every meal. Regurgitation of food that is trapped in the esophagus can occur, especially when the esophagus is dilated.

Primary achalasia is also called *idiopathic achalasia* since the cause is unknown. An autoimmune cause has been proposed because the predominant cell type of the inflammatory infiltrate in the myenteric plexus is the T lymphocyte, which is known to be involved in other autoimmune diseases. There is also a high prevalence of certain class II histocompatibility antigens in patients with achalasia, which are also known to be associated with other autoimmune disorders.

A number of other diseases can cause so-called *secondary achalasia*. One of the most common is cancer in the proximal stomach that may directly infiltrate and destroy esophageal myenteric neurons. A number of other malignancies have been described as a cause of secondary achalasia. They appear to produce immune-mediated myenteric neural damage as part of a paraneoplastic syndrome.

Besides failure of LES relaxation, both primary and secondary peristalsis is also impaired in achalasia. The inhibitory innervation is crucial in generating an initial wave of inhibition in the circular smooth muscle of the esophagus, which is responsible for the peristaltic sequencing of the esophageal contractions as well as relaxation of the LES. In animal models as well as humans, drugs that interfere with NO, the primary inhibitory neurotransmitter in the esophagus, produce motility changes that mimic achalasia.

Regurgitation occurs because of retention of large volumes of saliva and ingested food in the esophagus. Characteristically, regurgitation occurs when the patient assumes the recumbent position at bedtime. Infrequently, regurgitation is complicated by aspiration pneumonia.

Once a diagnosis of achalasia is made, it is necessary to distinguish primary (idiopathic) achalasia from secondary achalasia. Achalasia secondary to cancer at the esophagus-gastric junction needs to be especially considered in patients with clinical evidence of achalasia that presents with recent onset and rapidly progressive dysphagia associated with marked weight loss.

Infrequently, the symptoms of achalasia may be confused with those of GERD, especially if the patient describes chest pain of a burning quality. However, a careful history should help differentiate the two conditions. It is particularly important to clarify the nature of the patient's regurgitation, which arises from the stomach in acid reflux disease and from the esophagus in achalasia. If there is any doubt, the barium X-ray findings, endoscopy, and manometry will clearly differentiate the two disorders.

Esophageal Manometry

The peristaltic activity of the esophagus can be studied by esophageal manometry. In this test, a catheter assembly consisting of a number of pressure sensitive catheters is passed into the esophagus so that one orifice of the catheter is each at: (a) Pharynx, (b) UES, (c) upper, middle and lower regions of esophagus, (d) LES and (e) stomach. Each catheter is perfused with water and connected to the pressure transducers of an ink writing polygraph.

As a bolus of water is swallowed, it sets up a peristaltic wave which is recorded as a sequence of pressure waves down the catheter assembly. Esophageal manometry is of gold standard for the diagnosis of achalasia of esophagus (Fig. 4.3), scleroderma and other motility disorders of esophagus.

Diaphragmatic (Hiatal) Hernia

Functional Anatomy

The esophagus passes through the diaphragmatic hiatus in the crural part of the diaphragm to reach the stomach. The diaphragmatic hiatus itself is approximately 2 cm in length and chiefly consists of musculotendinous

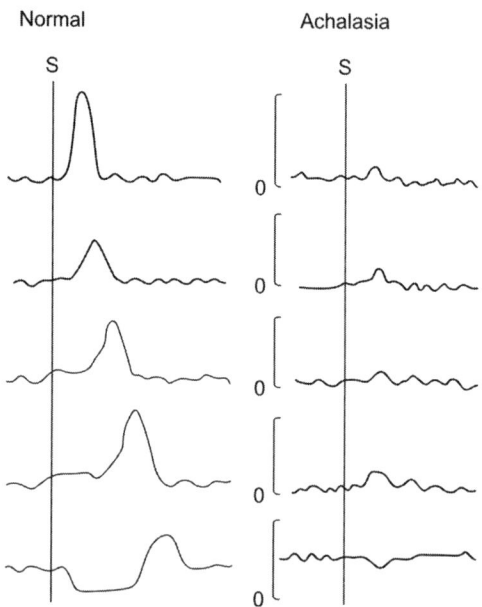

Fig. 4.3: Manometric recording of esophageal peristalsis in a normal individual and a patient of primary achalasia. S = swallow. Note the absence of peristaltic pressure rise in the body of esophagus and absence of relaxation of LES in the patient's record.

slips of the right and left diaphragmatic crura arising from either side of the spine and passing around the esophagus before inserting into the central tendon of the diaphragm. The size of the hiatus is not fixed, but narrows whenever intra-abdominal pressure rises, such as when lifting a heavy weight or coughing.

The upper part of the LES normally lies within the diaphragmatic hiatus, while the lower section normally is intra-abdominal. At this level, the visceral peritoneum and the phrenoesophageal ligament cover the esophagus. The phrenoesophageal ligament is a fibrous layer of connective tissue arising from the crura, and it maintains the LES within the abdominal cavity. Any sudden increase in intra-abdominal pressure also acts on the portion of the LES below the diaphragm to increase the sphincter pressure. An acute angle, the angle of His (Fig. 4. 4A) is formed between the cardia of the stomach and the distal esophagus and functions as a flap at the gastroesophageal junction and helps prevent reflux of gastric contents into the esophagus.

Hiatal Hernia

A hiatal hernia occurs when a portion of the stomach prolapses through the diaphragmatic esophageal hiatus. Hiatal hernia has been described in earlier in medical literature; its diagnosis has assumed importance only in the last century or so because of its association with gastroesophageal

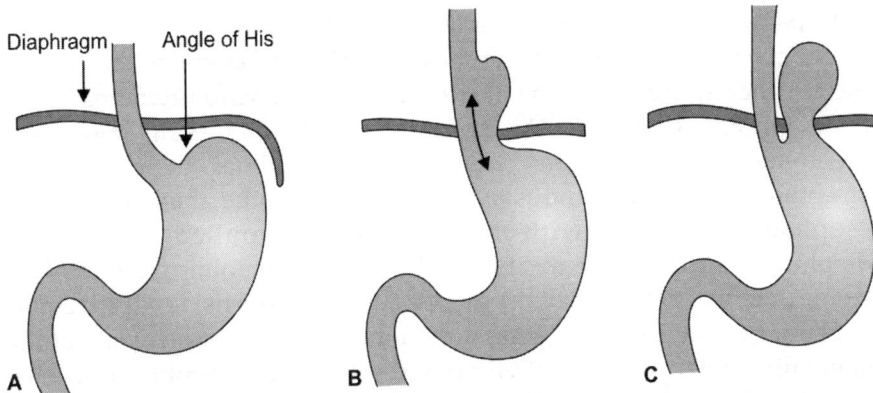

Fig. 4.4: Normal esophageal-stomach relationship: (A) Note the angle of His, (B) shows a sliding hiatal hernia with disappearance of angle of His, (C) shows a paraesophageal hernia, with intact angle of His.

reflux disease (GERD) and its complications. Hiatal hernias are more common in Western countries. The frequency of hiatus hernia increases with age, from 10% in patients younger than 40 years to 70% in patients older than 70 years.

Diaphragmatic hernias may be congenital or acquired. Acquired hiatal hernias are divided further into nontraumatic and traumatic hernias. The most common types of hernias are those acquired in a non-traumatic fashion. By far, most hiatal hernias are asymptomatic and are discovered incidentally. On rare occasion, a life-threatening complication, such as gastric volvulus or strangulation, may present acutely. Hiatus hernias are also divided into 2 types, (1) sliding hiatal hernia and (2) para-esophageal hiatal hernia. A mixed variety with coexisting sliding and para-esophageal components is possible.

Sliding hiatal hernia by far is the most common type of hiatal hernia. It occurs when the gastroesophageal junction, along with a portion of the stomach, migrates into the mediastinum through the esophageal hiatus. The majority of patients such patients are asymptomatic. However, some of such patients suffer from gastroesophageal reflux disease.

Sliding hiatal hernia interferes with the reflux barrier mechanism in several ways. As the LES moves into the chest, it no longer is exposed to positive intra-abdominal pressure and, therefore, is less effective as a sphincter. In fact, the sphincter moves into an area of low pressure, which interferes with the sphincter activity. In addition, the widening hiatus affects the competence of the diaphragmatic crura. The angle of His is lost, making regurgitation of gastric contents more likely (Fig. 4.4B). These changes not only predispose to reflux of gastric contents into the esophagus, but also prolong the acid contact time with the epithelium of the esophagus.

In paraesophageal hernia, the widened hiatus permits the fundus of the stomach to protrude into the chest, anterior and lateral to the body of the esophagus; however, the gastroesophageal junction remains below the diaphragm (Fig. 4.4C). As the hiatus widens, increasing amounts of the greater curvature of the stomach and, sometimes, the gastric-colic omentum, follows. The fundus eventually comes to lie above the gastro-esophageal junction, with the pylorus being pulled towards the diaphragmatic hiatus. In this type of hernia, the anatomic relation of the stomach to the lower end of the esophagus (angle of His) tends to remain unchanged, so gross acid reflux does not occur. Paraesophageal hernias generally tend to enlarge with time, and sometimes the entire stomach is found within the chest. There is risk of these paraesophageal hernias becoming incarcerated, leading to strangulation or perforation. This complication is potentially lethal, and surgical intervention is necessary. Because of the high mortality associated with this condition, elective repair is often advised wherever a paraesophageal hernia is found.

Predisposing factors for the development of hiatus hernia include the following:

- Muscle weakening and loss of elasticity associated with ageing.
- Loss of muscle tone around the diaphragmatic opening with age.
- Hiatal hernias are more common in women. This may be related to the intra-abdominal forces exerted in pregnancy.
- Fiber-depleted diet of the western world leads to a state of chronic constipation and straining during bowel movement.
- Obesity predisposes to hiatus hernia because of increased abdominal pressure.
- The presence of ascites also is associated with hiatal hernias.

Gastroesophageal Reflux Disease (GERD)

The reflux of products of gastric digestion (chyme containing acid, pepsin or even bile) into the esophagus produces a substernal burning sensation that moves up and down the chest. These symptoms are usually described as *"heart burn."* If the reflux material reaches the pharynx, the patient notices a sour or even bitter taste. Regurgitation of the material into the airways may provoke cough or even choking sensation. Sudden filling of the mouth with warm salty fluid (water brash) results from hypersecretion of saliva triggered by the acid reflux. The repeated exposure to the reflux material produces esophageal erosions, ulceration or even cancer of the lower end of esophagus.

Pathophysiology

The etiology of GERD seems to be multifactorial.

A. Low LES Pressure

Even in empty stomach, the intragastric pressure exceeds the intra-esophageal pressure. Straining, coughing or sneezing causes a marked increase in intra-abdominal and intragastric pressures, especially after a large meal. Despite the favorable pressure gradient, gastroesophageal reflux does not normally occur. The gastroesophageal junction acts as a barrier to prevent reflux of contents from the stomach into the esophagus by a combination of mechanisms forming the *antireflux barrier*. The components of this barrier include:
- Diaphragmatic crura,
- LES baseline pressure and its intra-abdominal segment
- Angle of His.

The presence of a hiatal hernia compromises this reflux barrier not only in terms of reduced LES pressure but also reduced esophageal acid clearance. Patients with hiatal hernias also have longer transient LES relaxation (tLESR) episodes particularly at night time (*see* below). These factors increase the esophageal mucosa acid contact time predisposing to esophagitis and related complications.

The LES is tonically closed at rest, maintaining an average pressure of about 20 mmHg, and serves to prevent gastroesophageal reflux. To allow passage of a bolus, LES pressure falls within 1.5 to 2.5 seconds of a swallow and remains low for 6 to 8 seconds as the peristaltic contraction transverses the esophageal body. Two main groups of peripheral neurons mediate active contraction and relaxation of the LES, acetylcholine being the excitatory neurotransmitter and nitric oxide and VIP as the main inhibitory neurotransmitters.

Gastroesophageal reflux occurs when LES pressure is lower than intragastric pressure. Ingestion of food is often associated with a drop in LES pressure, resulting in large part from the secretion of hormones such as secretin and cholecystokinin (CCK), particularly with fat intake. LES pressure is decreased by chocolate, alcohol, and caffeine. During pregnancy, LES pressure is low because of high concentrations of circulating estrogen and progesterone, particularly the latter. Pharmacological agents such as dopamine, nitroglycerin, anti-cholinergics and beta-adrenergic agonists also decrease LES tone. All these medications can potentially predispose to gastroesophageal reflux.

B. Transient Lower Esophageal Sphincter Relaxation (tLESR) Episodes

Evidence exists that episodes of transient lower esophageal sphincter relaxation are the most frequent mechanism of reflux in patients showing normal LES pressure (> 10 mm Hg). tLESRs:
- are independent of swallowing

- are not accompanied by esophageal peristalsis
- are accompanied by diaphragmatic inhibition
- persist longer than swallow-induced LES relaxation (> 10 sec)

The dominant stimulus for tLESRs is distention of proximal stomach. tLESR is the dominant mechanism of belching. tLESR can be experimentally induced by gaseous distention of stomach. It is a vagally-mediated reflex response. The vagal afferent receptors are located in the gastric cardia. The afferent impulses reach nucleus of tractus solitarius and subsequently to dorsal motor nucleus of vagus. The efferent neurons project on the inhibitory neurons localized in the myenteric plexus of distal esophagus. The tLESR response consists not only of LES relaxation but also diaphragmatic crural inhibition. The frequency of tLESRs increases with assumption of erect posture. Transient LES relaxation occurs largely in the postprandial period.

C. Other Factors

Gastric emptying: Delayed emptying is common in GERD patients. It has been demonstrated that approximately 25% of patients of GERD have gastric emptying time greater than 4 hours.

Sleep: Many of the physiologic changes that occur with sleep favor development of GERD. These changes include:
  i. Increased acid secretion that can even be seen as "nocturnal breakthrough" in GERD patients on proton pump therapy.
  ii. A marked decrease in acid clearance with enhanced proximal migration of acid in the esophagus owing to loss of gravitational effects in the supine position, decreased frequency of swallowing and therefore of primary peristalsis, and decreased saliva production.
  iii. Changes in the gastric slow-wave electrical activity that could predispose to decreased gastric emptying.

Obesity: The relationship of obesity to GERD is controversial. Obesity has been found to be a risk factor for GERD, but the relationship may in large part be determined by the presence of hiatus hernia in obese patients. Weight loss may or may not be associated with improvement in GERD symptoms.

To conclude, for gastroesophageal reflux to occur, one or more of the following factors have to be present:
- Low basal LES tone
- Frequent episodes of tLESRs
- Hiatus hernia
- Excessive gastric filling
- Delayed gastric emptying

- Ingestion of foods that lower LES pressure, e.g. dietary fat, alcohol coffee.
- Increased intra-abdominal pressure due to obesity or pregnancy.

Esophagitis in GERD

In patients with gastroesophageal reflux, a greater duration of exposure of the esophagus to a pH < 4 leads to increases the severity of esophagitis and its complications. Both the LES mechanisms that produce excess reflux of acid and the esophageal body motility disorders that result in prolonged acid exposure to the mucosa contribute to the duration of the exposure. After an initial acid-pepsin injury to the lower esophagus, a vicious cycle sets in. Both a low LES pressure and disturbed esophageal motility are more common and pronounced in patients with more severe esophagitis. Evidence is accumulating that inflammation affects nerves and muscle to alter LES pressure and esophageal body motility. Inflammation seems to produce both a decrease in cholinergic excitatory and an increase in NO inhibitory activity in the esophagus.

Barrett's esophagus is a well-recognized premalignant condition for the development of esophageal adenocarcinoma, and it results from chronic gastroesophageal reflux disease. It is characterized by a metaplastic transformation of the typically squamous epithelium native of the esophagus, to a *columnar type highlighted by the presence of goblet cells on histological evaluation.* On endoscopy, Barrett's esophagus is visualized as pale squamous epithelium merging into the darker columnar-cell-lined esophagus (Fig. 4.5). The condition entails a 30- to 50-fold greater risk of developing adenocarcinoma.

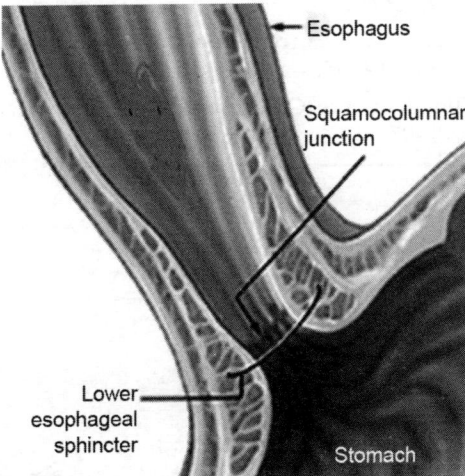

Fig. 4.5: Endoscopic image of Barrett's esophagus with pale squamous epithelium merging into the darker columnar-cell-lined esophagus

From a pathophysiological point of view, BE results from esophageal response to acid-induced injury. Initially, the acid-induced injury is healed by repair by stratified squamous epithelium. Repeated and prolonged acid-injury induces in some patients, not all, an intestinal metaplastic process by which the stratified squamous epithelium is replaced by intestinal columnar epithelium with crypts and goblet cells. This change, called Barrett's esophagus, affects a variable length of the lower esophagus. The metaplastic change offers greater tolerance to gastric acid-pepsin, but predisposes to the development of esophageal adenocarcinoma.

The entire esophagus is normally lined with squamous cells. The cancer starting in these cells is called squamous cell carcinoma. This type of cancer can occur anywhere along the length of the esophagus. At one time, squamous cell carcinoma was more common type of esophageal cancer, making up to 90% of all esophageal cancers. This has changed over time, and now squamous cell carcinoma makes up less than 50% of esophageal cancers. Adenocarcinoma is more common in the lower esophagus.

The relationships among GERD, BE, and esophageal adenocarcinoma are clearly established. Duration and severity of GERD symptoms increases risk not only for BE, but also for esophageal adenocarcinoma. However, it has also been shown that 40% of patients with esophageal adenocarcinoma deny having had GERD symptoms. It may be correlated with the fact that significant number of BE patients do not report symptoms of GERD.

Further Reading

Diamant, NE **Pathophysiology of gastroesophageal reflux disease.** *GI Motility online* 2006 doi:10.1038/gimo21

Eckardt, AJ; Eckardt VF. **Current clinical approach to achalasia.** *World J Gastroenterol* 2009; 15: 3969–75.

Kahrilas, PJ. "**Clinical practice. Gastroesophageal reflux disease.**". *New Engl J of Med.* 2008; 359: 1700–07.

5

Disorders of Stomach

FUNCTIONAL ANATOMY AND PHYSIOLOGY

The anatomical divisions of the stomach (Fig. 5.1A) consist of cardia, fundus, body, pyloric antrum and pylorus.

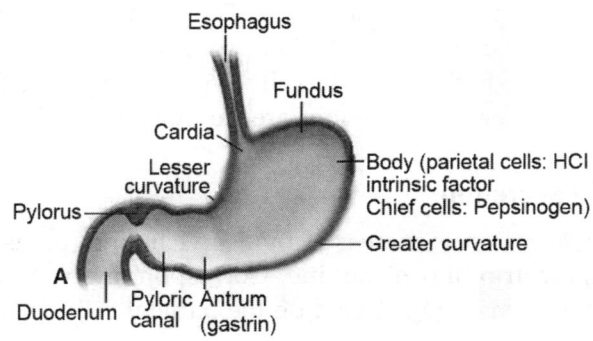

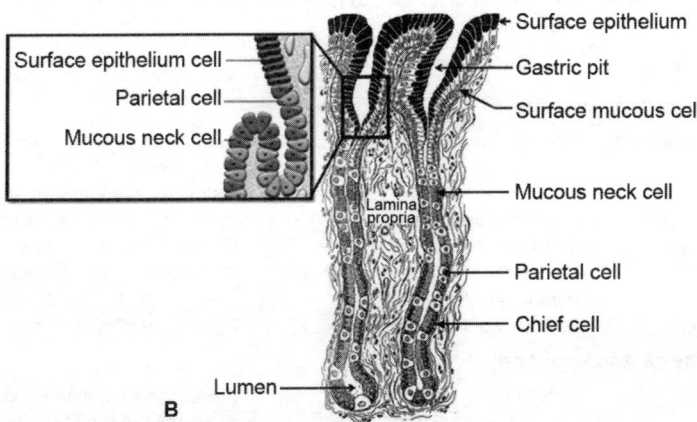

Fig. 5.1: (A) Gross anatomy of the stomach and (B) histology of glands of body of the stomach.

Innervation

The stomach receives both parasympathetic and sympathetic innervations. The preganglionic parasympathetic fibers reach the stomach through the vagi and form extensive synapses with intrinsic ganglia which constitute the Meissner's (submucosal) plexus as well as Auerbach's (myenteric) plexuses. The postganglionic parasympathetic fibers innervate the secretory components as well as the smooth muscle in the wall of the stomach. Parasympathetic stimulation increases the secretion of parietal cells and chief cells of gastric glands, directly and indirectly by stimulation of G cells. Gastric motility is increased by parasympathetic stimulation. Sympathetic fibers chiefly supply the blood vessels and smooth muscle in the wall of the stomach. Sympathetic stimulation decreases gastric motility.

Secretory Functions of Stomach

Mucosal glands of the fundus and body of the stomach (Fig. 5.1B) secrete gastric juice rich in acid and pepsinogen. Mucosa of the pyloric regions secretes bicarbonate-rich soluble mucus. The surface of the entire gastric mucosa is lined by columnar cells that produce viscid bicarbonate-rich mucus that adheres to the cells. The cell source and the main functions of the constituents of gastric secretions are summarized in Table 5.1.

Gastric Acid Secretion

Gastric acid secretion is increased by acetylcholine (parasympathetic stimulation), gastrin and histamine. Correspondingly, three types of receptors have been demonstrated on the parietal cells... M_3 muscarinic

Table 5.1: The cell source and chief functions of various constituents of gastric juice and endocrine gastric secretions

Constituent	Cell source	Chief function
Exocrine gastric secretion		
Hydrochloric acid	Oxyntic (parietal cells)	Sterilizes upper GIT, activates pepsinogen. Helps in intestinal iron absorption.
Intrinsic factor	Oxyntic (parietal cells)	Intestinal absorption of vitamin B_{12}
Pepsinogen	Chief cells	Protein digestion (as pepsin).
Mucus	Mucus cells in fundus and body Pyloric glands	Protection of gastric mucosa.
Bicarbonate	Surface epithelial cells	Protection of gastric mucosa.
Endocrine gastric secretion		
Gastrin	G cells (in pyloric antrum)	Increased secretion of oxyntic and chief cells of the stomach and exocrine pancreatic acini
Somatostatin	D cells (all over gastric mucosa)	Suppression of acid secretion

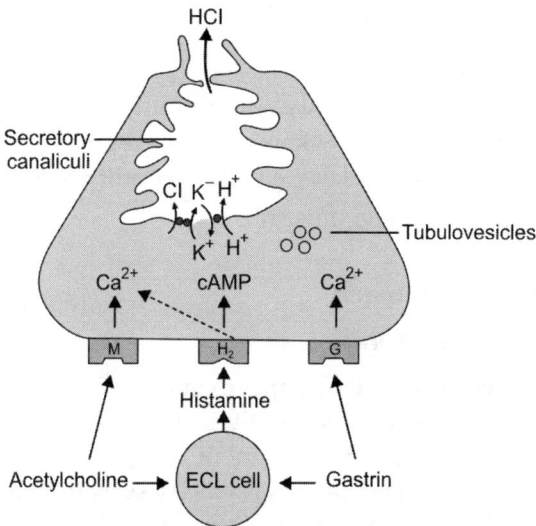

Fig. 5.2: Mechanism of secretion of gastric hydrochloric acid.

receptors for acetylcholine, G receptors for gastrin and H_2 receptors for histamine. Intracellular mediators for these receptors include Ca^{++} (for M_3 and G receptors) and CAMP for H_2 receptors (Fig. 5.2). The effects of gastrin and vagal stimulation on gastric acid secretion are intimately related. Vagal stimulation increases acid secretion by:

i. M_3 receptor stimulation
ii. enhancing the sensitivity of G cells to gastric distention
iii. lowering the parietal cell threshold for response to circulating gastrin.

The physiological role of histamine in gastric acid secretion is not clear. Histamine is the most potent stimulus for gastric acid secretion. Histamine-secreting mast cells and enterochromaffin like (ECL) cells are located in close proximity to the parietal cells. Because H_2-receptor blockers inhibit vagal and gastrin stimulated acid secretion, histamine is thought to be final mediator of acid secretion. However, H_2-receptor blockers reduce the meal-stimulated acid secretion by approximately 75% only in contrast to almost complete inhibition of acid secretion by a proton pump inhibitors.

Histamine H_2 receptor antagonists act by blocking the effect of histamine on parietal cells. Proton pump inhibitors act by inhibiting the enzyme in parietal cells that catalyzes acid production for release into the gastric lumen. G cells, enterochromaffin-like cells, and parietal cells are all regulated by release of the inhibitory peptide somatostatin from somatostatin (S) cells, which are distributed throughout the stomach. The effect of *H. pylori* infection on acid secretion depends on which part of the stomachis most inflamed because this determines which of these regulatory cells are affected most.

Blockers of Acid Secretion

1. *Receptor blockers*
   - Gastrin-receptor, blockers, e.g. proglumide
   - Acetylcholine-receptor blockers, e.g. pienzepine
   - Histamine-receptor blockers, e.g. H_2-receptor antagonists
2. *Proton pump blockers*, e.g. omeprazole

Motor Functions of Stomach

1. *Storage of Ingested Food*

Empty stomach has a capacity of approximately 50 ml only. As food is ingested, the gastric capacity gradually increases. At the end of a meal, the stomach may contain 1000–1500 ml of food, water and gastric juice. The storage function of the stomach is chiefly served by the fundus and body regions, which undergo a *gradually increasing, vagally mediated, reflex receptive relaxation*. That is why; after vagotomy, the patients often complain of early satiety as well as postprandial epigastric fullness.

2. *Mixing, Grinding and Sieving Function*

Peristaltic waves passing down the body and pyloric part of stomach produce thorough mixing of food with the gastric juice. The food is macerated into a semiliquid chyme. The narrow pyloric sphincter acts like a sieve and allows particles less than 1 mm in size to leave the stomach in to the first part of duodenum.

3. *Regulation of Gastric Emptying*

Distention of stomach or increased gastrin secretion increases the strength of gastric peristalsis. On the other hand, presence of highly acid chyme, hyperosmolar chyme or fat-rich chyme in the *duodenum* decreases the strength of gastric peristalsis. These duodenal inhibitory influences on gastric emptying ensure that amount of chyme containing acid, and food particles is ideal for the proper digestion and absorption in the small intestine.

Estimation of Gastric Acid Output

Measurement of gastric acid output is not necessary to diagnose or exclude peptic ulcer. Endoscopy is the gold standard. Gastric acid is estimation is important for the diagnosis of (i) Zollinger-Ellison (Z-E) syndrome and (ii) Pernicious anemia. Gastric acid output can be estimated as: Basal acid output and maximum gastric output.

Basal acid output (BAO) is the acid secreted by the stomach in unstimulated (fasting) state. Four 15 minute collections of gastric juice are aspirated and added up. Normal values are ≤ 15 mEq H^+/ hr. Higher levels are suggestive of Zollinger-Ellison syndrome.

Maximum Acid Output (MAO)

Following a subcutaneous injection of pentagastrin, the acid secreted in one hour (four 15-minute collections) is estimated. Values less than 6.9 mEq H^+/ hr in males and less than 5 mEq H^+/hr in females are suggestive of pernicious anemia.

Plasma gastrin level is normally between 25 and 100 pg/ml. Fasting plasma gastrin level higher than 1000 pg/ml is diagnostic of Z-E syndrome.

PATHOPHYSIOLOGY OF PEPTIC ULCER

It is a physiological marvel that gastric juice can easily digest the swallowed pieces of meat but normally, it has no corrosive action on the gastric mucosa itself. Several factors seem to be involved in the protection of gastric mucosa from autodigestion. These factors, collectively known as **gastric mucosal barrier,** include:

a. **Mucous** secreted by surface epithelial cells and mucous neck glands which forms a water insoluble viscoelastic gel with poor diffusion coefficient for H^+.

b. **Bicarbonate** secreted by surface epithelial cells into the boundary zone between the epithelial cells and the mucus layer. The secretion of mucus and bicarbonate is believed to be mediated through prostaglandins.

c. **Tight junctions** between the adjacent cells of gastric surface epithelium.

d. **Rapid turnover** of surface epithelial cells, and rich blood supply.

e. **Prostaglandins.** Endogenous prostaglandins stimulate secretion of gastric mucus as well as gastric and duodenal mucosal bicarbonate. Prostaglandins also participate in the maintenance of gastric mucosal blood flow and integrity of mucosal barrier and promote epithelial cell renewal in response to mucosal injury.

Under normal conditions, a physiologic balance exists between peptic acid secretion and gastroduodenal mucosal defense. Mucosal injury which may lead to peptic ulcer occurs when the balance between the aggressive factors and the defensive mechanisms is disrupted. Aggressive factors, such as **NSAIDs, H. pylori, alcohol, cigarette smoking, psychogenic stress** (excessive acid, and pepsin) or Zollinger-Ellison syndrome can alter the mucosal defense and allow back diffusion of hydrogen ions and subsequent epithelial cell injury.

Cigarette smoking appears to be a risk factor for the development, maintenance, and recurrence of peptic ulcer disease. Smokers are about two times as likely to develop ulcer disease as nonsmokers. Smoking has an inconsistent effect on gastric acid secretion, but it does have other effects on upper gastrointestinal function that could contribute to the pathogenesis of peptic ulcer disease. These include (a) interference with the action of histamine-2 antagonists, (b) acceleration of gastric emptying of liquids, (c) promotion of duodenogastric reflux, (d) reduction in mucosal blood flow, and (e) inhibition of mucosal prostaglandin production. Because these effects are related directly to the act of smoking and cessation of smoking is associated with the prompt recovery of the respective functions, smokers will benefit immediately by stopping or reducing cigarette consumption. Cigarette smoking not only causes ulcer formation, but also in creases the risk of ulcer complications such as ulcer bleeding, stomach obstruction and perforation. Cigarette smoking is also a leading cause of ulcer medication treatment failure.

Mechanisms of injury differ distinctly between duodenal and gastric ulcers. Duodenal ulcer is essentially a *H. pylori*-related disease and is caused mainly by an increase in acid and pepsin load, and gastric metaplasia in the duodenal cap. Gastric ulcer, at least in Western countries, is most commonly associated with NSAID ingestion, although *H. pylori* infection might also be present. Chronic, superficial and atrophic gastritis predominate in patients with gastric ulcers, when even normal acid levels can be associated with mucosal ulceration. Basically in both conditions, ulcer is associated with an imbalance between protective and aggressive factors, with inflammation being a leading cause of this imbalance.

Role of Helicobacter Pylori

Helicobacter pylori is a bacillus responsible for one of the most common infections found in humans worldwide. *H. pylori* organisms are spiral-shaped gram-negative bacteria that are highly motile because of multiple unipolar flagella (Fig. 5.3). They are microaerophilic (need less oxygen) and potent producers of the enzyme urease. *H. pylori inhabit the mucus* adjacent to the gastric mucosa. The most common route of *H. pylori* infection is either oral-to-oral: kissing (stomach contents are transmitted from mouth-to-mouth) or fecal-to-oral (from stool to mouth) contact. Parents and siblings seem to play a primary role in transmission

Helicobacter pylori bacteria colonize the stomach and induce chronic gastritis. It is widely believed that in the absence of treatment, *H. pylori* infection—once established in its gastric niche—persists for life. In Western countries the prevalence of *Helicobacter pylori* infections roughly matches age (i.e. 20% at age 20, 30% at age 30, 80% at age 80, etc.). *Prevalence is higher in third world countries. Most individuals infected by H. pylori will never experience clinical symptoms despite having chronic gastritis.* Approximately 10–20% of those colonized by *H. pylori* will ultimately

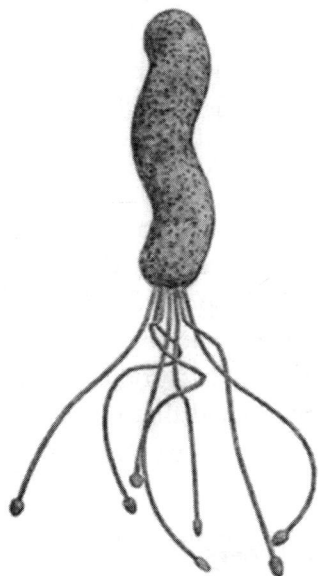

Fig. 5.3: *Helicobacter pylori* bacterium.

develop gastric and duodenal ulcers. A larger proportion of people will get non-specific discomfort, abdominal pain or gastritis. The severity of the inflammation is likely to underlie *H. pylori*-related diseases. Duodenal and stomach ulcers result when the consequences of inflammation allow the acid and pepsin in the stomach lumen to overwhelm the mechanisms that protect the stomach and duodenal mucosa from these caustic substances.

The type of ulcer that develops depends on the location of chronic gastritis, which occurs at the site of *H. pylori* colonization. *In those with duodenal ulcer, H. pylori colonizes the antrum.* The inflammatory response to the bacteria causes destruction of somatostatin-producing D cells in the pylorus. Consequently, the G cells in the antrum secrete more of the hormone gastrin, which travels through the bloodstream to the fundus and body of the stomach. Gastrin stimulates the parietal cells to secrete more acid into the stomach lumen. Chronically increased gastrin levels eventually cause the number of parietal cells to also increase, further escalating the amount of acid secreted. The increased acid load damages the duodenum, and ulceration may eventually result.

In contrast, gastric ulcers are often associated with normal or reduced gastric acid production, suggesting that the mechanisms that protect the gastric mucosa are defective. In these patients *H. pylori* colonize the corpus of the stomach, where the acid-secreting parietal cells are located. However, chronic inflammation induced by the bacteria leads to further reduction of acid production, and eventually atrophy of the stomach lining. Gastric atrophy may lead to gastric ulcer and increases the risk for stomach cancer.

Role of Stress

The development of acute gastric ulcers as a result of severe stress after major surgery or extensive burns is well known. Reduced gastric blood flow coupled with raised plasma cortisol levels seem to be primarily responsible for such ulcers.

Till 1980s, psychological stress was considered the chief cause of duodenal ulcer. The high stung type "A" individuals were considered special candidates for the development of duodenal ulcer. In 1990s, after the discovery of *H. pylori*, it began to be believed that psychogenic factors play no role in the development of chronic peptic ulcer disease. Over the years, it is now being appreciated that psychogenic stress acts as a co-factor with *H. pylori* in the production of hyperacidity leading to duodenal ulcer.

Complications of Peptic Ulcers

Hemorrhage

Mild to severe hemorrhage is the most common complication of peptic ulcer disease. It may occur even when the ulcer pain is not severe. Symptoms include hematemesis (fresh blood or "coffee ground" material); passage of bloody stools or black tarry stools (melena); and weakness, syncope, thirst, and sweating caused by blood loss. However, small amounts of blood in the stool may not be noticeable but, if persistent, can still lead to anemia.

Perforation

A peptic ulcer may penetrate the wall of the stomach. If adhesions prevent leakage into the peritoneal cavity, free penetration is avoided and confined perforation occurs. Ulcers on the front surface of the duodenum, or less commonly the stomach, can go through the wall, creating an opening to the free space in the abdominal cavity. Perforation often leads to catastrophic consequences. Erosion of the gastrointestinal wall by the ulcer leads to spillage of gastric or intestinal content into the abdominal cavity. Perforation at the anterior surface of the stomach leads to acute peritonitis, initially chemical and later bacterial peritonitis. The first sign is often sudden intense abdominal pain. Posterior wall perforation leads to pancreatitis; pain in this situation often radiates to the back.

Penetration

An ulcer may penetrate the muscular wall of the stomach or duodenum and continue into an adjacent organ, such as the liver or pancreas.

Gastric Outlet Obstruction

Gastric outlet obstruction is the third most frequent complication of peptic ulcer disease after bleeding and perforation. It can occur during the acute phase of the disease or in chronic disease.

Obstruction may be caused by scarring, spasm, or inflammation from an ulcer. Symptoms include recurrent, large-volume vomiting, occurring more frequently at the end of the day and often as late as 6 h after the last meal. Loss of appetite with persistent bloating or fullness after eating also suggests gastric outlet obstruction. Prolonged vomiting may cause weight loss, dehydration, and alkalosis.

Cancer

People with ulcers caused by *Helicobacter pylori* have 3 to 6 times the chance of developing stomach cancer later in life. There is no increased risk of developing cancer from ulcers that have other causes.

The association of *H. pylori* with gastric malignancy has been well documented in several epidemiologic studies. However, the course of progression from inflammation to cancer remains unclear. One model describes the stepwise progression of *H. pylori* infection to hypochlorhydria, chronic gastritis, atrophic gastritis, intestinal metaplasia, and gastric cancer. Increased production of the cytokine interleukin-1α has been linked to an increased risk of hypochlorhydria and gastric cancer in infected subjects.

Zollinger-Ellison Syndrome

The syndrome is caused by excessive gastric acid secretion, which results from a gastrin-producing gastrinoma. The tumors are thought to arise from the delta cells that are found in the pancreas and account for about 25 to 40% of gastrinomas. The remaining 50 to 70% arise from enteroendocrine cells in the small intestine. Gastrinomas located in the duodenum are usually multiple and small in size, and are less likely to become malignant than the solitary, sporadic pancreatic gastrinomas. About 55 to 90% of gastrinomas are malignant.

Gastrin not only directly stimulates parietal cell secretion but also causes expansion of the mass of parietal cells. The increase in parietal cells results in an increase in basal acid output and maximal acid output. This substantial secretion of acid results in gastroesophageal reflux disease (GERD) symptoms and damage to the mucosal lining of the GI tract, causing peptic ulcers. In addition, the excessive acid inactivates pancreatic enzymes, which contributes to the diarrhea, steatorrhea, and malabsorption syndrome.

INFANTILE HYPERTROPHIC PYLORIC STENOSIS

Pyloric stenosis, also known as infantile hypertrophic pyloric stenosis (IHPS), is the most common cause of intestinal obstruction in infancy. Although less common in Asian population, IHPS is by no means a rarity. It is 4 times more common in male children. Although it can occur any time from the day of birth to about 3 to 4 months of age, most common presentation is between the 3rd and 6th week of age. The presenting symptoms are almost always projectile non-bilious vomiting in a baby hitherto normal. The presence of an ovoid olive-shaped mass in the right upper quadrant area close to the epigastrium is a very important sign.

Pathophysiology

The lesion is characterized by gastric outlet obstruction and multiple anatomic abnormalities of the pyloric antrum. There is marked hypertrophy and hyperplasia of the mainly circular, but also longitudinal, muscle fibers of pylorus. The antropyloric muscle is abnormally innervated (*see* below). In addition, further luminal narrowing is caused by crowded and redundant mucosa. The mucosa usually is edematous and thickened (Fig. 5.4). In advanced cases, the stomach becomes markedly dilated in response to near-complete obstruction.

Nitric oxide has been demonstrated as a major inhibitory nonadrenergic, noncholinergic neurotransmitter in the GI tract, causing relaxation of smooth muscle of the myenteric plexus. Impairment of this neuronal nitric oxide synthase (nNOS) production has been implicated not only in IHPS, but also achalasia, diabetic gastroparesis, and Hirschsprung's disease.

The gastric outlet obstruction due to the hypertrophic pylorus impairs emptying of gastric contents into the duodenum. As a consequence, all

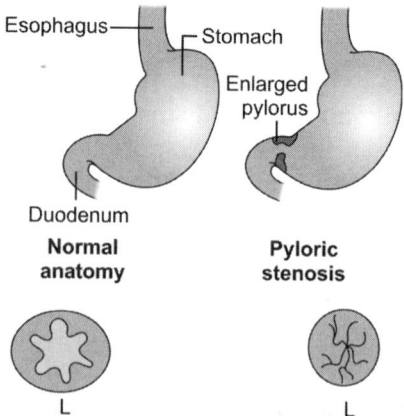

Fig. 5.4: The pyloric sphincter in a normal infant and in a case of hypertrophic pyloric stenosis. L = lumen of pylorus

ingested food and gastric secretions can only exit via vomiting, which can be of a projectile nature. The vomited material does not contain bile because the pyloric obstruction prevents entry of duodenal contents (containing bile) into the stomach. This results in loss of gastric acid (hydrochloric acid), leading to metabolic alkalosis. Persistent vomiting is accompanied by loss of not only acid but also fluids from the stomach. The resulting hypovolemia leads to a secondary hyperaldosteronism. The high aldosterone levels cause the kidneys to:

a. Retain Na^+ (to correct the intravascular volume depletion)
b. Excrete increased amounts of K^+ and H^+ into the urine, resulting in hypokalemia and further aggravation of alkalosis.

Further Reading

Eastwood GL. **The role of smoking in peptic ulcer disease.** J ClinGastroenterol. 1988;10 Suppl 1:S19–23.

Levenstein S. **Stress and peptic ulcer: life beyond helicobacter.** *BMJ* 1998; 316: 538

*www.uptodate.com/***Association between** *Helicobacter pylori* **infection and duodenal ulcer**

6

Disorders of Intestines

SMALL INTESTINE

The small intestine measures approximately 2.5–3 cm in diameter and 6 meters in length during life (in a cadaver, it is much longer because of the loss of smooth muscle tone). The ligament of Treitz demarcates duodenum from jejunum. Below the duodenum, the upper 40% of the small intestine is called the jejunum and the remaining 60% as ileum. There is no anatomic demarcation between jejunum and ileum. The villi, a characteristic feature of small intestinal mucosa are largest and most numerous in the duodenum and jejunum, and become fewer and smaller in the ileum. The ileum ends with the ileocecal valve (sphincter), which regulates the movement of chyme into the large intestine and prevents backward movement of material from the large intestine.

Small intestine is the site of final digestion and absorption of foodstuffs. Most of the digestive enzymes that act in the small intestine are secreted by the pancreas (Table 6.1). In addition bile salts are essential for proper digestion and absorption of dietary fats. The pancreatic and bile ducts open in the second part of duodenum. As a small bolus of chyme leave the stomach, its intimate mixing with pancreatic juice and bile helps in proper digestion and absorption. Presence of food in the upper small intestine is essential for the release of gastrointestinal hormones such as

Table 6.1: Principal digestive enzymes in the small intestine

Source	Enzyme	Substrate
Pancreas	Trypsin	Proteins
	Chymotrypsin	Proteins
	Carboxypeptidase	Proteins
	Lipase	Fats
	Amylase	Starch
Intestinal mucosa	Enterokinase	Trypsinogen
	Maltase	Maltose
	Lactase	Lactose
	Sucrase	Sucrose

Table 6.2: Site of absorption of various foodstuffs in the GIT

Stomach	Duodenum and jejunum	Ileum	Colon
Alcohol (some drugs)	Sugars Amino acids Water soluble vitamins Fat soluble vitamins Fatty acids Na^+ K^+ Ca^{++} Fe^{++} Cl^- Water	Vitamin B_{12} Bile salts Na^+ Water	Na^+ Cl^- Water

secretin and cholecystokinin which increase the secretion of pancreatic juice and bile. When the duodenum is bypassed (e.g. Billroth II operation) malabsorption commonly occurs. The optimum pH for the activity of pancreatic enzymes is 6–7. Such pH is achieved by neutralization of the highly acidic chyme that leaves the stomach by the alkaline pancreatic and bile juices.

The intestinal digestion of foodstuffs results in production of monosaccharides, amino acids and fatty acids. These products and various other components of food such as vitamins, minerals and water are absorbed in specific parts of the small intestine (Table 6.2). This knowledge becomes important when a part of the small intestine is to be resected as a treatment of some disorder (e.g. Crohn's disease). Extensive resection of small intestine is most likely to result in intestinal malabsorption (short bowel or short gut syndrome). Short bowel syndrome usually develops when less than 2 meters of the small intestine left after surgery.

Defense Mechanisms of the Small Intestine

1. *Gastric Acid*

Gastric acid is primarily responsible for killing the bacteria swallowed in raw, uncooked vegetables and fruit. Gastric acid is the chief cause of low bacteria populations in the proximal small intestine, particularly anaerobic bacteria. Reduced gastric acid secretion, because of atrophic gastritis or peptic ulcer surgery, markedly increases the bacteria in the stomach and upper small intestines.

2. *Small Intestinal Motility*

Migrating motor complexes (MMC) (or migrating myoelectric complexes) are waves of activity which sweep through the intestines in a regular cycle during fasting state. These motor complexes help trigger peristaltic waves which facilitate transportation of indigestible substances such as bone, fiber and foreign bodies from the stomach, through the small intestine past the ileocecal sphincter into the colon. The MMC originates in the stomach roughly every 75–90 minutes during the interdigestive phase (between meals) and is responsible for the rumbling experienced when hungry.

MMC also serves to transport bacteria from the small intestine to the large intestine, and to inhibit the migration of colonic bacteria into the terminal ileum. Anatomical defects can reduce peristaltic efficacy; for example, blind pouches result in a stagnant portion of the intestine, e.g. blind loop, and small bowel diverticuli. Impaired motility in the small intestine is a characteristic feature of scleroderma.

3. *Mucosal Barrier*

The tight junctions between the adjacent epithelial cells constitute an important anatomic barrier. Moreover, the epithelial cells are covered with a layer of mucus secreted by goblet cells and surface epithelial cells, which entraps the bacteria. The constant renewal of epithelial cells (every 48 hours) ensures that the bacteria are swept down with very little chance of deep tissue invasion. This protective mechanism is disrupted in disorders such as celiac disease, tropical sprue, etc.

4. *Immunological Barrier*

The lymphoid tissue associated with gastrointestinal mucosa constitutes about 25% of the total lymphoid tissue of the body. Recent studies have shown a unique class of immunocytes called M cells (microfold cells) among the small intestinal mucosal epithelial cells. M cells differ from the adjacent enterocytes in that they lack microvilli on the apical surface. Instead, they possess broad microfolds that give the cells the name. M cells are far less abundant than enterocytes (Fig. 6.1). M cells are believed to act as antigen sampling system. Primary function of M cells seems to be rapid uptake of the antigen/microorganism, processing it and presentation to the immune system located in the lamina propria of the mucosa. Thus, M cells promote effective immune responses. M cell damage seems to be responsible for increased rate of bacterial invasions in patients with chronic inflammatory disorders of the intestines.

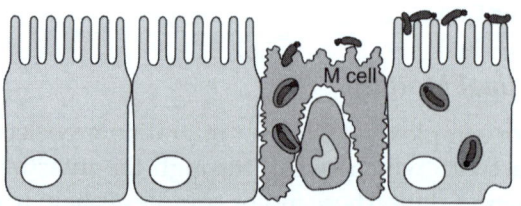

Fig. 6.1: The M cell among enterocytes.

5. *Normal Intestinal Florae*

For example: *Lactobacillus*—protect the gut from bacterial overgrowth by maintaining a low pH. Abnormal communications may produce pathways that allow enteric bacteria to pass between the proximal and distal bowel.

Malabsorption Syndrome

Intestinal malabsorption may occur because of a variety of causes involving inadequate digestion of foodstuffs, inadequate absorption or both.

Inadequate Digestion

a. Inadequate intestinal pancreatic enzyme concentration: Chronic pancreatitis
b. Inadequate intestinal bile salt concentration
   - Parenchymal liver disease
   - Intrahepatic or extrahepatic biliary obstruction
   - Intestinal bacterial overgrowth
c. Multifactorial: postgastrectomy

Inadequate Absorption

a. Inadequate absorptive surface: extensive small intestinal resection
b. Primary mucosal absorptive defect
   - Lactase deficiency
   - Celiac disease
   - Tropical sprue

Diarrhea is the most common presenting symptom of intestinal malabsorption. Basically it is osmotic diarrhea. As a result of inadequate digestion/absorption of foodstuffs, a greater solute and water load is presented to the colon. Moreover, presence of fatty acids causes irritation of the colon. Steatorrhea is another common presenting symptom. This term refers to presence of excessive amount of fat in the stools. The stools are bulky, foul-smelling, have oily appearance and float on toilet water. Flatus, another common symptom is produced by bacterial fermentation of unabsorbed carbohydrates in the colon. The pathophysiological basis of various clinical features of malabsorption syndrome is summarized in Table 6.3.

Lactose Intolerance

Lactose intolerance syndrome is a group of symptoms that develop on consumption of milk or milk products. Typical symptoms consist of abdominal bloating, abdominal cramps, flatulence, nausea, barborygmi (rumbling stomach) and diarrhea. These symptoms develop between 30 minutes to 2 hours of intake of lactose-containing food.

Table 6.3: Pathophysiological mechanism of various clinical features of malabsorption syndrome

Organ system	Clinical feature	Pathophysiological mechanism
GI tract	Diarrhea	(i) Malabsorption of food stuffs in the small intestine leads to greater solute and water load on the colon.
		(ii) Irritation of colon an fatty acids
	Flatus	Bacterial fermentation of unabsorbed carbohydrates.
	Abdominal pain	Distension or inflammation of bowel or chronic pancreatitis.
	Glossitis, cheilosis, stomatitis	Deficiency of vitamins and iron.
General	Generalized weakness	Loss of calories and vitamins in feces, anorexia.
Hemopoietic	Anemia	Impaired absorption of iron, folic acid and vitamin B_{12}.
	Bleeding	Vitamin K malabsorption, hypoprothrombinemia.
Musculoskeletal	Bone pains	Protein depletion: osteoporosis. Vitamin D deficiency: osteomalacia.
	Tetany	Hypocalcemia, hypomagnesemia.
Nervous system	Night blindness, xeroophthalmia	Vitamin A deficiency.
	Peripheral neuropathy	Vitamin B_1 and B_{12} deficiency.

In most of the mammals, the concentration of lactose, a brush small intestinal border enzyme, begins to decline after weaning. However, in some human populations, particularly Europeans, the production of the enzyme persists even in adulthood. The incidence of milk intolerance varies from 5% in Europeans to over 90% in some Asian and African populations.

In lactase deficient individuals, small amounts of milk (or milk products) are often tolerated. The severity of symptoms increases with the increase in lactose load. In lactase deficiency state, the dietary lactose passes unabsorbed into the colon, where it undergoes bacterial fermentation to produce gases such as hydrogen, carbon dioxide and methane. Presence of lactose in the colon also produces diarrhea by osmotic effect on luminal water.

The clinical diagnosis of lactase intolerance can be confirmed by hydrogen breath test after oral administration of 25 g of lactose. Intestinal biopsy to demonstrate the deficiency of lactase is seldom resorted to. Lactase intolerance should not be confused with milk allergy to milk proteins.

Lactase deficiency has been classified as follows:
1. *Primary* lactase deficiency. Symptoms usually begin after the age of 2 years. More often, symptoms manifest in late adolescents or adults.
2. *Secondary or transient* lactase deficiency. It results secondary to an injury to small intestinal mucosa by acute gastroenteritis, diarrhea or intestinal parasites.

3. ***Congenital*** lactase deficiency is very rare. This autosomal recessive disorder is apparent from birth.

Celiac Disease (Non-tropical Sprue; Gluten-sensitive Enteropathy)

This disorder is caused by an abnormal intestinal mucosal response to gluten, the high molecular weight protein found in wheat and wheat products. The exact mechanism is not clear. Deficiency of any specific peptidase has not been demonstrated. Gluten is believed to produce intestinal mucosal damage by an immunological reaction. Serum of patients with celiac disease contains antibodies to gliadin, an alcohol-soluble peptide fraction of gluten. The concept of immune nature of the disorder is supported by the association of other autoimmune diseases such as Type I diabetes mellitus and autoimmune thyroiditis.

Histological examination of jejunal biopsy reveals loss of villi leading to blunting and flattening of mucosal surface, elongation of crypts and dense infiltration of lamina propria by lymphocytes (Fig. 6.2). The symptoms and histological picture of jejunum can be reversed by intake of gluten-free diet.

Tropical Sprue

Tropical sprue is an intestinal malabsorption syndrome with specific geographical distribution. It affects residents or visitors of tropics including Indian subcontinent, Southeast Asia, Northern South America, Caribbean islands and Africa. The small intestinal histological picture is similar to celiac disease (villus-blunting and crypt hyperplasia) but for two differences: (i) total flattening of mucosa is rare and, (ii) though upper small intestine is predominantly affected; the distal small intestine up to the terminal ileum may be involved. That explains more common occurrence of megaloblastic anemia, because of folic acid and vitamin B_{12} deficiency in tropical sprue. The exact etiology of tropical sprue is not known. Much evidence points towards gastrointestinal infections, but

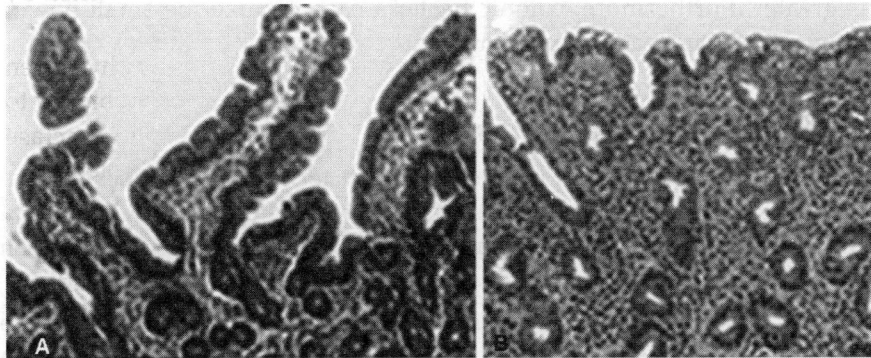

Fig. 6.2: Histological structure of jejunal biopsy: (A) Normal and (B) a case of celiac disease

no specific pathogen has been identified. Stool culture shows coliform bacteria such as Klebsiella, *E.coli* and Enterobacter. The speculation is primarily based on the fact that administration of broad spectrum antibiotics results in prompt recovery.

Small Bowel Syndrome

The jejunum has taller villi, deeper crypts, and greater enzyme activity compared to the ileum. Therefore, under normal conditions, about 90% of digestion and absorption of foodstuffs is accomplished in the proximal 100–150 cm of the jejunum. If a significant portion or all of the jejunum is resected, the absorption of proteins, carbohydrates, and most vitamins and minerals may be affected in spite of mucosal adaptation in that occurs in the ileum. Enzymatic digestion suffers because of the irreplaceable loss of intestinal hormones produced by the jejunum. Consequently, biliary and pancreatic secretions decrease. Gastrin levels rise, causing hypersecretion of gastric juice. The resultant high acid output from the stomach may injure the small bowel mucosa. Additionally, the low intraluminal pH creates unfavorable conditions for optimal activity of the pancreatic enzymes that are present. Diarrhea may then result if a large osmotically active solute load of unabsorbed nutrients is delivered to the ileum and colon.

Ileal resection severely decreases the capacity to absorb water and electrolytes, in spite of the fact that colonic water absorption can be increased to as much as 5 times its normal capacity following small bowel resection. In addition, the terminal ileum is the site of absorption of bile salts and vitamin B_{12}. Loss of significant lengths of ileum almost invariably results in diarrhea. Continued loss of bile salts following resection of the terminal ileum leads to fat malabsorption, steatorrhea, and loss of fat-soluble vitamins. Retention of the ileocecal valve plays a pivotal role in massive small bowel resection. If the ileocecal valve can be preserved, intestinal transit is slowed, allowing more time for absorption. If the ileocecal valve is lost, transit time is shorter, and loss of fluid and nutrients is greater. Furthermore, colonic bacteria can colonize the small bowel, worsening diarrhea and nutrient loss.

Bacterial Overgrowth Syndrome

Bacterial overgrowth syndrome (BOS) is a term that describes clinical manifestations that occur when the normally low number of bacteria that inhabit the stomach, duodenum, jejunum, and proximal ileum significantly increases or becomes overtaken by other pathogens.

Low concentrations of various bacteria live within or attached to intestinal luminal surface. These bacteria are thought to be present soon after birth and throughout later life living in symbiosis with the human host. This relationship is thought to be vital for normal digestive processes, immunity, and intestinal development.

In a normal person, the bacterial count in the upper small intestine is less than 10^3 organisms/ml aspirate. When the defense mechanisms of the small intestine, discussed earlier breakdown, the bacterial count may increase above 10^{10} organisms/ml aspirate. The bacteria usually found are those normally present in the colon. The overgrowth of the bacteria causes direct or indirect alteration in bile salt metabolism, and other metabolic defects. The bacteria *deconjugate the bile salts* leading to:
  a. Decreased concentration of bile salts,
  b. Absorption of deconjugated bile acids in the jejunum. It further decreases the intraluminal concentration of bile salts in the jejunum. (Bile salts are normally absorbed in the ileum).

Consequently, both intestinal digestion and absorption of fat suffers. Deconjugated bile acids directly inhibit carbohydrate transporters. The unabsorbed sugars ferment into organic acids, thereby reducing the intraluminal pH and producing osmotic diarrhea. The deconjugated bile acids also damage intestinal enterocytes and induce water secretion by the colonic mucosa. All these changes produce malabsorption syndrome. Uptake of vitamin B_{12} by the bacteria accounts for particularly low plasma levels of the vitamin and symptoms of pernicious anemia. In chronic ALS, iron deficiency results from deficiency of gastric acid and upper intestinal bypass.

Postgastrectomy Malabsorption Syndrome

In such cases, malabsorption is basically due to maldigestion caused by:
1. Decreased stimulation of exocrine pancreas since chyme bypasses duodenum
2. Inadequate mixing of chyme with bile and pancreatic juice
3. Stasis of intestinal contents in the afferent loop leading to bacterial overgrowth.

Diabetic Steatorrhea

The occurrence of diarrhea and steatorrhea in diabetes mellitus is well documented. One or more of the following may be implicated:
1. Associated exocrine pancreas insufficiency.
2. Coexisting celiac sprue
3. Abnormal bacterial proliferation in small intestine
4. Autonomic neuropathy

COLON

Colon or the large intestine is a tube about 6 cm in diameter and 1.5 meters in length. Alkaline mucus (pH 8) is the chief secretion of colon. Absorption of water and electrolytes is the chief function of the large intestine. The colonic lumen contains a large number of bacteria which synthesize vitamin K, folic acid and a number of other vitamins included in B complex, which are absorbed in blood circulation.

Large intestine cannot absorb carbohydrates, amino acids or fatty acids. These products reach the colon in patients with inadequate digestion/absorption of foodstuffs in the small intestine (maldigestive/malabsorption syndrome). The fermentation of undigested carbohydrates by the colonic bacteria produces large amount of gases (flatus). Undigested fats are hydrolyzed by the bacteria in to fatty acids, which cannot be absorbed. Fatty acids act as irritant to the colonic mucosa, producing diarrhea. Undigested proteins are broken down by the bacterial deaminases. Thus, even in a case with severe maldigestion, the stools contain the degraded products rather than macromolecules of carbohydrates, fats or proteins as such.

Diarrhea

Diarrhea is characterized by increased water content of the feces, which is usually accompanied by increased frequency of defecation. In the Western world, average normal fecal weight is 200 g/day, with firm to hard consistency of stools. In India and most other developing countries, where fiber-rich carbohydrates constitute the staple diet, the bulk and water content of feces is larger. Therefore, it has been suggested that diarrhea may be defined as a condition in which fecal mass and its water content are greater than usual. Diarrhea may be due to:

a. Abnormalities in Small Intestines

- Endotoxins
- Maldigestion/malabsorption of food stuffs

b. Abnormalities in the Colon

- Infections
- Irritable bowel syndrome
- Ulcerative colitis
- Crohn's disease

  From pathophysiological point of view, diarrhea may be classified as:
- Secretory
- Exudative
- Osmotic
- Malabsorptive
- Motility disorder

1. Secretory Diarrhea

Out of approximately 9 liters of water entering the human lumen (as food, water, and GIT secretions), only 1–1.5 L of water reach the colon. In the colon, most of it is reabsorbed and approximately 200 ml is excreted with feces per day. If challenged by excessive fluid load from the small intestine, the colon has the maximum absorptive capacity of 6 liters per day. Such a situation arises typically due to endotoxins produced by *V. cholerae* or in patients suffering from malabsorption syndrome.

Endotoxins of *V. cholerae* produce uncontrolled secretory activity in the epithelial cells of the small intestinal mucosa. The fluid loss in the stools may be as high as 1 L per hour. Unless promptly treated, volume depletion, dehydration, hyperkalemia and hyperchloremic metabolic acidosis may lead to death within hours of onset of diarrhea. The endotoxin does not affect gastric or colonic function. Even in the small intestine, the absorptive function is normal. Thus, oral fluid therapy is sound, logical and efficacious.

2. Exudative Diarrhea

This type of diarrhea is due to outpouring of plasma proteins, blood, mucus or pus from the sites of colonic mucosal ulceration. Exudative diarrhea is the hallmark of ulcerative colitis and infective diarrhea caused by *E. histolytica*, Shigella or Solmonella. In this type of diarrhea, frequency of defecation may be large, but the volume of stools passed each time is such that the total volume of stools passed per day is less than 1 L per day. Tenesmus, sense of rectal urgency followed by passage of small volume of stools is noteworthy features of exudative diarrhea. Tenesmus is characterized by a continued sensation of needing to pass tools, accompanied by pain, cramping and straining.

3. Osmotic Diarrhea

This type of diarrhea is due to the presence of poorly absorbed solutes in the gastrointestinal tract. These solutes withdraw large amount of water into the lumen of the gut by osmotic effect. Such type of diarrhea is seen in lactose intolerance.

4. Malabsorptive Diarrhea

This type of diarrhea is characterized by passage of large, bulky, greasy and foul-smelling stools. Basically, it is osmotic type of diarrhea.

5. Motility Disorder Diarrhea

Diarrhea of irritable bowel syndrome and hyperthyroidism belong to this category.

Irritable Bowel Syndrome

Irritable bowel syndrome (IBS) is said to be the commonest reason for referral to a gastroenterologist. It is called a functional disorder because it is not associated with any specific biochemical, structural or serological abnormality. Characteristic clinical symptoms of IBS include lower abdominal pain related to the bowel movements, changing bowel habits (e.g. diarrhea, constipation or alternation between the two), abdominal bloating, a sense of incomplete rectal evacuation and passage of mucus. Exact pathophysiology of IBS is not known. Following are outlines of some of the theories in this regard.

- Visceral hypersensitivity because of chronic stress.
- Functional imbalance between release and reuptake of serotonin in the serotonergic neurons of enteric nervous system
- Low grade infection following acute gastroenteritis
- Some cases labeled IBS may actually be mild cases of celiac disease. The American College of Gastroenterology recommends that all patients with symptoms of IBS be tested for celiac disease.

Inflammatory Bowel Disease

Inflammatory bowel disease (IBD) is the term used to include two chronic conditions of uncertain etiology, namely ulcerative colitis (UC) and Crohn's disease (CD). Both are characterized by recurrent episodes of abdominal pain, often with diarrhea. Intestinal ulceration and bleeding can be complications of severe mucosal inflammation in both UC and CD. Although ulcerative colitis and Crohn's disease have distinct histopathological picture, a significant percentage of patients have indeterminate findings. Crohn's disease is also referred to a regional enteritis, terminal ileitis, or granulomatous ileocolitis.

The pathogenesis of Crohn's disease and ulcerative colitis is still unclear. Both autoimmune and immune-mediated phenomena seem to be involved. Immune-mediate phenomena include a variety of abnormalities of humoral and cell-mediated immunity, and a generalized enhanced reactivity against intestinal bacterial antigens in both CD and UC. It is currently believed that loss of tolerance against the indigenous enteric flora is the central event in IBD pathogenesis. Various complementary factors probably contribute to the loss of tolerance to commensal bacteria in IBD. The immune response disrupts the intestinal mucosa and leads to a chronic inflammatory process.

In ulcerative colitis, inflammation begins in the rectum and extends proximally in an uninterrupted fashion to the proximal colon, eventually involving the entire length of the large intestine. The small intestine is never involved. The rectum is always involved in ulcerative colitis, and no "skip areas" (i.e., normal areas of the bowel interspersed with diseased areas) are present. Ulcerative colitis primarily involves the mucosa and the submucosa, with formation of crypt abscesses and mucosal ulceration. The mucosa typically appears granular and friable. In more severe cases, pseudopolyps form, consisting of areas of hyperplastic growth with swollen mucosa surrounded by inflamed mucosa with shallow ulcers. As the disease becomes chronic, the colon becomes a rigid foreshortened tube that lacks its usual haustral markings, leading to the lead pipe appearance observed on barium enema radiograph. The characteristic histological findings are acute and chronic inflammation of the mucosa (infiltration by polymorphonuclear leukocytes and mononuclear cells), crypt abscesses, distortion of the mucosal glands, and goblet cell depletion (Fig. 6.3A).

The most consistent clinical feature of UC is the presence of blood and mucus mixed with stool, accompanied by lower abdominal cramping which is most intense during the passage of bowel movements. The presence of diarrhea with blood and mucus as opposed to the absence of blood is used clinically to differentiate between UC and irritable bowel syndrome.

Crohn's disease, in contrast to UC, can involve any part of the gastrointestinal tract from the oropharynx to the perianal area. Diseased segments frequently are separated by intervening normal bowel, leading to the term "skip areas." Inflammation can be transmural, often extending through to the serosa, resulting in sinus tracts or fistula formation. Histological findings include mall superficial ulcerations over a Peyer's patch and focal chronic inflammation extending to the submucosa, sometimes accompanied by non-caseating granuloma formation (Fig. 6.3B). The most common location is the ileocecal region, followed by the terminal ileum alone; diffuse small bowel, or isolated colonic disease in decreasing order of frequency. Gastrointestinal symptoms depend on the location, extent, and severity of involvement. Extensive

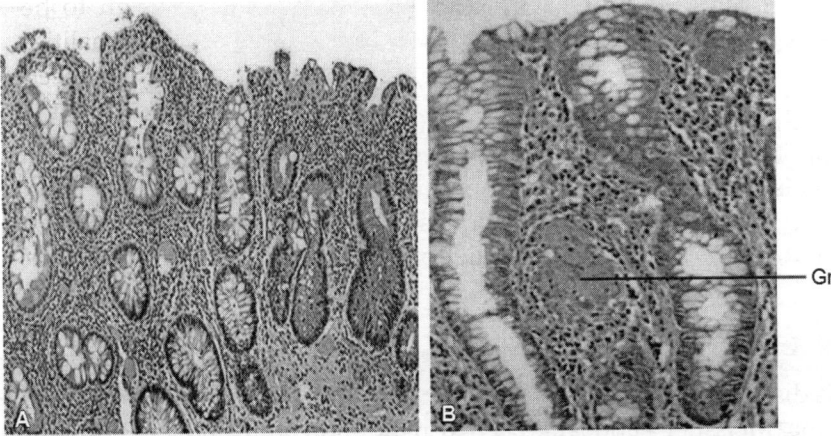

Fig. 6.3: Histolopathological picture of ulcerative colitis (A) and Crohn's disease (B). Gr = granuloma.

small bowel disease causes diffuse abdominal pain, anorexia, diarrhea, and weight loss and may result in lactose malabsorption. Colonic CD may mimic UC, presenting with diarrhea with blood and mucus associated with crampy lower abdominal pain that is often relieved by defecation.

Because of malabsorption of fat and bile salts, the incidence of gallstones and kidney stones is increased in Crohn's disease. Gallstones are formed because of increased cholesterol concentration in the bile, caused by a reduced bile salt pool. Patients who have Crohn's disease with ileal disease or resection also are likely to form calcium oxalate kidney stones. With the fat malabsorption, unabsorbed long-chain fatty acids bind calcium in the lumen. Oxalate in the lumen normally is bound to calcium. Calcium oxalate is poorly soluble and poorly absorbed. However, if calcium is bound to mal-absorbed fatty acids, oxalate combines with sodium to form sodium oxalate, which is soluble and is absorbed in the colon (enteric hyperoxaluria).

The differences in intestinal complications between ulcerative colitis and Crohn's disease depend on the characteristically dissimilar behavior of the inflammation associated with these diseases. Therefore, complications involving the small intestine, such as malabsorption, occur only in Crohn's disease and not in ulcerative colitis. Small intestinal bacterial overgrowth in Crohn's disease can result from an intestinal stricture. In Crohn's disease of the duodenum and jejunum, malabsorption of nutrients can cause malnutrition, weight loss, and diarrhea; whereas in Crohn's disease of the ileum, malabsorption of bile salts can cause diarrhea and malabsorption of vitamin B_{12} can lead to anemia.

Extraintestinal manifestations of inflammatory bowel disease (IBD) include iritis, episcleritis, arthritis, and skin involvement, as well as pericholangitis and sclerosing cholangitis. These extraintestinal manifestations are observed in up to 20–40% of patients with IBD.

Cancer Risk

Cancer of the small intestine, where Crohn's disease usually occurs, is an exceedingly rare disease. The potential risk of cancer of the colon, as a complication of ulcerative colitis or Crohn's disease (in cases in which colon is involved) is well known. The incidence is significantly greater than in the average population but usually occurs in those cases in which the entire colon has been involved for at least 10 years.

HIRSCHSPRUNG'S DISEASE

This disorder results from a congenital absence of intramural ganglionic plexus (Meissner's and Auerbach's) in the anorectum and variable length of distal colon. The disorder is also known as congenital aganglionosis of the distal bowel. Aganglionosis begins with the anus, which is always involved, and continues proximally for a variable distance. The precise mechanism underlying the development of Hirschsprung's disease is unknown.

Enteric ganglion cells are derived from the neural crest. During normal development, neuroblasts can be seen in the small intestine by the 7th week of gestation and will reach the colon by the 12th week of gestation. One possible etiology for Hirschsprung disease is a defect in the migration of these neuroblasts down their path to the distal intestine. Alternatively, normal migration may occur with a failure of neuroblasts to survive.

Additionally, the observation that the smooth muscle cells of aganglionic colon are electrically inactive when undergoing electrophysiologic studies also points to a myogenic component in the development of Hirschsprung's disease.

Normal motility is primarily under the control of intrinsic neurons. These ganglia control both contraction and relaxation of smooth muscle, with relaxation predominating. Extrinsic control is mainly through the cholinergic and adrenergic fibers. The cholinergic fibers cause contraction, and the adrenergic fibers mainly cause inhibition. Bowel function remains adequate despite a loss of extrinsic innervation.

Under normal circumstances, the ganglia appear to act as a final common path for both sympathetic and parasympathetic influences. Their absence may perhaps produce the uncoordinated contractions of the affected bowel. Spasm, lack of propulsive peristalsis, and mass contraction of the aganglionic segment have all been well documented, in addition to the lack of relaxation of the bowel and the spasm of the internal sphincter. The clinical results of these pathophysiological events is partial or total colonic obstruction.

Further Reading

Bamias, G; Nyce, MR; Rue, S; Cominelli, F. **New Concepts in the pathophysiology of inflammatory bowel disease.** *Ann Intern Med 2005 ; 143:895–904.*

Camilleri, M. **Etiology and pathophysiology of irritable bowel syndrome and chronic constipation.** *Adv Stud Med 2005; 5: S955–S964.*

Eagon, JC; Miedema, BW; Kelly, KA. **Postgastrectomy syndromes.** *Surg Clin North Am. 1992;72:445–65.*

Hendrickson, BA; Gokhale, R, Cho, JH. **Clinical aspects and pathophysiology of inflammatory bowel disease.** *Clinical Microbiology Reviews. 2002; 15:79–94.*

Kucharzik, T, et al. **Role of M cells in intestinal barrier function.** *Ann N Y Acad Sci. 2000;915:171–183.*

Ovens, RS; Greenson JK. **The pathology of malabsorption: current concepts.** *Histopathology 2007;50:64–82.*

7
Disorders of Pancreas

Acinar cells of exocrine pancreas (Fig.7.1A) produce a huge variety of digestive enzymes (*see* Table 6.1). Such enzymes are produced in inactive forms and packed in the cytoplasm of acinar cells as stable vesicles called zymogen granules. Another type of granules that are present in most of the cells including pancreatic acinar cells called lysosomal granules. These granules are involved in the breakdown of intracellular organelles. In the acinar cells these granules are kept segregated from the zymogen granules. During normal digestion, the zymogen granules pour the inactive digestive enzymes into the pancreatic ductules. The digestive enzymes are activated only in the lumen of the upper small intestine.

ACUTE PANCREATITIS

Acute pancreatitis remains a common disorder with potentially devastating consequences. Although most episodes are mild and self limited, up to a fifth of patients develop a severe attack that can be fatal.

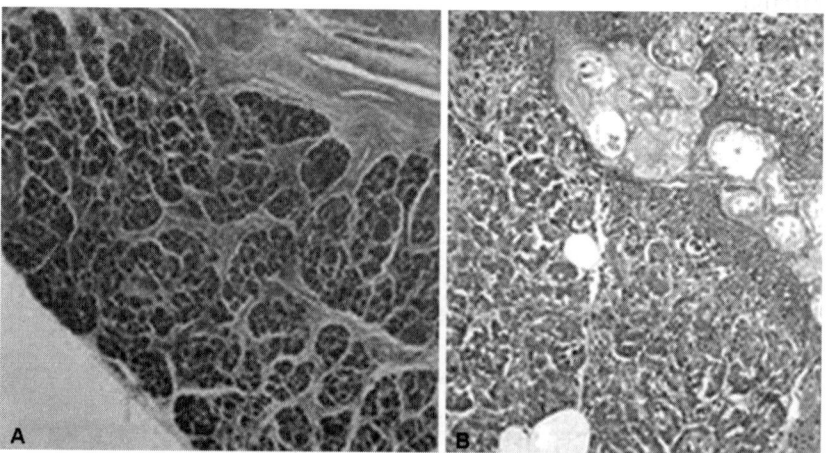

Fig. 7.1: Histological picture of acute pancreatitis (B) as compared to normal architecture (A).

Acute pancreatitis is an acute inflammatory process of the pancreas that can involve peripancreatic tissues or remote organ systems, or both. It may occur as an isolated attack or recur in distinct episodes with reversion to normal histology between attacks. By definition, acute pancreatitis is reversible; it is distinguished from chronic pancreatitis by the absence of continuing inflammation, irreversible structural changes, and permanent impairment of exocrine and endocrine pancreatic function. It can be difficult to distinguish between acute pancreatitis and an acute exacerbation in chronic pancreatitis.

One of the very first events in the development of acute pancreatitis is premature activation of digestive enzymes within the acinar cells, by the contents of lysosomal granules, particularly cathepsin B. The activated enzymes, primarily trypsin, but also chymotrypsin and elastase cause necrosis of the acinar cells. Subsequently, the activated digestive enzymes diffuse into the interstitial and endothelial spaces and begin autodigestion of the gland. Tissue breakdown products potentiate vascular injury, with local recruitment of cytokine and arachidonic acid metabolite-secreting leukocytes. These agents produce edema and oxidative stress. The increase in vascular permeability promotes thrombosis and hemorrhage. The pathological process may progress to pancreatic ischemia and necrosis. Increased vascular permeability can lead to bacterial translocation into the pancreatic bed and result in infected pancreatic necrosis (necrotizing pancreatitis), a life-threatening complication of acute pancreatitis. In more severe cases, systemic inflammatory response syndrome, renal failure, shock, myocardial stress, fever, or acute respiratory distress syndrome may develop.

Activated enzymes and cytokines that enter the peritoneal cavity cause a chemical burn and third spacing of fluid; those that enter the systemic circulation cause a systemic inflammatory response that can result in acute respiratory distress syndrome and renal failure. The systemic effects are mainly the result of increased capillary permeability and decreased vascular tone, which result from the released cytokines and chemokines. Phospholipase A_2 is thought to injure alveolar membranes of the lungs.

Alcoholic Pancreatitis

Alcohol is a well-known precipitant of acute pancreatitis, although the incidence of acute pancreatitis in heavy alcohol consumers is not more than 5% per year. Therefore, it seems there are some other factors, environmental or genetic, that influence the development of acute pancreatitis in alcoholics. Furthermore, alcoholic acute pancreatitis has the highest associated risk of overall mortality, with the odds of death increased 90% as compared with biliary pancreatitis. The exact mechanism by which alcohol causes acute pancreatitis is still not clear. It has been suggested that products of alcohol metabolism such as acetaldehyde and oxygen radicals are responsible for the rupture of membranes of the zymogen and lysosomal granules.

Alcoholics are usually admitted with an acute exacerbation of chronic pancreatitis. Occasionally, however, pancreatitis can develop in a patient with a weekend binging habit, and several case reports have described a large alcohol load precipitating a first attack. Distinguishing between the two most common etiologies of acute pancreatitis, gallstones and alcohol, has important implications for treatment.

Potential Complications of Acute Pancreatitis

- Hypovolemia
- Pancreatic necrosis
- Extra-pancreatic necrosis
- Acute respiratory distress syndrome
- Acute renal failure
- Adynamic ileus
- Circulatory shock
- Sepsis

Biliary Pancreatitis

Biliary pancreatitis, synonymous with gallstone pancreatitis, is a form of acute pancreatitis caused by the passage of gallstones through the cystic duct and into the distal common bile duct and temporarily lodging at the sphincter of Oddi, where they can obstruct the biliary and pancreatic ducts. It is thought that acinar cell injury is secondary to increasing pancreatic duct pressures caused by the gallstone. Incidence is highest in patients with small gallstones, or microlithiasis, as these stones are more likely to escape the gallbladder and transit the cystic duct to reach the common bile duct.

Post-endoscopic retrograde cholangiopancreatography (Post-ERCP) pancreatitis is probably the third most common cause of pancreatitis. Prospective studies have shown the risk is at least 5%. The risk is increased if the endoscopist is inexperienced, the patient is thought to have sphincter of Oddi dysfunction, or manometry is performed on the sphincter of Oddi.

Abdominal trauma causes an elevation of amylase and lipase levels in 17% of cases and clinical pancreatitis in 5% of cases. Pancreatic injury occurs more often in penetrating injuries (e.g., from knives, bullets) than in blunt abdominal trauma (e.g., from steering wheels, horses, bicycles).

CHRONIC PANCREATITIS

Chronic pancreatitis (CP) is defined as a progressive inflammatory disease of the pancreas, characterized by irreversible morphologic changes and gradual fibrotic replacement of the gland. Most people with chronic

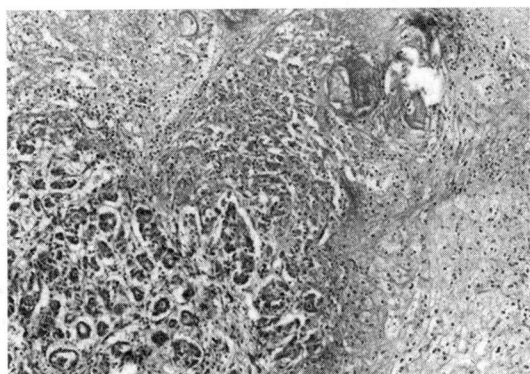

Fig. 7.2: Chronic pancreatitis.

pancreatitis have abdominal pain, although some people have no pain at all. The pain may get worse when eating or drinking, spread to the back, or become constant and disabling. In certain cases, abdominal pain goes away as the condition advances, probably because the pancreas is no longer making digestive enzymes or nerve endings have been destroyed. Other symptoms include nausea, vomiting, weight loss, and fatty stools.

People with chronic disease often lose weight, even when their appetite and eating habits are normal. The weight loss occurs because the body does not secrete enough pancreatic enzymes to break down food, so nutrients are not absorbed normally. Poor digestion leads to fecal loss of fats, proteins, and carbohydrates. If the insulin-producing cells of the pancreas (islet cells) have been damaged, diabetes may also develop at this stage.

On gross examination, the pancreas may be enlarged or atrophic, with or without cysts or calcifications. The ducts may be dilated, irregular, or strictured. Essential pathologic features include irregular and patchy loss of acinar and ductal tissue, chronic inflammation (monocyte and lymphocyte infiltration), ductal changes, and fibrosis (Fig. 7.2).

Heavy and prolonged alcohol use is the most common cause of CP. In contrast to other causes, alcohol-related CP is associated with more severe pain, more extensive calcification and ductal changes, and more rapid progression to endocrine and exocrine insufficiency. Most patients experience recurrent episodes of acute pancreatitis for several years before CP develops.

The necrosis-fibrosis theory of chronic pancreatitis differs from other theories in that it emphasizes that acute and chronic pancreatitis represents a spectrum of disease. Inflammation from acute pancreatitis leads to scarring and extrinsic compression of the pancreatic ductules. Obstruction results in stasis, atrophy, and stone formation.

Of patients with chronic pancreatitis, 10 to 30% possess no clear risk factors for the disease. Idiopathic chronic pancreatitis has a bimodal age presentation. Early-onset idiopathic chronic pancreatitis manifests with severe abdominal pain in childhood, with relatively a few structural and functional changes. Late-onset idiopathic chronic pancreatitis manifests in middle and late adulthood, often with minimal pain and pronounced exocrine insufficiency.

Whatever the etiology of chronic pancreatitis, pancreatic fibrogenesis appears to be a typical response to injury. This involves a complex interplay of growth factors, cytokines, and chemokines, leading to deposition of extracellular matrix and fibroblast proliferation. A major advance in understanding the underlying cellular mechanisms of pancreatic fibrogenesis is in the primary role of pancreatic stellate cells. Stimulated by alcohol and oxidative stress, activated stellate cells migrate to the periacinar areas to deposit collagen and fibronectin. Stellate cells are also stimulated by specific cytokines, many of which are emitted during the inflammatory phase of acute pancreatitis. Transforming growth factor beta-1 has received considerable attention as an important mediator of pancreatic fibrosis.

Further Reading

Marshal JB. **Acute pancreatitis: A review with emphasis on newer developments**. *Arch Intern Med 1993;153:1185–98.*

Mergener K; Baillie, J. **Acute pancreatitis**. *BMJ 1998;316:44–8.*

Stevens T; Conwell, DL; Zuccaro G. **Pathogenesis of chronic pancreatitis: an evidence based review of past theories and recent developments**. *Am J gastroenterol 2004; 99:2256–70.*

8

Disorders of Liver

FUNCTIONAL ANATOMY

Histologically, liver is made up of hepatic lobules. Each lobule consists of a central vein, centrifugally radiating blood sinusoids separated from each other by a double layer of hepatocytes and portal tracts are the periphery of each lobule (Fig. 8.1). A bile canaliculus runs between the two adjacent cords of hepatocytes. Each portal tract contains a terminal branch each of hepatic artery, portal vein and bile duct. Blood from branches of hepatic artery and portal vein enters the sinusoids to be drained into central vein, a tributary of hepatic vein. The hepatic vein drains blood into inferior vena cava. The bile canaliculus drains bile synthesized by hepatocytes into a tributary of bile duct in the portal tract.

The hepatic sinusoids have relatively wide lumen, and lined by a discontinuous layer of endothelial cells. Highly phagocytic Kupffer cells

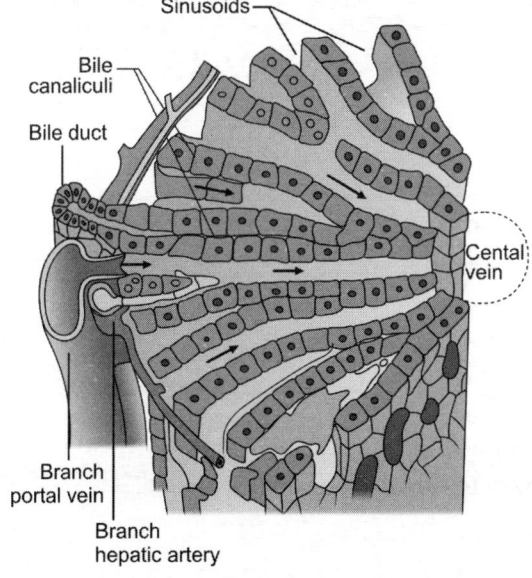

Fig. 8.1: A hepatic lobule.

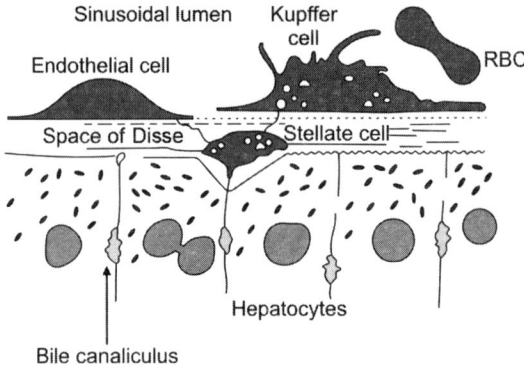

Fig. 8.2: Ultrastructure of liver showing the location of space of Disse and stellate cell and Kupffer cell.

lie on the luminal side of endothelial cells. Kupffer cells provide 80% of the total phagocytic activity of the body. A small space exists between the sinusoidal endothelial cell lining and hepatocytes. The space, known as the space of Disse, contains reticular fibers and occasional perisinusoidal stellate cell, whose functions include storage of vitamin A (Fig. 8.2). In recent years, stellate cells have been implicated in the pathogenesis of liver cirrhosis.

Functions of the Liver

A. *Functions of Parenchymal Cells*

1. Metabolism of
   - Carbohydrates
   - Fats
   - Proteins
   - Vitamin D
2. Synthesis of
   - Bile
   - Plasma proteins
   - Coagulation factors
3. Storage of
   - Glycogen
   - Proteins
   - Vitamin B_{12}
4. Excretion of bilirubin
5. Inactivation/detoxification of
   - Hormones
   - Drugs
   - Toxic products

B. *Function of Non-parenchymal Liver Cells*

1. Kupffer cells: Uptake of
   - Lipoproteins
   - IgG complexes
   - Old erythrocytes, bacteria, viruses
2. Endothelial cells: Lipoprotein uptake
3. Stellate cells: Storage of vitamin A

Carbohydrate Metabolism (Fig. 8.3)

Maintenance of blood glucose level within the normal range is one of the most important functions of the liver. In the *postprandial state*, blood glucose level begins to rise but soon brought back to normal by the following insulin-mediated reactions in liver, skeletal muscle and adipose tissue:

a. Glycogen synthesis in liver and skeletal muscle.
b. Increased breakdown of glucose by glycolysis and citric acid cycle in liver and skeletal muscle to yield energy.
c. Fatty acid synthesis in liver for storage in adipose tissue.
d. Synthesis of non-essential amino acids in liver.

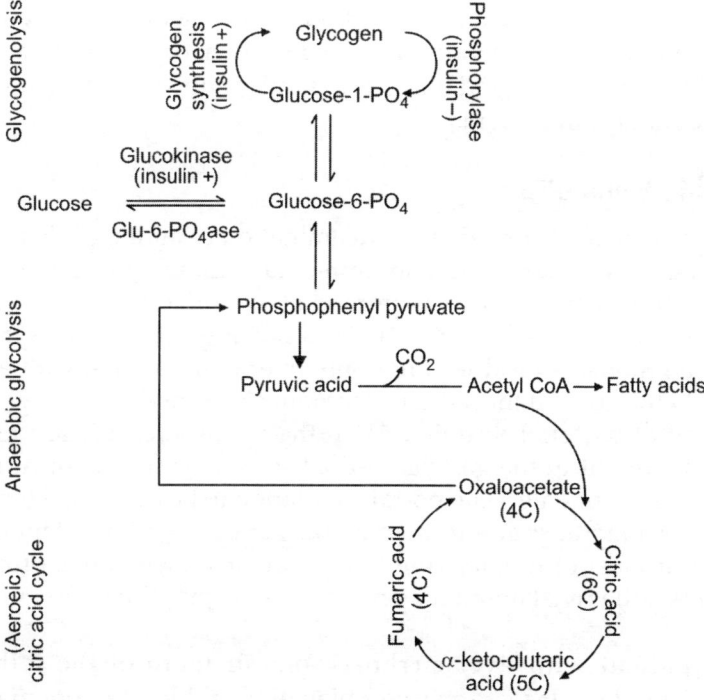

Fig. 8.3: Carbohydrate metabolism.

In fasting state, e.g. in between the meals or after overnight fast, continued utilization of glucose by peripheral tissues tends to lower blood glucose level. Under such conditions, liver helps to maintain blood glucose level by glycogenolysis as well as by gluconeogenesis. These reactions are mediated by shutting off insulin secretion coupled with increased glucagon secretion.

Glycogen stores of liver are exhausted after one day of fasting. Poor hepatic parenchymal cell function often results in hypoglycemia in patients with acute fulminating hepatitis. It may also be seen in end-stage of liver cirrhosis. In such cases with diminished hepatic cell mass, hyperglycemia or lactacidosis may also occur due to poor capacity of the hepatocytes to handle a load of glucose or lactate.

Protein Metabolism

Liver is an important site of synthesis as well as degradation of proteins. Liver synthesizes proteins not only for its own needs but also synthesizes a number of "export proteins" such as albumin, blood clotting factors and transport proteins (transferrin, ceruloplasmin, haptoglobin, transcortin, etc.).

Liver is the chief site for amino acid catabolism by two major reactions: transamination and oxidative deamination. Transamination involves transfer of an amino ($-NH_2$) group from an amino acid to a keto acid resulting in the formation of another amino acid and a keto acid. Transamination reactions occur in many other organs such as heart, skeletal muscle, kidney and brain. Transamination results in synthesis of "non-essential" amino acids.

Ammonia Metabolism

Liver is the chief site of oxidative deamination of amino acids resulting in production of a keto acid and ammonia. Ammonia is a highly toxic product, but in the liver, it is immediately converted into relatively harmless product, urea. In man, liver is the only site of urea synthesis, though ammonia is produced not only liver, but also many other sites, especially the gut and the kidney. Ammonia is formed in the large gut by the action of bacterial deaminases on the unabsorbed dietary proteins and urea present in the gastrointestinal secretions (Fig. 8.4). Ammonia formed in the gut enters the portal circulation to be converted to urea in the liver. Ammonia is also formed in the kidney as an important urinary buffer, but most of it enters the renal tubular lumen and captures H^+. Only very little renal ammonia enters the systemic circulation via renal veins.

In a patient with liver cirrhosis, one or more of the following mechanisms may lead to marked elevation of blood ammonia level, precipitating hepatic encephalopathy:

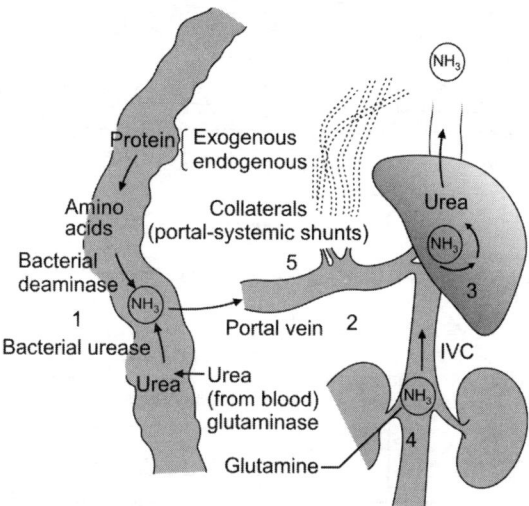

Fig. 8.4: Sources and metabolism of ammonia in normal individuals (steps 1–4) and in a patient with liver cirrhosis with porto-caval collaterals step 5).

- Severe depression of hepatocellular function.
- Excessive intake of dietary proteins.
- Gastrointestinal bleeding.
- High blood urea level (hepatorenal syndrome).
- Porto-systemic shunts.
- If alkalosis and hypokalemia supervenes, ammonia produced in the kidney enters the systemic circulation since H^+ is not available to capture ammonia.

Lipid Metabolism (Fig. 8.5)

Liver is the chief site of anabolic, catabolic and transport reactions of lipids. Dietary fats consist mainly of triglycerides of long chained fatty acids as well as a small amount of cholesterol esters and phospholipids. Dietary fats are hydrolyzed in the small intestine, incorporated into chylomicrons by the intestinal epithelial cells and transferred via lymphatics to blood circulation.

The enzyme lipoprotein lipase is present in the endothelial lining of blood vessels in many organs, especially the liver and adipose tissue. The hepatic lipoprotein activity increases free fatty acid (FFA) levels in hepatocytes. Dietary carbohydrates can also be converted into FFA in hepatocytes. In the hepatocytes, some FFA are oxidized in citric acid cycle to yield energy, but mostly are converted to lipids such as triglycerides, cholesterol and cholesterol esters and "exported" to other tissues for storage (e.g. triglycerides storage in adipose tissue cells) or utilization as tissue lipids. Before the lipids formed the hepatocytes can be released

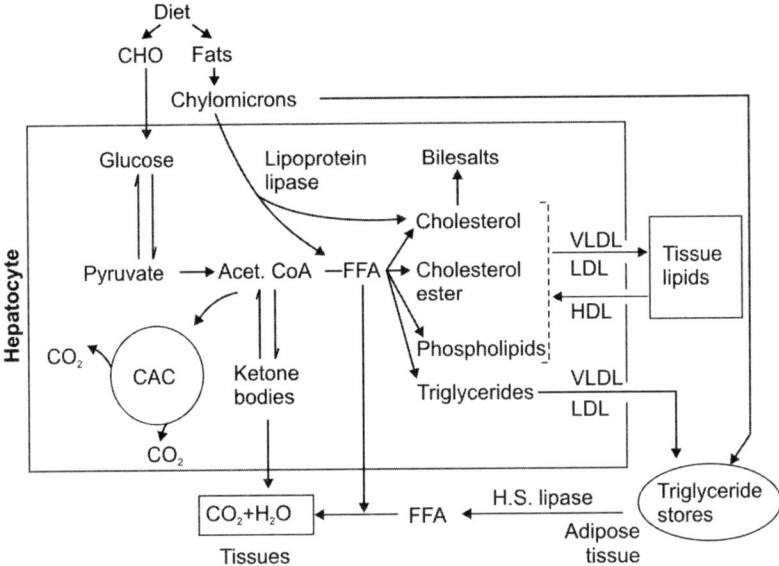

Fig. 8.5: Lipid metabolism.

into blood circulation, they need to be incorporated into lipoproteins for transport in plasma water. Very low density lipoproteins (VLDL) and low density lipoproteins (LDL) are vehicles of transport of triglycerides and cholesterol esters to non-hepatic tissues including storage sites in adipose tissue. Liver also synthesizes high density lipoproteins (HDL), which transfer cholesterol esters released from tissue cells back to liver for excretion/catabolism.

The plasma chylomicrons represent the exogenous triglycerides freshly absorbed from the intestine on their way to liver or adipose tissue. The endogenous lipids synthesized by the liver are transported to the tissues as VLDL or LDL.

An enzyme, hormone sensitive lipase, causes mobilization of FFA from triglycerides stored in adipose tissue. The enzyme is inhibited by insulin, but activated by glucagon, catecholamines, growth hormone and glucocorticoids. Tissues use FFA as a substrate for energy production. Liver also converts some FFA into ketone bodies. Ketone bodies utilization occurs mostly in extra-hepatic tissues. Under normal circumstances, utilization of FFA and ketone bodies keep pace with their generation. Hence, their plasma levels remain low. In diabetes mellitus, starvation or intake of high-fat-low carbohydrate diet, excessive production of FFA results in ketonemia, ketonuria and metabolic acidosis.

Detoxification/Inactivation Function

Water-soluble endogenous waste products or therapeutically administered drugs are easily excreted by the kidney. However, lipid-soluble waste products, hormones and drugs tend to accumulate in the body, unless they are metabolized to less toxic products and/or converted to water-soluble derivatives, which can be excreted in bile or urine.

Detoxification mechanisms of the liver may be divided into two phases:
  i. Phase I reactions involve chemical modification of the substance by oxidation, reduction, hydroxylation, methylation, etc. Such reactions mostly lead to inactivation of the toxic substance, but still it remains lipid-soluble and cannot be excreted.
  ii. Phase II reactions convert lipid-soluble inactivated substances to their water-soluble derivatives (glucuronide, sulfate, acetyl derivatives, etc.) which can be excreted in bile or urine.

In a patient with liver disease, there may be varying degree of impairment of hepatic uptake, detoxification or excretion of many drugs such as anticonvulsants, anti-inflammatory, tranquillizers, cardioactive drugs (propranolol, lidocain) and many antibiotics. Therefore, such patients have a decreased dosage requirement of these drugs. More importantly, there is narrowing of the range between their therapeutic and toxic doses.

Inactivation or modification of several hormones occurs in the liver. That is why several hormonal imbalance disorders may be observed in patients with chronic liver disease. Imbalance in plasma testosterone: estrogen ratio has been implicated in the development of feminization of males with chronic liver disease. Because of hepatocellular failure, a large percentage of testosterone fails to undergo hepatic degradation. Instead, it is converted to estrogen in the peripheral tissues, thereby lowering plasma testosterone: estrogen ratio.

PATHOPHYSIOLOGY OF JAUNDICE

Bilirubin Metabolism

Destruction of senescent red blood cells in the tissue macrophages (in spleen, liver, bone marrow, etc.) results in catabolism of hemoglobin to heme (and globin) and subsequently to bilirubin. Approximately 80% of bilirubin arises from this source. The remaining 20% bilirubin arises from catabolism of heme derived from ineffective erythropoiesis in the bone marrow, a normal phenomenon, and from heme present in compounds such as myoglobin, cytochromes and catalases. In all, approximately 200–250 mg of bilirubin is formed each day. Bilirubin released from the tissue macrophages is called unconjugated bilirubin. It a lipid soluble pigment transported in blood tightly bound to albumin. In the liver, the hepatocytes convert it into water-soluble compounds called conjugated bilirubin (bilirubin mono- and di-glucuronide). The hepatic metabolism of bilirubin involves three distinct steps:

- Hepatic uptake
- Conjugation reactions
- Excretion into bile canaliculi.

In various congenital or acquired hepatic diseases, one or more of these 3 steps may get deranged leading to accumulation of bilirubin in blood.

Hepatic Uptake

Hepatic uptake of bilirubin involves its dissociation from albumin, carrier-mediated transport across the hepatic cell membrane, followed by binding to a cytoplasmic protein called ligandin.

Conjugation Reactions

Conjugation of bilirubin with glucuronic acid occurs with the help of an enzyme bilirubin glucuronyl transferase. The reaction seems to occur in two stages; resulting in initial formation of bilirubin monoglucuronide (BMG) followed by formation of bilirubin diglucuronide (BDG). The bile contains both types of conjugated bile pigments, but BDG predominates (85%).

Impairment of either of the hepatic uptake or conjugation reaction leads to accumulation of unconjugated bilirubin in the blood.

The enzyme glucuronyltransferase activity is low at birth, but increases to the adult level within 15 days. That explains the development of mild icterus in most of the newborn babies, which resolves without any treatment (*physiological jaundice of the newborn*). In premature babies, the physiological jaundice may become severe enough to warrant treatment. Congenital absence of the glucuronyltransferase results in hereditary (congenital) unconjugated hyperbilirubinemias (Gilbert's syndrome, Crigler-Najjar disease).

Excretion into Bile

Only conjugated bilirubin is excreted into the bile canaliculi. Excretion requires an active transport system. *This rate-limiting step in the overall hepatic metabolism of bilirubin is predominantly affected in hapatocellular disease.* The active transport system may be congenitally absent due to a hereditary defect (Dubin-Johnson syndrome, Rotor syndrome). The excretory function seems to be mildly affected by high plasma levels of estrogens and progesterone. That explains mild cholestatic jaundice seen in some cases of pregnancy (recurrent jaundice of pregnancy), or those on contraceptive pills. Methyl testosterone also impairs the excretory function and hence should not be administered in patients with liver disease.

In viral hepatitis, all the three steps of hepatic metabolism in the liver are affected, but the impairment of excretory function predominates, i.e.

the blood contains mainly the excess of conjugated bilirubin. Extrahepatic obstruction of the biliary tract, e.g. by a gallstone, a stricture in the bile duct, or a tumor of the head of the pancreas also produce predominantly conjugated hyperbilirubinemias.

Conjugated bilirubin cannot be absorbed in the intestines. In the large gut, bacterial degradation converts it to stercobilinogen (= urobilinogen), a water soluble colorless product. Some of the urobilinogen is absorbed into the portal blood to reach the systemic circulation. Being water soluble it is excreted into the urine by the kidneys. The remaining stercobilinogen (40–280 mg/day) is excreted in the feces. On exposure to air, stercobilinogen is oxidized to stercobilin which gives brown color to the feces.

In obstructive jaundice, since bilirubin does not reach the intestines, stercobilinogen and urobilinogen excretion in the feces and urine is very low. That accounts for the pale chalky-color of the stools of such patients.

Conjugated bilirubin is water-soluble; if present in the blood, it can be excreted by the kidneys into the urine (bilirubinuria). Bilirubin imparts dark brown color to the urine, an important clinical sign of conjugated hyperbilirubinemias (hepatic and post-hepatic jaundice). Classification of jaundice based on the pathophysiology of bilirubin metabolism is given in Table 8.1.

Liver Function Tests

Normal functions of the liver are huge and diverse. Equally wide is the spectrum of hepatic disorders that may disrupt hepatic function. That is why; even a battery of tests cannot be recommended which may be used in every clinical setting. Some of the tests have to be selected which may help in the differential diagnosis in a given case.

A. Tests based on Bilirubin Metabolism

1. Serum Bilirubin

Raised serum bilirubin level is one of the most commonly recorded evidence of liver disease. However, serum bilirubin level may be elevated due to a non-biliary disorder (e.g. hemolytic anemia, increased ineffective erythropoiesis), or it may be normal in some types of hepatic disorders (e.g. early stages of liver cirrhosis). By spectrophotometric analytic method, two types of bilirubin can be identified in the plasma/serum:

   i. A water soluble fraction that gives direct reaction with diazo reagent. It is known as conjugated bilirubin or direct bilirubin. This fraction consists of mono- and di-glucuronides of bilirubin.

   ii. A lipid soluble fraction that gives an "indirect" reaction with diazo reagent. It consists of unconjugated type of bilirubin. The test report gives levels of direct bilirubin (normal ≤ 0.25 mg/dL) and total bilirubin (direct + indirect; normal ≤ 1 mg/dL).

Table 8.1: Differential diagnosis of jaundice

Prehepatic jaundice	Hepatic jaundice		Posthepatic jaundice
	Decreased uptake/ conjugation	Decreased excretion	
Excessive hemolysis	Hepatocellular disease	Hepatocellular disease	Gallstones
Excessive ineffective erythropoiesis	Neonatal jaundice	Cholestatic jaundice of pregnancy	Stricture
	Sepsis	Recurrent benign intrahepatic jaundice	Tumor
	Drugs	Drugs	
	Gilbert's syndrome	Oral contraceptives	
	Crigler-Najjar syndrome	Dubin-Johnson syndrome	
		Rotor syndrome	

2. Urinary Bilirubin

Only water soluble, conjugated type of bilirubin can pass through the kidney filter. Therefore, bilirubinuria indicates presence of elevated plasma conjugated bilirubin levels. Bilirubinuria occurs even with a minimal degree of obstructive jaundice and may be detected even before jaundice is clinically evident.

3. Urinary Urobilinogen

An increase in the urobilinogen excretion in urine is a sensitive indicator of hepatocellular dysfunction. It is a good indication of alcoholic liver damage, well compensated cirrhosis or malignant disease of the liver. In viral hepatitis it increases in the initial stage. It is markedly increased in patients with excessive hemolysis.

B. Serum Enzymes Assays

1. Enzymes that Detect Hepatocellular Necrosis: Aminotransferases

The aminotransferases (formerly called transaminases) are the most frequently utilized and specific *indicators of hepatocellular necrosis*. The two enzymes commonly tested are: *aspartate aminotransferase (AST,* formerly called serum glutamate oxaloacetic transaminase—SGOT) and *alanine amino-transferase (ALT,* formerly known as serum glutamic pyruvate transaminase—SGPT). These enzymes catalyze the transfer amino group of the amino acids aspartate and alanine respectively to the keto group of α-ketoglutaric acid. ALT is primarily localized to the hepatic cells but the AST is present in a wide variety of tissues such as the heart, skeletal muscle, kidney, brain and liver.

The activity of these enzymes in the plasma at any moment reflects the relative rate at which they enter and leave circulation. Their plasma activity does not reflect any specific function of the liver.

Interpretation of Mild, Moderate and Severe Elevation of Serum Aminotransferases

1. *Severe (> 20 times, 1000 U/L):* AST and ALT levels are increased to some extent in almost all liver diseases, but the highest elevations occur in severe viral hepatitis, drug or toxin induced *hepatic necrosis* and circulatory shock. Although enzyme levels may reflect the extent of hepatocellular necrosis, they do not correlate with eventual outcome. In fact, declining AST and ALT may indicate either recovery or poor prognosis in fulminating hepatic failure.

$$\text{Aspartate} + \alpha\text{-ketoglutarate} \xrightarrow{AST} \text{Oxaloacetate} + \text{glutamate}$$
$$\text{Alanine} + \alpha\text{-ketoglutarate} \xrightarrow{ALT} \text{Pyruvate} + \text{glutamate}$$

2. *Moderate (3–20 times):* The AST and ALT levels are moderately elevated in acute hepatitis, chronic hepatitis, drug induced hepatitis, alcoholic hepatitis and acute biliary tract obstruction. The ALT is usually more frequently increased as compared to AST except in chronic liver disease. In uncomplicated acute viral hepatitis, the very high initial levels approach normal levels within 5 weeks of onset of illness and normal levels are obtained in 8 weeks in 75% of cases.

3. *Mild (1–3 times):* These elevations are usually seen in sepsis induced neonatal hepatitis, drug toxicity, myositis, Duchene muscular dystrophy and even after vigorous exercise.

   AST: ALT ratio is sometimes useful in differentiating between causes of liver damage. When greater than 2.0, it is more likely to be associated with alcoholic hepatitis. When less than 1.0, it is more likely to be associated with viral hepatitis.

Other Enzymes Tests of Hepatocellular Necrosis

Other enzymes sometimes tested for hepatic function include glutamate dehydrogenase, isocitrate dehydrogenase, lactate dehydrogenase and sorbitol dehydrogenase. None of these tests has proved to be more useful in practice than the aminotransferases.

2. *Enzymes that Detect Cholestasis*
i. *Alkaline Phosphatase (ALP):* This enzyme arises from the bone, intestines, liver and placenta. In the absence of bone disease and pregnancy, elevated levels of serum alkaline phosphatase indicate impaired biliary function. The increase in the activity of this enzyme is due to greater production by the biliary tract epithelium and hepatocytes than regurgitation of the enzyme due to obstruction. Slight to moderate (up to 2 folds) may occur in parenchymal liver disorders. Very high levels (10 folds or higher) occur with extrahepatic biliary obstruction or intrahepatic cholestasis. *Normal serum alkaline phosphatase level almost rules out intra- or extra-hepatic cholestasis.*

ii. *Serum 5-nucleotidase:* Level of serum 5-nucleotidase is raised along with that of alkaline phosphatase in liver disease. This enzyme has a biliary origin and hence levels are not elevated in bone disease.

iii. *Gamma-glutamyltransferase (gamma-glutamyltranspeptidase, GGT):* GGT is increased in most diseases that cause acute damage to the liver or bile ducts but is usually not helpful in distinguishing between different causes of liver damage. For this reason, use of GGT is controversial, and guidelines published by the National Academy of Clinical Biochemistry and the American Association for the Study of Liver Diseases do not recommend routine use of GGT. These guidelines suggest that it can be useful in determining the cause of a high ALP, because GGT is elevated in liver disease but not bone disease.

C. Tests of the Liver's Biosynthetic Capacity

i. *Serum proteins:* The liver is the major source of most the plasma proteins. The parenchymal cells are responsible for synthesis of albumin, fibrinogen and other coagulation factors and most of the α- and β-globulins.

Albumin: Albumin is quantitatively the most important plasma protein synthesized by the liver and is a useful indicator of hepatic function. Normal plasma values range from 3.5 to 4.5 g/dl. Because the half life of albumin in plasma is as long as 20 days, the plasma albumin level is not a reliable indicator of hepatic protein synthesis in acute liver disease. Plasma albumin level is affected not only in liver disease but also by nutritional status or renal disease. Hypoalbuminemia is not specific for liver disease and may occur in protein malnutrition, nephrotic syndrome and chronic protein losing enteropathies.

The plasma albumin levels are typically depressed in patients with cirrhosis and ascites. In such patients, with or without ascites, the plasma albumin level correlates with prognosis.

The plasma albumin levels tend to be normal in diseases such as acute viral hepatitis, drug related hepatotoxicity and obstructive jaundice.

Albumin levels below 3 g/dl in a case with acute hepatitis should raise the suspicion of a chronic liver disease like cirrhosis which usually reflects decreased albumin synthesis.

ii. *Prealbumin:* The plasma prealbumin level is 0.2–0.3 g/L. The levels fall in liver disease presumably due to reduced synthesis. Because of its short half life, changes may precede alteration in serum albumin. Determination of prealbumin has been considered particularly useful in drug-induced hepatotoxicity.

iii. *Plasma ceruloplasmin:* Normal plasma levels are 0.2–0.4 g/L. It is synthesized in the liver and is an *acute phase protein*. The plasma concentration *rises* in infections, rheumatoid arthritis, pregnancy, liver disease (except Wilson disease) and obstructive jaundice. Plasma ceruloplasmin is an important diagnostic marker in Wilson disease, in which its level is usually low.

iv. *Procollagen III peptide:* The plasma concentration of this peptide appears to increase not only with hepatic fibrosis but also with inflammation and necrosis. Serial measurement of plasma procollagen III may be helpful in the follow up of chronic liver disease.

v. *α-1 antitrypsin:* It is a glycoprotein synthesized by the liver and is an inhibitor of serine proteinases, especially elastase. Its normal concentration is 1–1.6 g/L. It is an acute phase protein; serum levels increase with inflammatory disorders, pregnancy and use of oral contraceptive pills.

vi. *α-Fetoprotein:* This protein, the principal one in fetal plasma in early gestation, is subsequently present at very low levels (<25 mg/L). It is increased in *hepatocellular carcinoma* (HCC) and more than 90% of such patients have raised levels. Raised values are also found in other liver diseases such as chronic hepatitis, in regeneration phase of acute hepatitis and in hepatic metastasis. α-fetoprotein elevation is less frequent when HCC arises in non-cirrhotic liver. Serial determination is of value in cirrhotic patients. A rise in the values should raise the suspicion of HCC.

vii. *Prothrombin time (PT):* Clotting is the end result of a complex series of enzymatic reactions that involve at least 13 factors. The liver is the major site of synthesis of 11 blood coagulation proteins. Most of these are present in excess and abnormalities of coagulation only result when there is substantial impairment in the ability of the liver to synthesize these factors. The standard method to assess is the one stage prothrombin time of quick, which evaluate the extrinsic coagulation pathway.

Prolonged PT is not specific for liver diseases and is seen in various deficiencies of coagulation factors, DIC, and ingestion of certain drugs.

In acute and chronic hepatocellular disease, the PT may serve as a *prognostic indicator*. In acute hepatocellular disease worsening of PT suggests an increased likelihood of acute hepatic failure. The PT is a predictor of outcome in cases of acetaminophen overdosage and acute alcoholic hepatitis. Prolongation of PT is also suggestive of poor long-term outcome in chronic liver disease.

If the PT returns to normal or improves by at least 30% within 24 hr of a single parenteral injection of vitamin K1 (5–10 mg), it may be surmised that parenchymal function is good and that hypovitaminosis K was responsible for the original prolongation of PT. Patients with parenchymal disease by contrast will show only minimal improvement.

Summary

A single liver function test is of little value in screening for liver disease as many serious liver diseases may be associated with normal levels and abnormal levels might be found in asymptomatic healthy individuals. The use of battery of liver function tests however constitutes a highly sensitive procedure. The number of false negatives must be reduced by this technique. The use of battery of liver tests is also associated with high specificity, especially when more than one test is abnormal. The pattern of enzyme abnormality, interpreted in the context of the patient's characteristics, can aid in directing the subsequent diagnostic work-up.

Alcohol liver Disease

Chronic heavy drinking may lead to:
- Alcoholic fatty liver
- Alcoholic hepatitis
- Alcoholic cirrhosis (Laennec's cirrhosis)

In alcoholic liver disease, the total amount and duration of ethanol ingested rather than the type of alcoholic drink ingested determines the results. For example, 360 ml of beer (5% alcohol) and 45 ml of whisky contain the same amount of ethanol. Women appear to develop alcohol induced liver injury at lesser levels of consumption than men. The role of concurrent malnutrition is controversial, but malnutrition seems to augment the detrimental effects of alcohol. The cause of malnutrition in alcoholics is not merely economic. Even when economic problem is not present, alcoholism tends to produce malnutrition. In chronic alcoholics, alcohol itself may provide over 50% of total caloric requirements, which otherwise would have been provided by food containing proteins, vitamins and minerals.

Liver is the main site of alcohol metabolism. In the hepatocytes, alcohol is first oxidized to acetaldehyde, which is further oxidized to acetate (Fig. 8.6). Both of these reactions increase the concentration of NADH

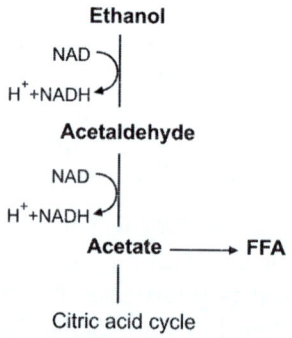

Fig. 8.6: Biochemical basis of alcohol induced hepatic injury.

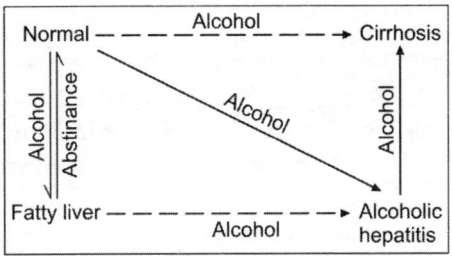

Fig. 8.7: Possible pathways of liver cirrhosis in alcoholics.

which inhibits the operation of citric acid cycle. Therefore, rather than undergoing further oxidation to CO_2 and water, acetate is diverted to fatty acid synthesis. There is inhibition of fatty acid oxidation as well. Excessive concentration of acetaldehyde seems to inhibit biosynthesis and secretion of lipoproteins, the form in which fatty acids can be exported from the liver. Therefore, triglycerides accumulate in the hepatocytes, producing "fatty liver" (Figs 8.8 and 8.9). Fatty liver may develop in any alcoholic after a bout of heavy drinking, but it is a reversible process. This condition presents clinically as a tender hepatomegaly with many non-specific symptoms such as malaise, weakness, anorexia, nausea, and abdominal discomfort. Elevated levels of hepatic enzymes may be the only laboratory finding. Jaundice is present in 15% of patients admitted to the hospital because of these symptoms of fatty infiltration of the liver. With total abstinence, the condition can return to normal within 2–4 weeks. However, continued alcohol consumption may result in more advanced forms of liver disease, either alcoholic hepatitis or cirrhosis (Fig. 8.7).

Alcoholic Hepatitis

Some 10–15% of chronic alcoholics develop alcoholic hepatitis. Alcoholic hepatitis is characterized by hepatocyte ballooning, hepatocyte necrosis

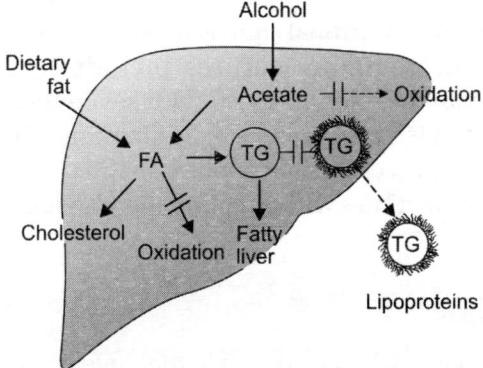

Fig. 8.8: Mechanism of production of fatty liver.

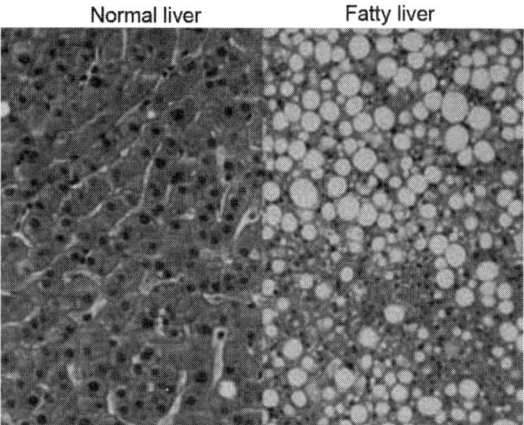

Fig. 8.9: Fatty liver.

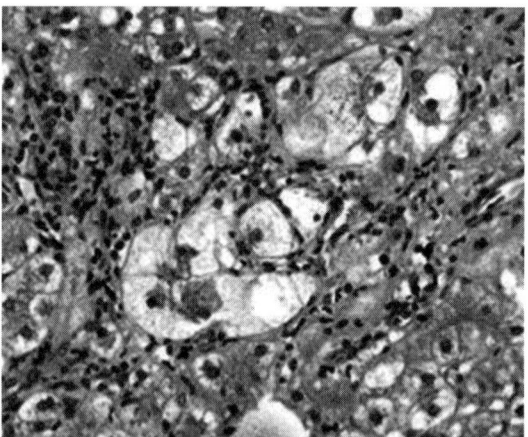

Fig. 8.10: Alcoholic hepatitis.

and polymorphonuclear infiltration (Fig. 8.10). Deposition of collagen fibers around the central vein and in perisinusoidal area sets the stage for progression to cirrhosis. Cardinal sign of alcoholic hepatitis is rapid onset of jaundice. Other common features include fever and ascites. Encephalopathy may develop in those with severe hepatitis. Alcoholic hepatitis usually persists and progresses to cirrhosis if heavy alcohol use continues. If alcohol use ceases, alcoholic hepatitis resolves slowly over weeks to months, sometimes without permanent sequelae but often with residual cirrhosis.

Alcoholic Cirrhosis

The pathological hallmark of cirrhosis is the development of scar tissue that replaces normal parenchyma, blocking the portal flow of blood

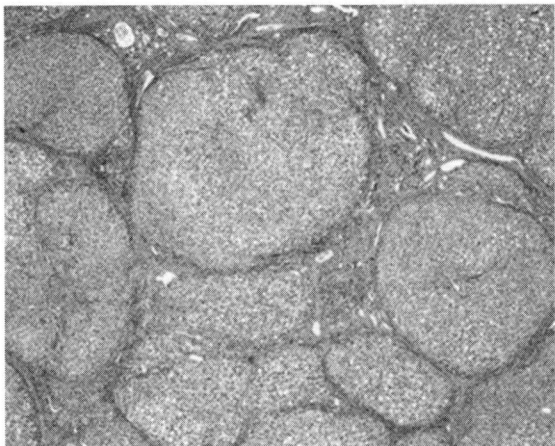

Fig. 8.11: Liver cirrhosis.

through the organ and disturbing normal function. The fibrous tissue bands (septa) separate hepatocyte nodules; which eventually distort the entire liver architecture (Fig. 8.11), and obstruct the normal hepatic blood flow (portal hypertension). The spleen becomes congested, which leads to hypersplenism and increased sequestration of platelets. Portal hypertension is responsible for most severe complications of cirrhosis.

The development of hepatic fibrosis reflects an alteration in the normally balanced processes of extracellular matrix production and degradation. Extracellular matrix, the normal scaffolding for hepatocytes, is composed of collagens, glycoproteins, and proteoglycans. Recent research has shown the pivotal role of stellate cell(Fig. 8.2), a cell type that normally stores vitamin A, in the development of cirrhosis. Stellate cells, located in the perisinusoidal space, are essential for the production of extracellular matrix. Stellate cells may become activated into collagen-forming cells by a variety of paracrine factors. Such factors may be released by hepatocytes, Kupffer cells, or sinusoidal endothelium following liver injury. As an example, increased levels of the cytokine transforming growth factor beta-1 (TGF-beta-1) are observed in patients with chronic hepatitis C and those with cirrhosis. TGF-beta-1, in turn, stimulates activated stellate cells to produce type I collagen.

Increased collagen deposition in the space of Disse (the space between hepatocytes and sinusoids) and the diminution of the size of endothelial fenestrae lead to the capillarization (decreased permeability) of sinusoids. Activated stellate cells also have contractile properties. Both capillarization and constriction of sinusoids by stellate cells contribute to the development of portal hypertension.

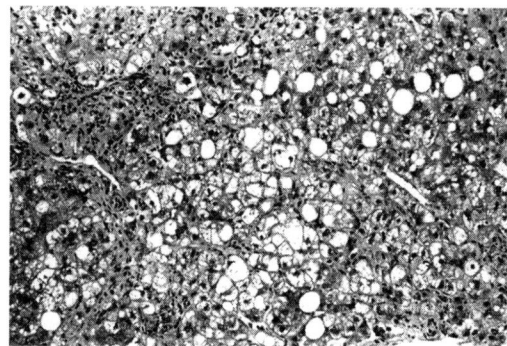

Fig. 8.12: Nonalcoholic steatohepatitis (NASH). Fat-filled hepatocytes and chicken-wire fibrosis are characteristic histologic features.

NONALCOHOLIC FATTY LIVER DISEASE

Non-alcoholic fatty liver disease (NAFLD) is one cause of a fatty liver, occurring when fat is deposited (steatosis) in the liver not due to excessive alcohol use. It is related to insulin resistance and the metabolic syndrome and may respond to treatments originally developed for other insulin-resistant states (e.g. diabetes mellitus type 2). Nonalcoholic steatohepatitis (NASH) is the most extreme form of NAFLD, and is regarded as a major cause of cirrhosis of the liver of unknown cause (Fig. 8.12). Most patients with NAFLD have few or no symptoms. Patients may complain of fatigue, malaise, and dull right-upper-quadrant abdominal discomfort. Mild jaundice may be noticed although this is rare. More commonly NAFLD is diagnosed following abnormal liver function tests during routine blood tests.

The exact cause of NAFLD is still unknown. However, both obesity and insulin resistance probably play a strong role in the disease process. The exact reasons and mechanisms by which the disease progresses from one stage to the next are not known. A "second hit", or further injury seems to be required for the progression from hepatic steatosis to hepatitis. Oxidative stress, hormonal imbalances, and mitochondrial abnormalities are potential causes for this "second hit" phenomenon.

At present, nonalcoholic fatty liver disease (NAFLD) has become the most common liver disease worldwide. The prevalence of simple fatty liver in obese persons has been estimated to be approximately 90% and that of NASH in obese persons to be 20%. Indian men seem to special predisposition to develop nonalcoholic fatty liver disease.

Fat accumulates in the liver when the rate of delivery of fatty acids to hepatocytes exceeds the metabolic capacity to process them. Liver accumulation of fat in patients with DM or with the insulin resistance syndrome is mainly related to increased lipolysis of adipose tissue, with increased flux of free fatty acids to the liver that exceeds the liver's capacity to export VLDL.

LIVER CIRRHOSIS

- Pathogenically, liver cirrhosis should be regarded as the final common pathway of chronic liver injury, which can result from any form of intense, repeated and prolonged liver cell assaults.
- The end result is the formation of broad bands of fibrous tissue separating regenerative nodules that do not maintain the normal organization of hepatic lobules.

Cirrhosis is defined histologically as a diffuse hepatic process characterized by fibrosis and the conversion of normal liver architecture into structurally abnormal nodules. Cirrhosis represents the final common outcome of a wide variety of chronic liver diseases. The progression of liver injury to cirrhosis may occur over weeks to years. Cirrhosis is most commonly caused by alcoholism, hepatitis B and C, and nonalcoholic fatty liver disease. Patients with hepatitis C may have chronic hepatitis for as long as 40 years before progressing to cirrhosis.

As cirrhosis can be caused by many different entities, which injure the liver in different ways, some cause-specific histopathological abnormalities can be observed in. For example, in chronic hepatitis B, there is infiltration of the liver parenchyma with lymphocytes; in cardiac cirrhosis there are erythrocytes and a greater amount of fibrosis in the tissue surrounding the hepatic veins; in primary biliary cirrhosis, there is fibrosis around the bile duct, the presence of granulomas and pooling of bile; and in alcoholic cirrhosis, there is infiltration of the liver with neutrophils.

Often a poor correlation exists between histological findings and the clinical picture. Some patients with cirrhosis are completely asymptomatic and have a reasonably normal life expectancy. Other individuals have a multitude of the most severe symptoms of end-stage liver disease and have a limited chance for survival. Common signs and symptoms may stem from decreased hepatic synthetic function (e.g., coagulopathy), decreased detoxification capabilities of the liver (e.g., hepatic encephalopathy), or portal hypertension (e.g., variceal bleeding).

There are many clinical features of cirrhosis of liver, any one or more can be a presenting feature. The pathophysiological consequences of cirrhotic liver can be categorized into:

- Disturbance of bilirubin metabolism in the liver.
- Effects of hepatocellular insufficiency.
- Effects of portal hypertension.
  1. *Jaundice:* It results from decreased uptake/conjugation/excretion of bilirubin by the liver
  2. *Bruising and bleeding:* It results from deficient production of clotting factors by the hepatocytes as well as thrombocytopenia.

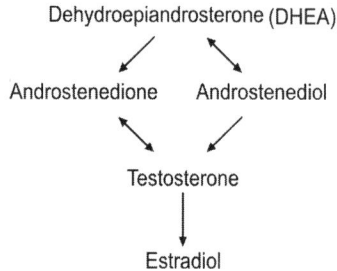

Fig. 8.13: Mechanism of development of gynecomastia in liver cirrhosis.

3. *Gynecomastia:* It involves benign proliferation of glandular tissue of male breasts presenting with a rubbery or firm mass extending concentrically from the nipples. Gynecomastia can occur in up to 70% of males with liver cirrhosis. This is due to increased plasma estradiol concentration. Because of defective hepatocellular function, a large percentage of testosterone fails to undergo hepatic degradation. Instead, it is converted to estrogen in the peripheral tissues (Fig. 8.13); which lowers plasma testosterone: estrogen ratio.

4. *Hypogonadism:* It is manifested as impotence, infertility, loss of sexual drive, and testicular atrophy. Clinical and histological evidence of testicular atrophy is found in 50% of the cirrhotics. Leydig cell dysfunction is reflected in reduced plasma testosterone levels. Hypogonadism occurs less frequently in nonalcoholic cirrhotics, except in end-stage hepatic failure. The exact cause of hypogonadism is not clear. It is believed to be related to primary gonadal injury by chronic alcoholism.

5. *Spider angiomata or spider nevi* are found slightly beneath the skin surface, often containing a central red arteriole resembling spider's body and reddish extensions which radiate outwards like a spider's web. These occur in about 1/3 of cases of cirrhosis. Spider nevi are usually associated with increased estrogen: testosterone ratio

6. *Palmar erythema:* It is due to exaggerations of normal speckled mottling of the palm, related to altered sex hormone metabolism.

7. *Greater sensitivity to medications:* In patients with liver cirrhosis, there may be varying degree of impairment of hepatic uptake, detoxification or excretion of certain drugs such as anticonvulsants, inti-inflammatory drugs, tranquillizers, cardioactive drugs (lignocain, propranolol) and antibiotics. Therefore, these patients have a decreased dosage requirement as well as narrowing of the range between their therapeutic and toxic levels.

8. *Hepatocellular carcinoma:* About 80 % of the cases of hepatocellular carcinoma have previous history of liver cirrhosis. In the remaining 20%, it can be attributed to chronic viral hepatitis (hepatitis B or hepatitis C virus).

9. *Portal hypertension.*

Portal Hypertension and its Complication

The portal vein draws blood from the spleen and from splanchnic vessels in the stomach, intestine and pancreas (Fig. 8.14). In the liver, the portal vein divides and subdivides into smaller vessels that ultimately open into the hepatic sinusoids. After numerous branching, a fine branch of hepatic artery also opens into the hepatic sinusoids. Blood from both sources enters a sinusoid at the portal triad end and leaves it through a tributary of central vein to enter the hepatic vein and finally the inferior into the vena cava. Normal portal venous pressure is very low (7–10 mmHg), because the hepatic sinusoids offer very little resistance to the blood flow. Portal hypertension can occur whenever there is obstruction to the portal blood flow.

Causes of Portal Hypertension

a. Extrahepatic presinusoidal causes:
   - Portal vein thrombosis
b. Intrahepatic causes:
   - Liver cirrhosis
   - Schistosomiasis
c. Extrahepatic postsinusoidal causes:
   - Congestive heart failure
   - Budd-Chiari syndrome
   - Constrictive pericarditis

Pathophysiology of portal hypertension in liver cirrhosis

Liver cirrhosis is the most common cause of portal hypertension. A number of factors are involved in the pathogenesis of portal hypertension:

a. A decrease in the total size of intrahepatic vascular bed secondary to destruction of hepatic parenchyma and disruption of hepatic sinusoids.

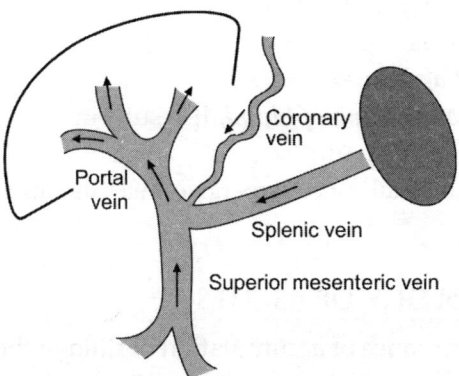

Fig. 8.14: Anatomy of portal vessels.

b. An increase in the resistance to blood flow in the remaining patent sinusoids due to perisinusoidal deposition of collagen. Portal vein thrombosis occurs in some patients of cirrhosis causing further increase in portal hypertension.
c. Increased hepatic vascular resistance in cirrhosis is not only a mechanical consequence of the hepatic architectural disorder, but a dynamic component also exists due to the active contraction of myofibroblasts, activated stellate cells, and vascular smooth-muscle cells of the intrahepatic veins.
d. Hyperdynamic circulation in the splanchnic vessels also contributes to the portal hypertension. Hyperdynamic circulation in the splanchnic area despite portal hypertension may seem incongruous. Actually in cirrhotics, the cardiac output is increased and *total* peripheral resistance is decreased. There is increased blood flow to the gastrointestinal tract and skeletal muscle. The fall in total peripheral resistance results from the opening of portal-systemic collaterals by portal hypertension. These collaterals act as a bypass for vasodilator metabolites produced in the GI tract in the postprandial state (but normally inactivated by the liver). Manifestations of splanchnic vasodilatation include increased cardiac output, arterial hypotension, and hypervolemia. This explains the rationale for treating portal hypertension with a low-sodium diet and diuretics to attenuate the hyperkinetic state.

Consequences of Portal Hypertension

1. *Development of portosystemic collaterals:* As much as 80 % of the portal blood may be diverted to the systemic circulation by the collaterals. These collaterals are seen as:
   - Gastroesophageal varices.
   - Perirectal varices (hemorrhoids)
   - Periumbilical collaterals in the abdominal wall (caput medusae).
2. *Splenomegaly, hypersplenism:*
   (thrombocytopenia, anemia, pancytopenia).
3. *Congestion of abdominal viscera.*
4. *Portosystemic shunting of blood.* It results in:
   - Hepatic encephalopathy
   - Impaired glucose tolerance, hyperglycemia (insulin bypasses liver).
5. *Ascites*

PATHOPHYSIOLOGY OF ASCITES

The most frequent cause of accumulation of fluid in the peritoneal cavity is liver cirrhosis. The initiating factors for the development of ascites in a cirrhotic are:

- Portal hypertension
- Hypoalbuminemia

Inappropriate salt and water retention is an additional factor that perpetuates ascites.

Role of Portal Hypertension and Hypoalbuminemia

To understand the mechanism of ascites in liver cirrhosis, one has to recapitulate the Starling forces involved in the formation and reabsorption of tissue fluids in the capillary beds. Briefly speaking, tissue fluid is formed at the arteriolar end of the capillary because the capillary hydrostatic pressure is greater than plasma protein oncotic pressure. Most of the tissue fluid thus formed is reabsorbed at the venous end of the capillary, where the hydrostatic pressure is lower than the plasma protein oncotic pressure. The residual tissue fluid and some filtered albumin return to the systemic circulation via the lymphatics. Any increase in venous pressure interferes with the reabsorption of tissue fluid. When the volume of formation of extracellular fluid exceeds the absorptive capacity of lymphatics, it accumulates in the extracellular spaces (edema). Hypoalbuminemia also favors extravasation of fluid out of capillaries by decreasing the plasma protein oncotic pressure.

In a patient with liver cirrhosis, both factors, high portal venous pressure and hypoalbuminemia, are present. Initially, it merely results in increased lymph production in the abdominal viscera, all of which is drained into the thoracic duct. In severe liver cirrhosis, the lymph flow in the thoracic duct may increase 10–20 folds above the normal levels. Fluid accumulates in the peritoneal cavity when the rate of formation of lymph exceeds the rate of reabsorption by the lymphatics. Lymph production is particularly increased in the liver, where it may be seen to "weep" freely from its surface. Due to destruction of hepatic architecture, hepatic lymph passes into peritoneal cavity instead of thoracic duct (Fig. 8.15, primary event).

Secondary Mechanisms

There is no doubt that patients with liver cirrhosis and ascites have elevated levels of plasma renin, angiotensin II, aldosterone and vasopressin, leading to significant salt and water retention in the body (Fig. 8.15). The secondary mechanism act to perpetuate ascites produced by the primary event discussed above. However, the pathogenesis of inappropriate Na^+ and water retention is debatable. The controversy is whether this is a primary abnormality responsible for ascites (overflow hypothesis) or a consequence of the development of ascites (underfill hypothesis).

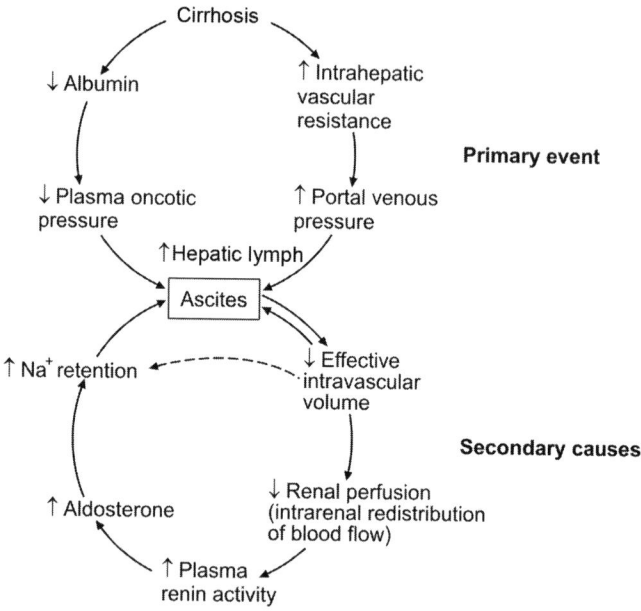

Fig. 8.15: Mechanism of ascites in cirrhosis. Primary event produces ascites. Secondary causes perpetuate it

According to *overflow hypothesis*, Na$^+$ and water retention is an essential component of liver cirrhotic disorder and it can be seen even before the development of ascites or edema. Evidence cited in support of this hypothesis is that ascites and edema are less common with primary biliary cirrhosis than in patients with Laennec's cirrhosis with comparable portal hypertension.

Underfill hypothesis is supported by a most of the research workers in this field. According to this hypothesis, the development of ascites is primarily caused by portal hypertension. The resulting decrease in effective intravascular volume triggers increased secretion of renin-angiotensin and vasopressin leading to salt and water retention.

Hepatic Encephalopathy

Hepatic encephalopathy is a complex neuropsychiatric syndrome seen in cases with severe hepatic failure. It is characterized by disturbances of consciousness and behavior, personality changes, asterixis (flapping tremor) and distinctive electroencephalographic changes.

A nomenclature has been proposed for categorizing hepatic encephalopathy:

- **Type A hepatic encephalopathy:** Describes encephalopathy associated with *acute* liver failure.

- **Type B hepatic encephalopathy:** Describes encephalopathy associated with portal-systemic *bypass* but no intrinsic hepatocellular disease.
- **Type C hepatic encephalopathy:** Describes encephalopathy associated with *cirrhosis and portal hypertension* or *portal-systemic shunts*. Type C hepatic encephalopathy is, in turn, subcategorized as episodic, persistent, or minimal.

Grading of the symptoms of hepatic encephalopathy is performed according to the so-called West Haven classification system:
- **Grade 0:** Minimal hepatic encephalopathy (previously known as subclinical hepatic encephalopathy). Lack of detectable changes in personality or behavior. Minimal changes in memory, concentration, intellectual function, and coordination. Asterixis is absent.
- **Grade 1:** Trivial lack of awareness. Shortened attention span. Impaired addition or subtraction. Hypersomnia, insomnia, or inversion of sleep pattern. Euphoria, depression, or irritability. Mild confusion. Slowing of ability to perform mental tasks. Asterixis can be detected.
- **Grade 2:** Lethargy or apathy. Disorientation. Inappropriate behavior. Slurred speech. Obvious asterixis. Drowsiness, lethargy, gross deficits in ability to perform mental tasks, obvious personality changes.
- **Grade 3:** Somnolent but can be aroused, unable to perform mental tasks, disorientation about time and place, marked confusion, amnesia, occasional fits of rage present; incomprehensible speech.
- **Grade 4:** Coma with or without response to painful stimuli.

Pathophysiology

The exact pathogenesis of hepatic encephalopathy is not clear. An essential factor is a severe hepatocellular dysfunction (acute hepatic failure) and/or intrahepatic or extrahepatic shunting of portal blood to systemic circulation bypassing detoxification function of the liver. Ammonia is one substance whose blood levels are mostly, but not always, elevated in patients with hepatic encephalopathy. Moreover, measures that decrease blood ammonia levels can improve symptoms of hepatic encephalopathy.

Ammonia has multiple neurotoxic effects. It can alter the transport of amino acids, water, and electrolytes across astrocytes and neurons. It can impair amino acid metabolism and energy utilization in the brain. Ammonia can also inhibit the generation of excitatory and inhibitory postsynaptic potentials. For over two decades, it has been postulated that hepatic encephalopathy is the result of *increased GABA concentration* in the blood. However, recent experimental work has not supported this hypothesis.

The development of encephalopathy may be a gradual terminal event in chronic hepatocellular failure, or may follow a well-defined precipitating event such as gastrointestinal bleeding, excessive dietary protein intake, sudden deterioration of renal function or alkalosis.

Hepatorenal Syndrome

Hepatorenal syndrome**(HRS)** is a life-threatening medical condition that consists of rapid deterioration in kidney function in individuals with cirrhosis or fulminant liver failure. HRS is usually fatal unless a liver transplant is performed, although various treatments, including dialysis, can help over short term.

While HRS can affect individuals with cirrhosis (regardless of cause), severe alcoholic hepatitis, or fulminant hepatic failure, it usually occurs when liver function deteriorates rapidly due to an acute injury, such as an infection, bleeding in the gastrointestinal tract, overuse of diuretic medications or large (over 5–6 L) abdominal paracentesis. HRS is a relatively common complication of cirrhosis, occurring in 20% of cirrhotics within one year of their diagnosis, and in 40% of cirrhotics within five years of the diagnosis.

The renal failure of HRS is a consequence of changes in renal blood flow, rather than direct damage to the kidney. The kidneys themselves appear normal to the naked eye and tissue is normal when viewed under the microscope. Moreover, the kidneys even function normally when placed in an otherwise healthy environment (such as if transplanted into a person with a healthy liver). Renal angiography in patients with HRS has revealed severe vasoconstriction in the outer segments of renal cortex whereas blood flow to deeper cortex and medulla is preserved. It seems, hepatorenal syndrome is caused by some humoral substance released from cirrhotic liver which disturbs the prostaglandin synthesis in the kidney.

There can be many causes of kidney failure in individuals with cirrhosis or fulminant liver failure. Consequently, it is a challenge to distinguish hepatorenal syndrome from other entities that cause renal failure in the setting of advanced liver disease, e.g. hypovolemic acute prerenal failure and acute tubular necrosis.

Further Reading

Blei AT, Córdoba J. **Hepatic Encephalopathy**. *Am J Gastroenterol 2001;96:1968–76.*

Briggs CD, Peterson M. **Investigation and management of obstructive jaundice**. *Surgery 2007;25:74–80.*

Collier J, Bassendine M. **How to respond to abnormal liver function tests**. *Clin Med 2002; 2:406–409.*

Lucas WB, Chuttani R. **Pathophysiology and current concepts in the diagnosis of obstructive jaundice**. *Gastroenterologist. 1995 Jun; 3:105–18.*

McCullough AJ. **Pathophysiology of nonalcoholic steatohepatitis**. *J Clin Gasteroenterol 2006; 40:S17–29.*

9

Heart Sounds and Murmurs

THE CARDIAC CYCLE

The heart sounds and murmurs can be discussed meaningfully only in context of the events during the cardiac cycle. Therefore, pressure changes in chambers of the heart during cardiac cycle need to be briefly discussed. The description given below applies to the left side of the heart (left atrium and left ventricle) (Fig.9.1). Events in the right side of the heart are essentially similar though pressure values are different (Table 9.1).

Atrial Systole (0.1 Sec)

Before the atrial systole begins, the mitral valve is open. Most of atrial blood has already been transferred to passively into the left ventricle.

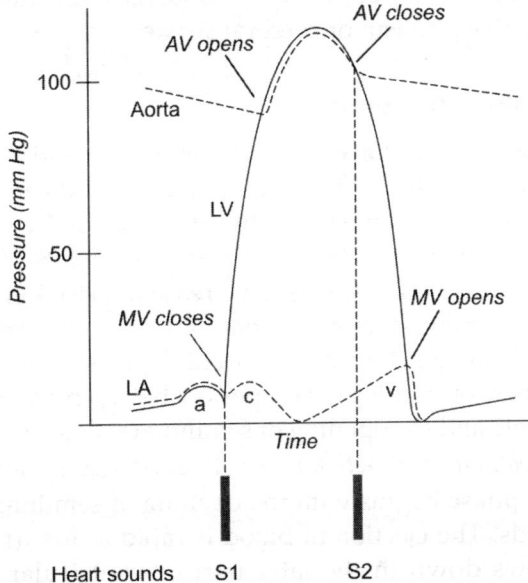

Fig. 9.1: The cardiac cycle. LA: left atrial pressure; LV: left ventricular pressure; MV: mitral valve; AV: aortic valve; S_1: first heart sound; S_2: second heart sound.

Table 9.1: Normal values of pressure in cardiac chambers during a cardiac cycle

Chamber	Peak pressure in systole (mm Hg)	Minimum pressure in diastole (mm Hg)
Left ventricle	120	5
Right ventricle	25	1
Right atrium	15	5
Right atrium	5	0

Atrial systole contributes only about 10% of the ventricular filling. However, when the heart rate is fast (e.g. during exercise) and duration of ventricular diastole is shortened, atrial systole contributes a higher percentage of ventricular filling.

The fact that atrial systole is not mandatory for ventricular filling is best illustrated in patients with atrial fibrillation, in whom there is no effective atrial systole. Though atrial fibrillation abolishes the contribution of atrial contraction to ventricular filling, it generally has relatively minor hemodynamic consequence at rest. However, it can significantly limit normal increases in ventricular stroke volume and cardiac output during exercise. Furthermore, in some cardiac diseases such as ventricular hypertrophy in which ventricular compliance is reduced and increased ventricular stiffness impairs passive filling, atrial contraction contributes significantly to ventricular filling even at rest. Therefore, in these patients, atrial fibrillation can significantly affect resting cardiac output. Of major concern with atrial fibrillation is the increased risk of thrombus formation within the atria (because of ineffective atrial contraction), and the release of these thrombi into the pulmonary or systemic circulation, which can lead to pulmonary embolism or cerebral stroke.

Ventricular Systole (0.3 Sec)

Isovolumic Contraction Phase: Ventricular systole begins just after the end of atrial systole. As the ventricular systole begins, the intraventricular pressure begins to rise, leading to an abrupt closure of AV valve. Closure of the AV valves coincides with the first heart sound (S_1) (Fig. 9.1). The intraventricular pressure continues to increase but ejection of blood into the aorta does not occur since semilunar valve is still closed. Semilunar valve opens only when the intraventricular pressure exceeds that in the aorta (approx. 80 mmHg). The period between the beginning of ventricular systole and the opening of semilunar valve (approx. 0.05 sec) is known as *isovolumic contraction phase* of ventricular systole.

The ejection phase begins with the opening of semilunar valve, and lasts 0.25 seconds. The ejection of blood is rapid at first (rapid ejection phase) and slows down in the later part of ventricular systole. The intraventricular pressure reaches its peak during the rapid ejection phase (Fig. 9.1 and Table 9.1). The amount of blood ejected out of ventricle in each systole is approximately 70 ml and another 50 ml of blood remains in the ventricle (end-systolic volume). Thus, of 120 ml of blood present in each ventricle at the end of diastole (end diastolic volume), only 70 ml are ejected during systole, giving normal ejection fraction of about 60% (normal range 55–70%). During exercise, or sympathetic stimulation, ejection fraction can be increased by decreasing the end-systolic volume. Ejection fraction can be calculated easily by echocardiography and constitutes an important component of cardiac function tests.

As the ventricle begins to relax, there is a steep fall in the intraventricular pressure. Therefore, the pressure gradient between the left ventricle and the aorta is reversed. Blood tends to regurgitate back into left ventricle, but is prevented by immediate closure of semilunar valve. The closure of semilunar valve produces second heat sound (S_2) (Fig. 9.1). The intraventricular pressure continues to decline till it falls below left atrial pressure, when the mitral valve opens. The duration between the closure of semilunar valve and opening of mitral valve is known as *isovolumic relaxation phase*.

Throughout the ventricular systole, the left atrium is being with blood from pulmonary veins. When the mitral valve opens, blood rushes into the left ventricle passively. Ventricular filling is rapid at first (rapid filling phase), but slows down in the later part of ventricular diastole (slow filling phase or diastasis). The next cardiac cycle begins with the next atrial systole.

HEART SOUNDS

First Heart Sound (S_1)

The first heart sound occurs at the beginning of ventricular systole (Fig. 9.2). S_1 is contributed by closure of both the mitral and tricuspid

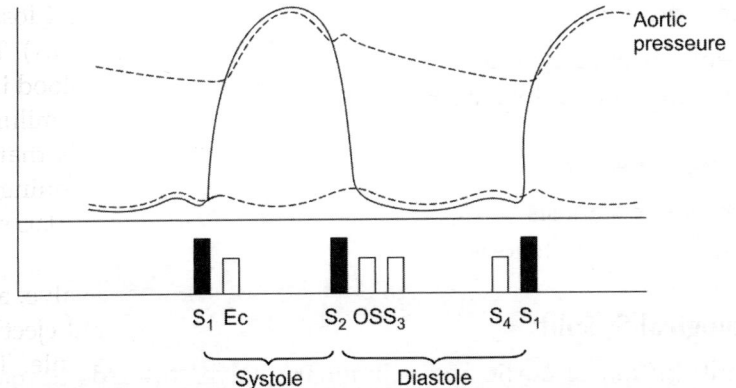

Fig. 9.2: Timing of the four normal and some abnormal heart sounds. Ec: ejection click; OS: opening snap.

valves, but mainly by mitral valve. Greater contribution of mitral valve to S_1 is because the higher pressure generated in the left ventricle at the beginning systole makes the mitral valve to snap shut. Intensity of S_1 is determined by the following:
- The position of mitral valve leaflets at the onset of ventricular systole. If the leaflets are already in apposition due to prolonged diastole (greater ventricular filling), they snap shut with lesser force. The reverse is also true. For example, in mitral stenosis, the mitral valve is fully open at the beginning of ventricular diastole, S1 is louder than normal.
- Rate of rise of left ventricular pressure.
- The presence of structural disease of the mitral valve.

S_1 is louder in
- Mitral stenosis
- Hyperdynamic circulation (anemia, pregnancy, thyrotoxicosis).

S_1 is Soft in
- Congestive heart failure
- Mitral regurgitation

Second Heart Sound (S_2)

S_2 demarcates the beginning of ventricular diastole (Fig. 9.2). It is produced by closure of both the aortic and pulmonary valves. The intensity of S_2 depends on:
- The velocity of blood trying to rush back from the great arterial trunks to the respective ventricle at the beginning of ventricular diastole, and
- The suddenness with which that motion is arrested by the closure of semilunar valves

S_2 is Accentuated in
- Systemic arterial hypertension
- Pulmonary arterial hypertension

S_2 is Diminished in
- Aortic valve stenosis
- Pulmonary valve stenosis

Physiological S_2 Split

The contribution of aortic and pulmonary valves towards S_2 may be designated as A_2 and P_2, respectively. During inspiration, splitting of two components of S_2 may occur normally. During inspiration, P_2 is delayed

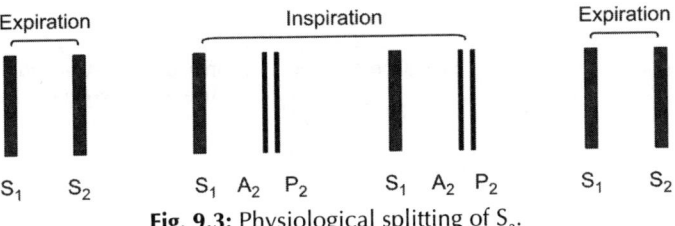

Fig. 9.3: Physiological splitting of S_2.

than A_2, since greater negative intrathoracic pressure promotes greater venous return leading to greater right ventricular load, and longer emptying time which delays closure of pulmonary valve. At the same time, increased capacity of pulmonary capillary bed decreases the left ventricular volume load, leading to shorter emptying time. Hence the aortic valve closes a bit earlier. During expiration, the situation is reversed and closure of the two valves is superimposed. Hence A_2 and P_2 occur simultaneously (Fig. 9.3).

Pathological S_2 Split

a. *Wide Splitting*

In this case splitting of S_2 is again heard in during inspiration, but the interval between A_2 and P_2 is wider than normal. It is usually caused by delayed closure of pulmonary valve as may occur in right BBB and pulmonary valve stenosis (Fig. 9.4B).

b. *Fixed Splitting*

This term refers to wide splitting of S_2 which persists throughout inspiration and expiration. It is seen in patients with septal defects (ASD or VSD) because right ventricular overload is present during inspiration as well as expiration (Fig. 9.4C).

c. *Paradoxical Splitting*

It refers to splitting of S_2 which is heard during expiration but disappears during inspiration (reverse of physiological splitting). Left BBB is the most common cause of paradoxical splitting. In such cases, the delay in the excitation of left ventricle causes aortic valve to close later than pulmonary valve during expiration. During inspiration, the delayed closure of aortic valve coincides with normally delayed closure of pulmonary valve. Therefore A_2 and P_2 are superimposed (Fig. 9.4D). Paradoxical splitting may also be caused by severe aortic outflow obstruction, when the ventricular ejection is prolonged.

Third Heart Sound (S_3)

Third heart sound is normally heard in some children and young adults. It coincides with rapid filling phase of ventricular diastole, when chordae

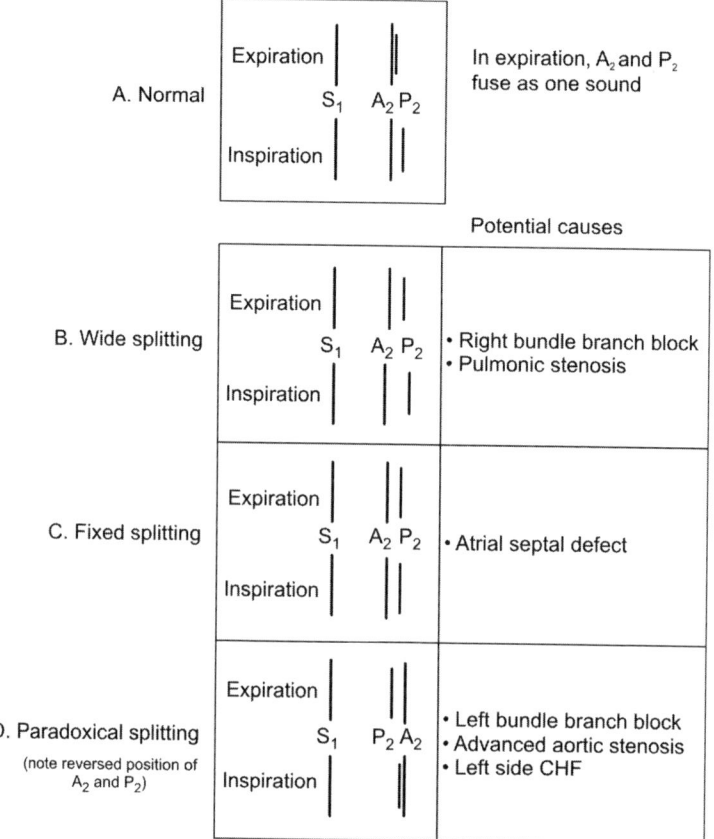

Fig. 9.4: Splitting patterns of second heart sound. S_1: first heart sound; A_2: aortic component of S_2. P_2: pulmonary component of S_2. (Use Fig 11.2 of pathophysiology)

tendineae become tense because of rapid expansion of the ventricles. When heard in middle age or old individuals, S_3 indicates a disease, e.g. congestive heart failure, or severe mitral or tricuspid regurgitation.

Pericardial knock is the name given to a high pitched heart sound that occurs earlier than S_3. It is often heard in patients with constrictive pericarditis, when the adherent pericardium halts ventricular filling abruptly.

A pathological S_3 is often referred to as *ventricular gallop*, because S_1, S_2 and S_3 are heard in a sequence.

Fourth heart sound (S_4)

Fourth heart sound coincides with atrial systole. It is not heard normally. When heard, it indicates a vigorously contracting atrium against a stiffened noncompliant ventricle, e.g. ventricular hypertrophy or myocardial ischemia. When heard, S_4 is often called *atrial gallop*.

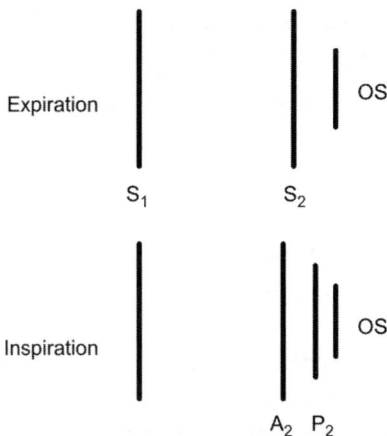

Fig. 9.5: Timing of OS, A_2 and P_2 in mitral stenosis.

Opening Snap

The opening of mitral and tricuspid valves is normally silent, but stenosis produces a sound when valve *opens*. The sound called opening snap, is heard shortly after S_2. It is a sharp high pitched sound that should not be confused with split S_2. Careful auscultation would reveal 3 closely timed sounds, A_2–P_2–OS in during inspiration and only S_2–OS during expiration (Figs 9.3. and 9.5).

Ejection Click

Ejection click is heard in patients with aortic or pulmonary valve stenosis or dilatation of pulmonary artery or aorta. It occurs just after S_1 and coincides with opening of aortic and pulmonary valves, when rapid ejection of blood begins in narrowed or dilated aorta/pulmonary artery.

MURMURS

Murmurs are generated by turbulent flow of blood, which may occur due to:
- Blood flow across a partial obstruction, e.g. stenosis of aortic or pulmonary valve.
- Excessive blood flow across a normal valve, e.g. hyperdynamic circulation (anemia, thyrotoxicosis)
- Ejection of blood into dilated chamber, e.g. aortic systolic murmur associated with aortic aneurysm.
- Regurgitation of blood across an incompetent valve, e.g. mitral or aortic valve regurgitation.
- Shunting of blood from a high pressure chamber to a low pressure chamber of the heart across an abnormal opening, e.g. atrial septal defect (ASD), ventricular septal defect (VSD) or patent ductus arteriosus (PDA).

A murmur may be described in terms of:
1. *Timing:* Systolic, diastolic or continuous.
2. *Intensity:* Grade 1/6 to 6/6

Grade	Description
Grade 1	Very faint
Grade 2	Soft
Grade 3	Heard all over the precordium
Grade 4	Loud, with palpable **thrill** (i.e. a tremor or vibration felt on palpation
Grade 5	Very loud, with thrill. May be heard when stethoscope is partly off the chest.
Grade 6	Very loud, with thrill. May be heard with stethoscope entirely off the chest.

3. *Location:* Site of murmur's maximum intensity in relation to auscultatory areas of the heart, e.g. mitral area, tricuspid area, aortic area or pulmonary area (Fig. 9.6).
4. *Shape:* It is the description of intensity variation of a murmur: uniform (pansystolic), increasing loudness (crescendo), decreasing loudness (decrescendo) or initial increase and then decrease in loudness (crescendo-decrescendo). The last one is also called star shaped after the shape of the murmur on a phonocardiogram.
5. *Quality:* Refers to unusual characteristics of a murmur, such as blowing, harsh, rumbling or musical
6. *Radiation:* Murmur may radiate to a specific area of precordium. Generally, a murmur radiates in the direction of blood flow.
7. *Effect of a manoeuver:* A change in character of the murmur during inspiration/expiration, Valsalva maneuvre, squatting or clenching of fist.

Accentuation of a murmur during inspiration (increased venous return to the heart) implies that its origin is in the right side of the heart. Valsalva maneuver, by diminishing both right and left ventricular filling, reduces

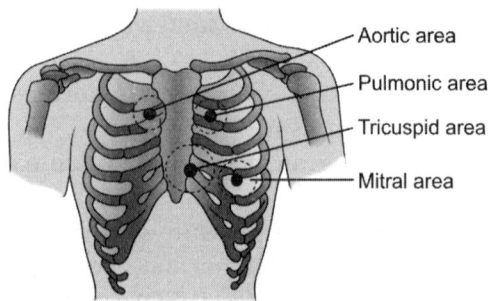

Fig. 9.6: Location of maximum intensity of various murmurs.

the intensity of most of the murmurs, but systolic murmurs of hypertrophic cardiomyopathy or mitral valve prolapse become louder and longer.

Standing position decreases the left ventricular volume and hence accentuates the systolic murmur of hypertrophic cardiomyopathy. Squatting makes most of the murmurs louder by increasing venous return to the heart, except that due to hypertrophic cardiomyopathy, or mitral valve prolapse. Sustained handgrip exercise, which increases the systemic arterial pressure and heart rate, often accentuates the murmurs of MR, AR, MS but diminishes those of AS or hypertrophic cardiomyopathy.

Systolic Murmurs (Fig. 9.7)

Systolic murmurs are the murmurs heard between S_1 and S_2. Systolic murmurs may be subdivided into three types:
- Pansystolic murmur
- Mid-systolic murmur
- Late systolic murmur

Pansystolic murmurs are heard when the turbulence blood flow occurs across a valve throughout systole, due to wide pressure gradient between two chambers. The murmur starts with S_1 and ends with S_2. Such a situation can arise between:
- Left ventricle and left atrium in MR
- Right ventricle and right atrium in TR or
- Left ventricle and right ventricle in VSD

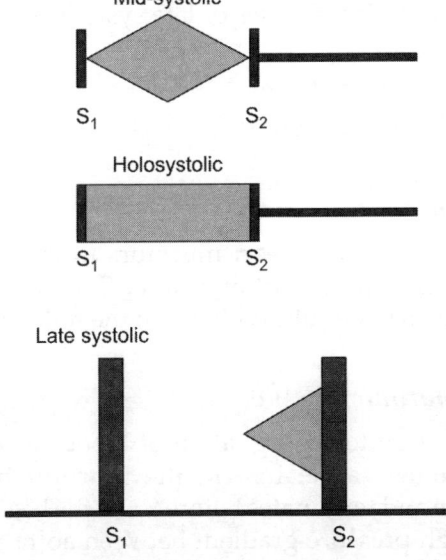

Fig. 9.7: Systolic murmurs.

Mid-systolic murmur (systolic ejection murmur) occurs when blood is ejected through a stenosed aortic or pulmonary valve. The murmur begins only when ejection begins, i.e. there is gap between S_1 and onset of murmur, corresponding to the isovolumic contraction phase of ventricular systole. The intensity of sound initially increases (crescendo) and then decreases (decrescendo) corresponding to the rapid ejection and reduced ejection phases of ventricular systole. The murmur ends just before S_2 (crescendo-decrescendo or star shaped murmur). Mid-systolic murmur may be heard in aortic and pulmonary areas in patients with hyperdynamic circulation. Causes of mid-systolic murmurs include:
- Aortic valve stenosis
- Pulmonary valve stenosis
- Atrial septal defect
- Fallot's tetrology (a large VSD)
- Anemia
- Pregnancy
- Hyperthyroidism

Late systolic murmur: Mitral valve prolapse the most common cause of late systolic murmurs. It can be heard best over the apex of the heart, usually preceded by click. If the prolapse becomes severe enough, mitral regurgitation may occur. Any maneuver that decreases left ventricular volume such as standing, sitting, valsalva maneuver, can produce earlier onset of clicks, longer murmur duration, and decreased murmur intensity. Any maneuver that increases left ventricular volume such as squatting, elevation of legs, hand grip, can delay the onset of clicks, shorten murmur duration, and increase murmur intensity. Papillary muscle dysfunction because of myocardial ischemia/infarction can also cause late systolic murmur and regurgitation. Causes or late systolic murmurs include:
- Mitral valve collapse
- Tricuspid valve prolapse (rare)
- Papillary muscle dysfunction

Diastolic Murmurs

Diastolic heart murmurs are heart murmurs heard during ventricular diastole. Diastolic murmurs start at or after S_2 and end before or at S_1. Diastolic murmurs may be subdivided into the following 2 types:

Early Diastolic Murmur (Fig.9.8)

Early diastolic are due to regurgitation of blood through incompetent aortic or pulmonary valve. In AR, the murmur begins at S_2, has decrescendo shape and terminates before S_1. At the beginning of diastole, (at S_2), there is high pressure gradient between aorta and left ventricle. Hence murmur displays maximum intensity at S_2. The intensity of

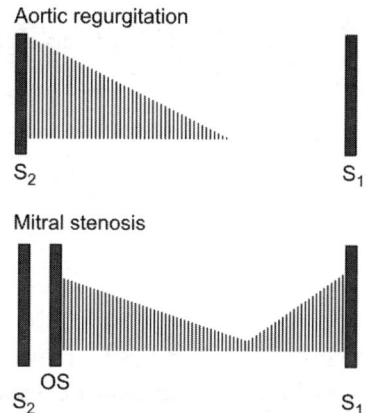

Fig. 9.8: Diastolic murmurs (OS: opening snap).

murmur decreases as the aortic pressure declines and the pressure gradient between aorta and left ventricle decreases. Causes of early (decrescendo) diastolic murmurs:
- Aortic valve regurgitation
- Pulmonary valve regurgitation

Mid-late Diastolic Murmurs (Fig. 9.8)

Mid-late diastolic murmurs result from turbulence in blood flow across stenosed mitral or tricuspid valve or less commonly from increased blood flow across the AV valves, e.g. severe anemia, thyrotoxicosis or pregnancy. The opening of a stenosed AV valve at the beginning of rapid filling phase produces a sound called opening snap (OS)

Continuous Murmurs

These murmurs are heard throughout the cardiac cycle, without any audible gap between systole and diastole. Thus, a murmur beginning with S_1 extends without any interruption through S_2 into diastole. Such a murmur is heard in patent ductus arteriosus because there is an abnormal communication between high pressure aorta and low pressure pulmonary artery. The murmur begins immediately after S_1, reaches a maximum at S_2 (when pressure gradient between aorta and pulmonary artery is greatest) and then decrescendos into next S_1 (Fig. 9.9).

The "to-and-fro" murmur of aortic stenosis with regurgitation should not be confused with continuous murmur. In this case, there is star shaped systolic murmur followed by early decrescendo diastolic murmur.

VALVULAR HEART DISEASE

Mitral Stenosis (MS)

Mitral stenosis is almost always caused by rheumatic heart disease. The symptoms usually manifest decades after the attack of acute rheumatic

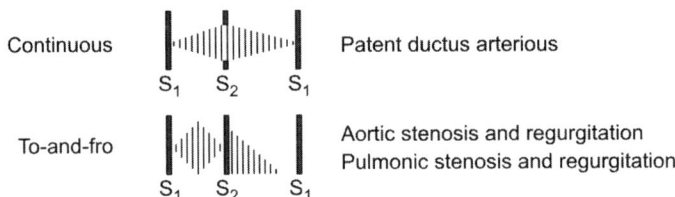

Fig. 9.9: Continuous murmur of PDA and to-and-fro murmur of aortic stenosis and regurgitation.

carditis. The normal cross section area of mitral valve in adults is 4–6 cm². If it narrows to 2 cm², a significant pressure gradient develops between left atrium and ventricle during diastole (normally zero) (Fig. 9.10). The left atrial pressure rises in order to propel blood against narrowed valve. Since left ventricular filling becomes more and more dependent on atrial systole, gradually left atrial wall undergoes hypertrophy and ultimately dilatation. Left ventricular pressure remains normal but cardiac output cannot increase when required. Hence, limitation of exercise tolerance and breathlessness on exertion are important symptoms.

Increased left atrial pressure is transmitted to the pulmonary circulation resulting in increased pulmonary venous and capillary pressure. Thus, the patient suffers from pulmonary congestion and pulmonary edema.

Pulmonary hypertension is a common complication of more advanced MS. Several factors contribute to the development of pulmonary hypertension in this setting:
- Passive backward transmission of the elevated left atrial pressure
- Pulmonary artery and arteriole vasoconstriction due to the elevated pulmonary venous pressures (reactive pulmonary hypertension)
- Hypertrophy of the pulmonary artery muscular layer as a result of the increased pressure

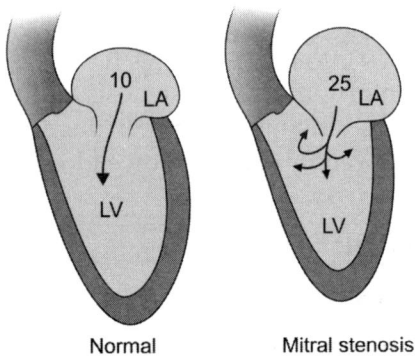

Fig. 9.10: Hemodynamic changes in mitral stenosis.

- Organic obliterative changes in the pulmonary vascular bed due to the chronically elevated pressures

Reactive pulmonary hypertension lessens pulmonary congestion and edema, but further decreases the cardiac output and increases the right ventricular pressure. Ultimately, right ventricular hypertrophy and right heart failure supervene.

The hypertrophy and dilatation of left atrium predisposes to the development of atrial fibrillation, which, in turn, predisposes to atrial thromboembolism.

Heart Sounds and Murmurs in MS

The auscultatory signs of MS include:
- Loud S_1
- Opening snap following S_2
- Mid-diastolic murmur
- Loud P_2

Normally, ventricular filling mainly occurs during diastole and mitral valve leaflets are floating over the pool of blood. Hence, they are already partially closed even before the beginning of ventricular systole. In MS, A-V pressure gradient is maintained throughout diastole, which keeps mitral valve open. The onset of ventricular systole abruptly slams the widely open leaflets of mitral valve, producing loud S_1.

P_2 is accentuated when pulmonary hypertension develops. When the stenotic leaflets of mitral valve are still flexible, the marked pressure gradient between left atrium and left ventricle at the onset of diastole causes the leaflets to open abruptly, producing an audible sound called opening snap. Turbulence of blood flow squirting the narrow valve produces a low pitched diastolic murmur beginning with OS and accentuated by atrial systole (just before S1).

Mitral Regurgitation (MR)

Proper closure of mitral valve during ventricular systole depends on many coordinated components: precise cooption of the two leaflets supported by chordae tendineae and papillary muscle as well as structural integrity of mitral annulus. MR may result from a defect in any of these components:
- Papillary muscle dysfunction due to ischemic heart disease.
- Mitral valve collapse due to myxomatous degeneration.
- Dilatation of mitral valve ring due to:
  - Rheumatic heart disease
  - Ischemic heart disease
  - Cardiac myopathy
  - Marked left ventricular enlargement

- Deformity of cusps
  - Rheumatic heart disease
  - Infective endocarditis

The basic hemodynamic abnormality in MR is the ejection of a part of ventricular stroke put back into left atrium (Fig. 9.11). At the onset of ventricular systole, as the ventricular pressure begins to increase, instead of isovolumic contraction, ventricular blood begins to be ejected back into low pressure left atrium through the incompetent mitral valve. With the onset of ejection phase, ventricular blood begins to be ejected into aorta, but regurgitation of blood into left atrium continues throughout ventricular systole. [Left atrial pressure is far lower than the left ventricular pressure throughout ventricular systole (Fig. 9.1).] Thus, a pansystolic murmur can be heard over the mitral area. Since, closure of mitral valve leaflets is not proper, S_1 is softer than normal.

During ventricular diastole, right ventricular output and regurgitated blood enter the ventricle together, producing a prominent S_3. When regurgitation is of a large magnitude, diastolic blood return from the atrium to the ventricle produces a third heart sound as well as a diastolic flow rumble. The extra amount of blood puts a large volume overload on the left ventricle. However, since left ventricular volume is reduced even before the aortic valve opens, ventricular stress is not significantly increased. Therefore, even though larger volume of blood is pumped by left ventricle in each beat, oxygen requirement does not increase significantly. That is why mitral regurgitation may be tolerated for many years before heart failure sets in.

Heart Sounds and Murmurs in MR

The auscultatory signs of MR include:
- Softer S_1
- Pansystolic murmur
- Prominent S_3
- Diastolic flow rumble (if regurgitation is severe)

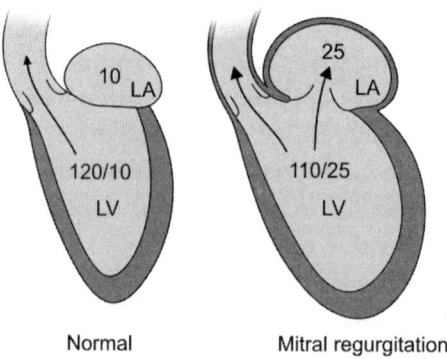

Fig. 9.11: Hemodynamic changes in mitral regurgitation.

The effect of MR on pulmonary circulation depends on the compliance of the left atrium. When mitral regurgitation develops suddenly, e.g. after myocardial infarction, left atrial compliance is normal and it cannot dilate quickly to accommodate extra regurgitated blood. Hence there is marked increase in left atrial pressure, elevated pulmonary capillary pressure, pulmonary congestion and pulmonary edema and tachycardia at exertion. When the condition worsens, patient develops dyspnea on exertion or even at rest.

When MR develops gradually, left atrium has time to undergo compensatory changes. It becomes a huge and abnormally compliant chamber. Therefore, left atrial pressure does not rise markedly, and pulmonary congestion and pulmonary edema are uncommon. However, because of the enlarged dilated left atrium, the patient become more prone to develop atrial fibrillation and thromboembolism.

Aortic Stenosis (AS)

Aortic valve stenosis may be due to:
- Congenitally deformed (bicuspid) valve
- Senile wear and tear and calcification of (otherwise, basically normal) valve
- Rheumatic heart disease

The normal area of aortic valve is approximately 3 cm^2. More than 50% decrease in orifice area results in a significant obstruction to the outflow of blood during ventricular systole. As a result, a gradient develops between the left ventricle and the aorta which may be as high as 100 mmHg (Fig.9.12). Decreased cardiac output produces a limitation to exercise tolerance. The turbulent outflow of blood across the narrow produces a diamond shaped mid-systolic murmur over the aortic area. The aortic component of P_2 is inaudible. Ejection click, caused by the impact of left ventricular outflow against the partially fused aortic valve leaflets, is more commonly associated with a mobile bicuspid aortic valve than an immobile calcified aortic valve.

To overcome the obstruction in the outflow of blood, the starling mechanism comes into action and restores cardiac output at rest to near normal. It also results in a gradual hypertrophy of left ventricle associated with stiffness of the ventricular wall. Consequently a larger percentage of atrial blood reaches the ventricle during atrial systole. This results in hypertrophy of left atrium and atrial gallop (audible S_4) over mitral area.

Heart Sounds and Murmurs in AS

Important auscultatory signs of AS include:
- Mid-systolic diamond-shaped murmur
- Ejection click

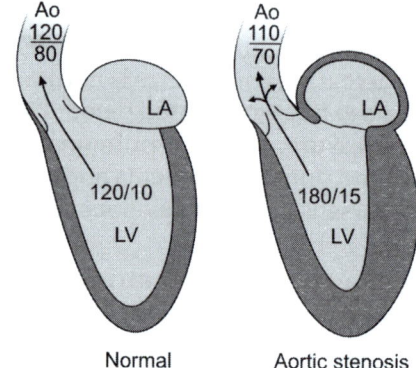

Fig. 9.12: Hemodynamic changes in aortic stenosis.

- Softer A_2 component in S_2
- Atrial gallop (at later stage)

In earlier stages, mean left atrial pressure is not increased since the rise in atrial pressure occurs mostly during atrial systole. However, with progress of the disease, left ventricular dysfunction leads to increased left atrial pressure followed by pulmonary congestion and congestive heart failure.

Angina and syncope are prominent features of AS. Angina can be attributed to at least three factors: (i) Increased oxygen demand by the hypertrophied myocardium, (ii) greater interference in coronary blood flow during systolic phase by generation of high intraventricular pressure, (iii) reduced diastolic pressure in aorta reduces the coronary blood flow even during diastolic phase of cardiac cycle. Sub-endocardium, where intramural pressure development is greatest, is more prone to develop infarction.

Syncope related to aortic stenosis is usually associated with exertion. Exertion causes relaxation of the body's blood vessel, lowering blood pressure. In aortic stenosis, the heart is unable to increase output to compensate for the drop in blood pressure during exertion. This results in insufficient cerebral blood flow and syncope during exercise.

Aortic Regurgitation (AR)

Aortic regurgitation (aortic valve incompetence) may be due to:
- Rheumatic heart disease
- Endocarditis
- Congenital deformity (bicuspid valve)
- Age-related wear and tear
- Dilatation of aortic root by aneurysm/dissection of aorta

In AR, a large volume of blood regurgitates back from the aorta into the left ventricle during diastole. In each systole, the left ventricle has to pump out this blood in addition to the right ventricular stroke output. Thus, left ventricle is subjected to volume overload (Fig. 9.13). The high stroke volume causes high systolic blood pressure, whereas the diastolic pressure is abnormally low because of regurgitation of blood. High pulse pressure (collapsing pulse) is one of the characteristic features of AR. The turbulent back flow of blood during diastole causes a prominent early decrescendo diastolic murmur starting with S_2. The murmur is best heard on third *left* intercostal space. A mid-systolic ejection murmur may also be because of increased stroke volume.

Important auscultatory signs of MR include:
- An early decrescendo diastolic murmur
- Mid-systolic flow murmur

Because left ventricular hypertrophy and dilatation are adequate to meet the demands of cardiac output, the patient is generally asymptomatic for many years. Gradually, fibrosis of left ventricular myocardium results in myocardial dysfunction leading to increased left atrial pressure, pulmonary congestion and congestive heart failure.

Tricuspid Valve Disorders

Tricuspid stenosis is a relatively uncommon manifestation of rheumatic heart disease. It results in an opening snap and a mid-diastolic murmur similar to that of MS, except that it is best heard over tricuspid area. Moreover, the intensity of murmur increases during inspiration. Jugular venous pulse shows a large "a" wave due to atrial contraction against narrowed tricuspid orifice.

Tricuspid regurgitation is common. It is usually functional rather than structural, i.e. because of pressure or volume overload on the right ventricle. The pansystolic murmur is soft, but its intensity increases during inspiration. More sensitive physical sign is a prominent "cv" wave in jugular venous pulse and a pulsatile liver (due to regurgitation of right ventricular blood into venae cavae).

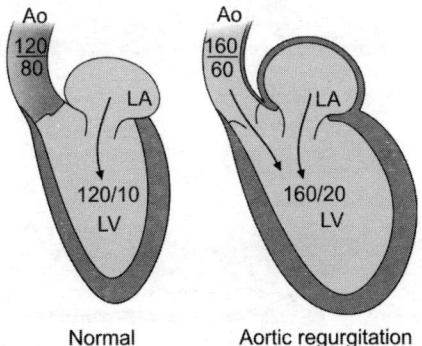

Fig. 9.13: Hemodynamic changes in aortic valve regurgitation.

Pulmonary Valve Disorders

Pulmonary stenosis is almost always due to a congenital defect. It produces a mid-systolic ejection murmur best heard on left upper sternum and radiating to the left shoulder. The intensity of murmur increases during inspiration. An ejection click may also be heard. Delayed right ventricular ejection may produce wide splitting of S_2.

Pulmonary regurgitation is rarely an isolated defect. It is usually associated with pulmonary artery dilatation due to pulmonary hypertension. It results in an early decrescendo diastolic murmur at left sternal border that is difficult to distinguish from AR.

Atrial Septal Defect (ASD)

This disorder results from the persistence of the direct communication between the two atria after birth (Fig. 9.14). The defect may vary from complete absence of interatrial septum with serious hemodynamic abnormalities to such a minor communication that the patient remains active and asymptomatic throughout life.

The right heart has low pressure chambers and right ventricle is more compliant than left ventricle. Therefore, communication between the two atria results in a left to right shunt of blood leading to a volume overload on the right ventricle. The result is:

a. A systolic flow murmur over pulmonary valve due to excessive blood volume passing through it.
b. Wide, fixed splitting of S_2 is an important auscultatory sign of ASD. Splitting of S_2 is due to delayed closure of pulmonary valve, because of volume overload. It is fixed split because the right ventricular

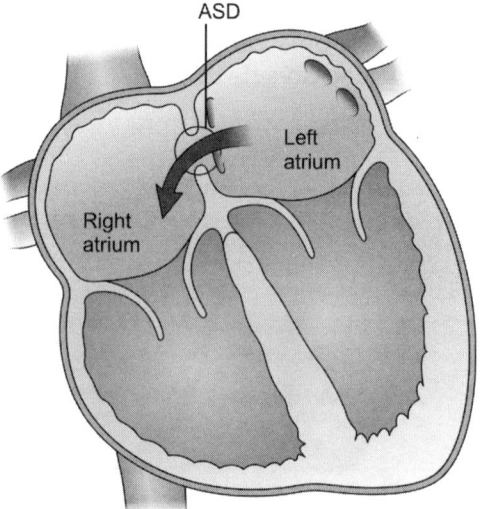

Fig. 9.14: Atrial septal defect.

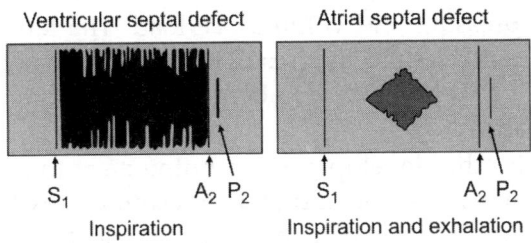

Fig. 9.15: Heart sounds and murmurs in VSD and ASD.

overload is present during inspiration as well as during expiration (Fig.9.15).

The symptoms commonly arise after fourth decade. The long-standing right ventricular overload results in right ventricular hypertrophy and dilatation. If pulmonary hypertension develops, the direction of shunt may be reversed. Therefore, transfer of venous blood to the left heart results in hypoxia and cyanosis. At this stage, both the pulmonary and tricuspid murmurs decrease in intensity.

Ventricular Septal Defect (VSD)

VSD is the most common congenital heart disease (Fig. 9.16). In this disorder, hemodynamic changes are more complex than in ASD. The communication between the two ventricles with marked pressure gradient results in shunting of blood from left to the right ventricle throughout ventricular systole. The patient has a pansystolic murmur which is best heard at the left sternal edge (Fig. 9.15). The right ventricle expands to

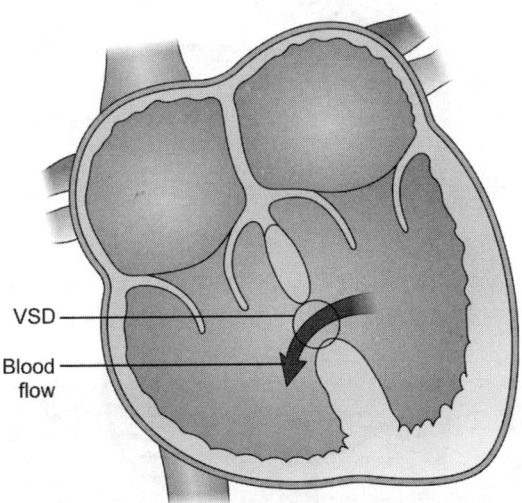

Fig. 9.16: Ventricular septal defect

accommodate pressure and volume overload. The left atrium dilates because of volume overload as a result of excessive venous return from pulmonary artery. Left ventricle undergoes hypertrophy in response to volume overload.

Subsequently, the development of pulmonary hypertension may reverse the shunt—it becomes a right to left shunt. Now the condition is called Eisenmenger syndrome. At this stage, the patient develops cyanosis and the systolic murmur disappears.

Patent Ductus Arteriosus (PDA)

PDA results from a failure of closure of ductus arteriosus, which normally occurs soon after birth (Fig. 9.17). Premature infants, particularly with birth weight less than 1.5 kg, are more prone to this disorder.

After birth, ductus arteriosus acts as a communication between high pressure aorta (70/40 mmHg) and pulmonary artery (20/10 mmHg). The pressure gradient persists throughout systole and diastole, resulting in a *continuous murmur* in the left hemithorax, louder in systole when pressure gradient is larger (Fig. 9.9).

The left to right shunt appears chiefly during diastole in ASD, chiefly during systole in VSD. In PDA, the gradient persists throughout the cardiac cycle. Hence, there is far greater volume overload on the pulmonary circulation and left side of the heart, which tends to produce heart failure earlier than in ASD or VSD.

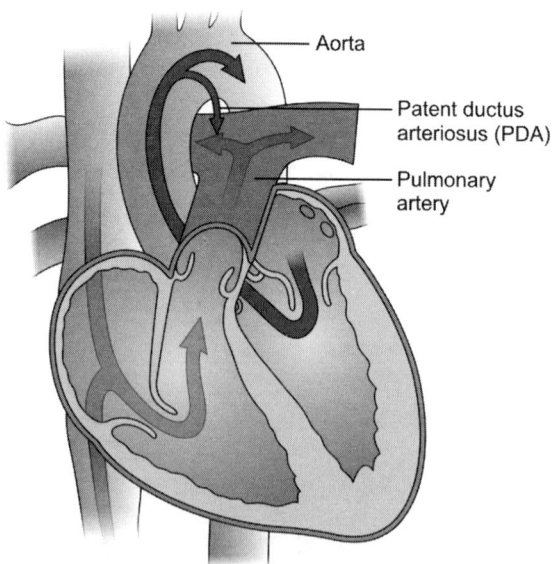

Fig. 9.17: Patent ductus arteriosus.

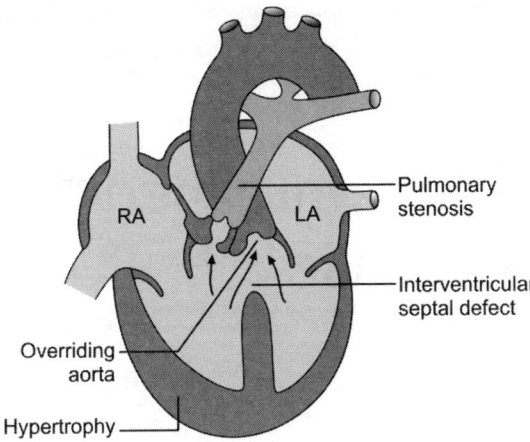

Fig. 9.18: Tetralogy of Fallot.

Tetralogy of Fallot (Fig. 9.18)

About 70% of infants with cyanotic congenital heart disease have tetrology of Fallot. The four characteristic features of the disorder are:
- A large VSD
- A large aortic root over riding the interventricular septum so that aorta receives blood from both the ventricles.
- A small right ventricular outflow tract.
- Right ventricular hypertrophy consequent to the three defects mentioned above.

Because of the fact that aorta over rides the septum and because of increased pulmonary outflow resistance, the right ventricular blood is diverted into aorta through VSD. The result is cyanosis, hypoxia and dyspnea on exertion. A systolic ejection murmur is produced by turbulent blood flow through the pulmonary valve.

Further Reading

Criley, JM; Criley, D. **The physiological origins of heart sounds and murmurs.** (1997) Lippincott Williams & Wilkins Philadephia.

www.learntheheart.com

www.uptodate.com/contents/auscult

10
Ischemic Heart Disease

PHYSIOLOGICAL ASPECTS OF CORONARY BLOOD FLOW

In most tissues, increased O_2 requirement is met with by greater oxygen extraction from the blood and by greater rate of blood flow per unit time. In cardiac muscle, even at resting heart rate, O_2 extraction is very high. Therefore, increased O_2 demand can be met with only increased rate of blood flow in the coronary artery. Under normal circumstances, a number of regulatory mechanisms provide a rate of coronary blood flow which exactly matches the metabolic (oxygen) demand, whether at rest or during exercise or exertion.

Myocardial oxygen demand is determined by:
- Heart rate
- Myocardial contractility (inotropic state)
- Ventricular wall tension

An increase in heart rate and/or contractility increases the myocardial oxygen demand. Negative chronotropic and inotropic drugs, such as β-blockers; decrease the O_2 demand of myocardium.

Myocardial wall tension is determined by the law of Laplace:

$$\text{Left ventricular tension} = \frac{P \times r}{n}$$

Where, P = transmural pressure
r = radius of left ventricle
n = thickness of left ventricle

Any increase in wall tension increases oxygen demand of the myocardium, e.g. increase in left ventricular systolic pressure in hypertension or aortic stenosis (conditions with increased afterload). As seen from the law of Laplace, ventricular tension is inversely proportionate to the thickness of the left ventricle. That is, hypertrophied heart shall have lower wall tension and oxygen demand. Thus, hypertrophy of heart in response to pressure or volume overload is a physiological adaptation to its increased oxygen demand. However, when ventricular hypertrophy progresses to dilatation, radius of the chamber increases. Therefore, left ventricular tension and hence oxygen demand increases. Any physiological or pharmacological mechanism that decreases preload or afterload or both shall decrease oxygen demand of the myocardium.

In dilated cardiomyopathy, the heart becomes greatly distended and the radius (r) of ventricle increases. Therefore to create the same pressure (P) during ejection of the blood much larger wall tension (T) has to be developed by the cardiac muscle. Thus dilated heart requires more energy to pump the same amount of blood as compared to the heart of normal size.

MYOCARDIAL OXYGEN SUPPLY

The myocardial oxygen supply depends on: (i) oxygen content of the arterial blood, and (ii) the rate of coronary blood flow. The oxygen content of arterial blood may be decreased because of decreased hemoglobin concentration or because of poor systemic blood oxygenation (hypoxic hypoxia). Thus, angina may be a presenting feature of a patient with severe anemia or lung disease. In the absence of anemia or lung disease, oxygen supply to the heart is determined by rate of coronary blood flow.

In most other organs, because of greater pressure, head, blood flow is greater during systole than diastole of the heart. However, in case of myocardium, the reverse is true. The coronary arteries that run on the surface of the heart are called epicardial coronary arteries. Branches of epicardial arteries that run into and supply blood to the myocardium are called subendocardial coronary vessels. During systole, myocardial contraction has a strangulating effect on the blood vessels passing through the cardiac muscle fibers. Because of this, blood flow in the subendocardial vessels stops. As a result, most myocardial perfusion occurs during diastole when the subendocardial coronary vessels are patent because of absence of extramural pressure (Fig. 10.1).

As explained above, in coronary circulation, perfusion pressure is chiefly determined by the diastolic blood pressure. That is the reason why myocardial oxygen supply is impeded in conditions where diastolic blood pressure is low, e.g. aortic regurgitation. Transmural pressure is greater in subendocardial region than in sub-epicardial region of myocardium. That explains the greater frequency of subendocardial left ventricular infarcts.

Although coronary vessels are supplied with sympathetic and parasympathetic nerve fibers, the coronary vascular resistance is chiefly determined by intrinsic metabolic factors rather than neural control. Local vasodilator metabolites such as adenosine (chiefly) and other products of anoxic metabolism (lactate, H^+, certain prostaglandins) regulate coronary blood flow by a direct action on vascular smooth muscle.

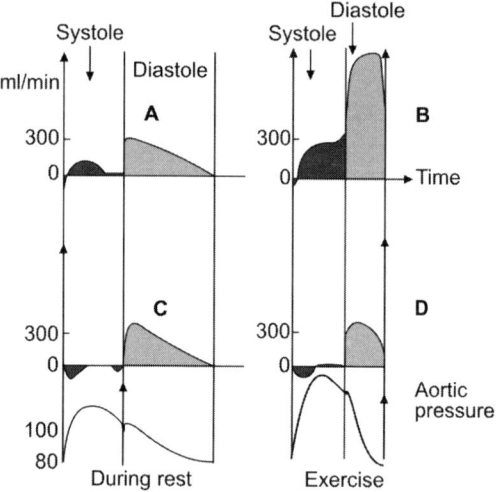

Fig. 10.1: Left coronary blood flow in systole and diastole at rest and during exercise. A, B: normal healthy person; C, D: a patient with coronary artery disease.

ATHEROSCLEROSIS

Atherosclerosis is characterized by lesions of tunica intima called atheromas or atheromatous (or fibro-fatty) plaques which protrude into and obstruct vascular lumens and weaken the underlying tunica media. Atheromas can lead to serious complications such as coronary artery disease, cerebrovascular accidents, peripheral arterial disease and aortic aneurism. Atherosclerosis develops primarily in large elastic arteries, e.g. aorta, carotid, iliac, or large or medium-sized muscular arteries such as coronary, renal and popliteal arteries.

Pathogenesis of Atherosclerosis

The mechanisms of atherogenesis remain uncertain. The "response-to-injury" theory is most widely accepted. Endothelial injury causes vascular inflammation and a fibroproliferative response follows. Probable causes of endothelial injury include oxidized low-density lipoprotein (LDL) cholesterol; infectious agents; toxins, including the byproducts of cigarette smoking and hyperglycemia. Circulating monocytes infiltrate the intima of the vessel wall, and these tissue macrophages act as scavenger cells, taking up LDL cholesterol and forming the characteristic foam cell of early atherosclerosis. These activated macrophages produce numerous factors that are injurious to the endothelium.

Hypercholesterolemia induces a number of changes on vascular-homeostasis, including a decrease in NO bioactivity, an increase in superoxide production, an increase in adhesion molecules and attenuation of endothelium-dependent vasodilatation. The combination of diabetes

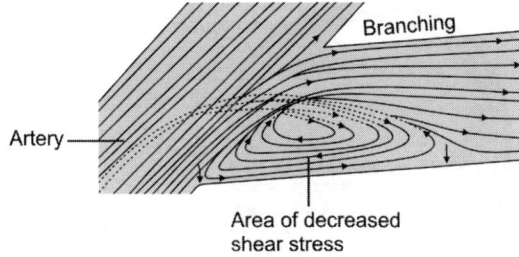

Fig. 10.2: Shear stress at the bifurcation of an artery.

and hypertension appears to have an additive effect on monocyte adhesion. It seems that cholesterol-induced endothelial dysfunction is related to the degree of LDL oxidation and not LDL concentration itself. Acute elevations of free fatty acids and triglycerides can attenuate vasodilator responses over the course of several hours.

Elevated serum levels of LDL cholesterol overwhelm the antioxidant properties of the healthy endothelium and result in abnormal endothelial metabolism of this lipid moiety. Oxidized LDL is capable of a wide range of toxic effects and cell/vessel wall dysfunctions that are characteristically and consistently associated with the development of atherosclerosis. These dysfunctions include impaired endothelium-dependent dilation and paradoxical vasoconstriction. These dysfunctions are the result of direct inactivation of nitric oxide by the excess production of free radicals.

The decrease in the availability of nitric oxide is also associated with increased platelet adhesion, increased plasminogen activator inhibitor, decreased plasminogen activator, increased tissue factor, decreased thrombomodulin, and alterations in heparin sulfate proteoglycans. The consequences include a procoagulant milieu and enhanced platelet thrombus formation.

The lesions of atherosclerosis do not occur in a random fashion. Hemodynamic factors interact with the activated vascular endothelium. Atherosclerotic plaques characteristically occur in regions of branching and marked curvature at areas of geometric irregularity and where blood undergoes sudden changes in velocity and direction of flow. Decreased shear stress and turbulence (Fig. 10.2) may promote atherogenesis at these important sites within the coronary arteries, the major branches of the thoracic and abdominal aorta, and the large conduit vessels of the lower extremities.

The earliest pathologic lesion of atherosclerosis is the fatty streak. The fatty streak is observed in the aorta and coronary arteries of most individuals by the age of 20 years. The fatty streak is the result of focal accumulation of serum lipoproteins within the intima of the vessel wall. Microscopy reveals lipid-laden macrophages, T lymphocytes, and smooth muscle cells in varying proportions.

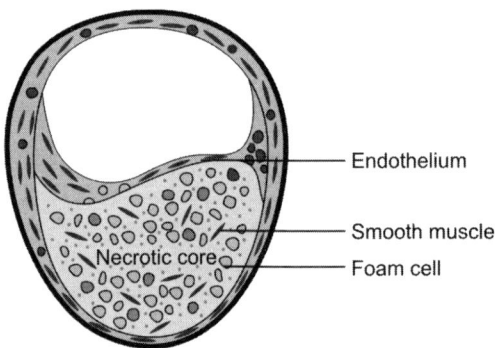

Fig. 10.3: Atherosclerotic plaque.

The fatty streak may progress to form a fibrous plaque (Fig. 10.3). Atherosclerotic plaque is the result of progressive lipid accumulation along with migration and proliferation of smooth muscle cells. Smooth muscle cells are responsible for the deposition of extracellular connective tissue matrix and form a fibrous cap that overlies a core of lipid-laden foam cells, extracellular lipid, and necrotic cellular debris. Growth of the fibrous plaque results in progressive luminal narrowing. Developing atherosclerotic plaques acquire their own microvascular network called vasa vasorum, which are prone to hemorrhage and contribute to progression of atherosclerosis. Denudation of the overlying endothelium or rupture of the protective fibrous cap may result in exposure of the thrombogenic contents of the core of the plaque to the circulating blood. This exposure constitutes an advanced or complicated lesion. The plaque rupture occurs due to weakening of the fibrous cap. A plaque rupture may result in thrombus formation, partial or complete occlusion of the blood vessel, and progression of the atherosclerotic lesion due to organization of the thrombus and incorporation within the plaque.

Effects of Atherosclerosis

The clinical response to ischemia associated with obstructive atherosclerosis is highly dependent on the regional circulation. For instance, in lower-extremity PAD, claudication and critical limb ischemia are the principal clinical manifestations, whereas in the carotid arteries, transient ischemic attacks and stroke are the principal clinical presentations. Obstructive disease in the renal circulation can result in hypertension or ischemic nephropathy or both. Abnormalities in renal function can also accelerate atherosclerosis elsewhere, particularly in the coronary arteries. Disease of the aorta can lead to obstruction or aneurysm formation; the latter is associated with rupture when the aneurysm reaches a critical size.

Atherosclerotic narrowing of coronary arteries produces its effects mainly by hypoperfusion of the myocardium, which may range from stable angina, unstable angina or myocardial infarction.

Stable Angina

In the normal individuals, by the local metabolite control, coronary arteriolar resistance decreases in proportion to the increase in O_2 demand of the myocardium. Thus, coronary blood flow increases in proportion to the oxygen demand of myocardium. When atherosclerotic narrowing (in one or more of the epicardial coronary arteries) is greater than 60–70%, coronary blood flow cannot increase in spite of presence of vasodilator metabolites (Fig. 10.4). Therefore myocardial ischemia results; which is commonly intermittent. Anginal pain occurs only at times of increased oxygen demand. Myocardial ischemia occurs during exertion or emotional excitement, but subsides by rest. Such a condition is known as *stable angina*.

In stable angina, pain may be localized to substernum or referred to left arm, neck, jaw or there may be feeling of heaviness or uselessness of left arm. The pain results from the effect of anoxic metabolites on the pain nerve endings in the myocardium.

Anginal pain may also be produced in some conditions in which O_2 supply to the heart is curtailed in the absence of any atherosclerotic narrowing of coronary vessels:
- Severe anemia
- Severe hypoxia
- Hypotension
- Low aortic diastolic pressure (aortic regurgitation)
- Severe aortic stenosis
- When oxygen demand is greater than what can be met by maximum coronary vasodilatation: Hypertrophic cardiomyopathy
- Severe aortic stenosis
- Hypertrophic cardiomyopathy

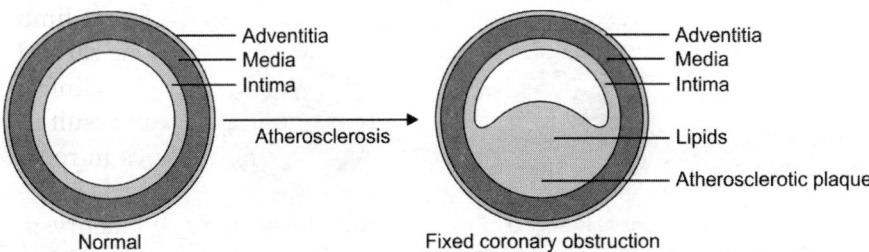

Fig. 10.4: Pathogenesis of stable angina

A very small percentage of angina patients may suffer from angina even though angiography does not reveal narrowing in any of the coronary arteries. Such anginal episodes, known as **variant angina,** *or* **Prinzmetal's angina,** are believed to be caused by severe coronary vasospasm. The mechanism that triggers the coronary vasospasm is not clear, but one of such episodes may progress to myocardial infarction, AV block, ventricular arrhythmias or even death.

Unstable Angina

In patients with stable angina, increased frequency and duration of anginal pain produced by lesser exertion or it may occur even at rest, but without ECG or enzymatic evidence of myocardial infarction, is known as unstable angina. These episodes reflect an acute reduction in coronary blood flow caused by thrombosis or spasm (Fig. 10.5).

If the patient is examined during the anginal episode, no physical abnormality may be detected. However, there can be tachycardia, dyspnea, pulmonary congestion (rales), atrial gallop or even ventricular arrhythmia. The pathophysiological mechanisms of the symptoms and signs of unstable angina are given in Fig. 10.6. Physiological basis of therapeutic agents used in the treatment of angina is given in Table 10.1.

If these symptoms and signs are accompanied by ECG and/or abnormality in serum enzymes (CK, SGOT, LDH), an acute myocardial infarction is said to have taken place.

Myocardial Infarction

When the myocardial ischemia progresses to a degree that irreversible necrosis of a part of myocardium occurs, an acute myocardial infarction (MI)

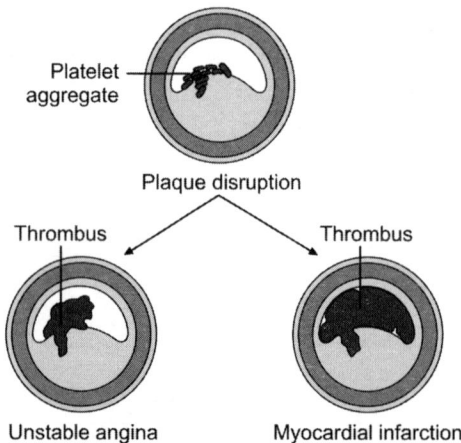

Fig.10.5: Pathological changes in coronary artery in unstable angina and myocardial infarction.

Ischemic Heart Disease

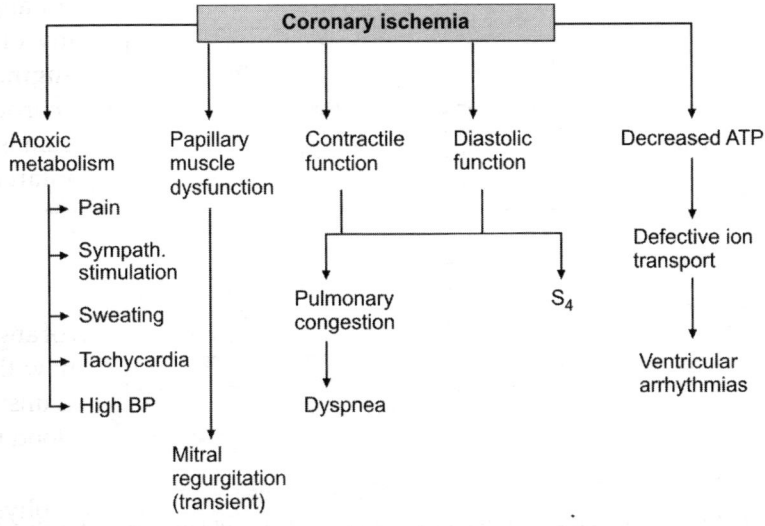

Fig. 10.6: Pathophysiology of symptoms and signs of myocardial ischemia.

Table 10.1:	Physiological basis of angina therapy	
Drugs		*Mode of action*
Organic nitrates	↓ Preload!	↓ Myocardial O_2 demand
	↑ Coronary perfusion	↑ Myocardial O_2 supply
	↓ Coronary vasospasm	↑ Myocardial O_2 supply
β-adrenergic blockers	↓ contractility	↓ Myocardial O_2 demand
	↓ Heart rate	↓ Myocardial O_2 demand
Calcium channel blockers	↓ Preload	↓ Myocardial O_2 demand
	↓ Afterload	↓ Myocardial O_2 demand
	↓ Contractility	↓ Myocardial O_2 demand
	↓ Heart rate	↓ Myocardial O_2 demand
	↓ Coronary spasm	↑ Myocardial O_2 supply

is said to have occurred. An acute MI almost always results from an acute thrombotic obstruction of an atherosclerotic coronary artery (Fig. 10.5). In acute MI, the pain has same characteristics as angina, but it is far more severe, lasts longer, may radiate more widely, and not relieved by rest or nitroglycerine. Pain may be due to accumulation of anoxic metabolites as well as products of tissue necrosis. The pain is accompanied by greater psychogenic effects, i.e. feeling of impending death. The pathophysiological mechanisms of various symptoms and signs of acute MI are depicted in Fig. 10.7.

Although chest pain is the most recognizable symptom, acute MI may occur in the absence of any pain. Such *silent infarcts* are particularly common in diabetics with autonomic neuropathy. Silent infarcts are detected subsequently either during a routine ECG checkup or by complications of acute MI such as arrhythmia, mitral regurgitation and cardiogenic shock, etc.

158   Pathophysiology

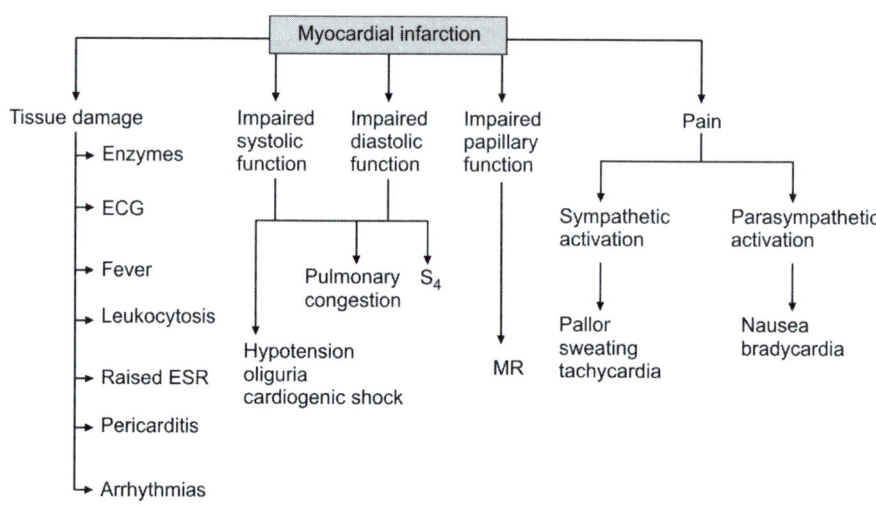

Fig. 10.7: Pathophysiology of symptoms and signs of acute myocardial infarction.

Cell membrane damage in acute MI leads to release of certain intracellular enzymes/proteins. Their concentration in plasma depends on the rate of release from the necrotic tissue as well as on the rate of their clearance. Therefore, rather than magnitude of elevation, temporal sequence of their rise and fall is more important as a diagnostic aid.

About 90% of patients who have an acute myocardial infarction develop some form of cardiac arrhythmia during or immediately after the event. In 25% of patients, such rhythm abnormalities manifest within the first 24 hours. In this group of patients, the risk of serious arrhythmias, such as ventricular fibrillation, is greatest in the first hour and declines thereafter. Most peri-infarct arrhythmias are benign and self-limited. However, those that result in hypotension, increase myocardial oxygen requirements, and/or predispose the patient to develop additional malignant ventricular arrhythmias should be aggressively monitored and treated. Acute myocardial infarction is characterized by generalized autonomic dysfunction that results in enhanced automaticity of the myocardium and conduction system. Electrolyte imbalances (e.g. hypokalemia and hypomagnesemia) and hypoxia further contribute to the development of cardiac arrhythmia. Moreover, the damaged myocardium acts as substrate for re-entrant circuits, due to changes in tissue refractoriness.

In peri-infarct period, disturbances of cardiac rhythm include:
- Sinus bradycardia
- Sinus tachycardia
- Supraventricular premature beats/tachycardia/fibrillation
- Ventricular premature beats/tachycardia/fibrillation
- AV block, BBB

Further Reading

Chilton, RJ. **Pathophysiology of coronary heart disease: A brief review.** *J Am Osteopath Assoc* 2004; 104 : Suppl5S-8S

Davies. PF. **Hemodynamic shear stress and the endothelium in cardiovascular pathophysiology.** *Nature Reviews Cardiology* 2009; 6, 16–26.

Falk, E. **Pathogenesis of atherosclerosis.** *J Am Collcardiol.* 2006; 47: C7-C12.

Grech, ED. **Pathophysiology and investigation of coronary artery disease.** *BMJ.* 2003 ; 32: 1027–30.

Hansson, GK. **Inflammation, atherosclerosis, and coronary artery disease.** *N Engl J Med* 2005; 352:1685–95.

Pepine, CJ; Nichols, WW. **The pathophysiology of chronic ischemic heart disease.***ClinCardiol.* 2007; 30: Suppl.1,4–9.

Thomsen, PEB, et al. **Long-term recording of cardiac arrhythmias with an implantable cardiac monitor in patients with reduced ejection fraction after acute myocardial infarction.** *Circulation* 2010; 122:1258–64.

11
Congestive Heart Failure

PHYSIOLOGICAL CONSIDERATIONS

As explained in Chapter 9, during a cardiac cycle, of 120 ml of blood present in each ventricle at the end of diastole (end diastolic volume—**EDV**), only 70 ml are ejected during systole (stroke volume) and another 50 ml of blood remains in the ventricle. The amount of blood that remains in the ventricle at the end of systole is called end-systolic volume (**ESV**). During exercise, or sympathetic stimulation, stroke volume can be increased by an increase in force of contraction of ventricles. This change is reflected as a decreasing in the end-systolic volume. The left ventricular is exposed to two types of load, known as preload and afterload. **Preload** is the tension on ventricular muscle before contraction determined by left ventricular end diastolic volume. **Afterload** is the pressure against which left ventricle pumps blood determined by aortic blood pressure (i.e. total peripheral resistance).

EDV represents preload on the heart. An increase in venous return to the heart results in increased EDV. An increase in EDV results in greater stretch of ventricular muscle (greater preload). Decreased ESV results from more forceful contraction of ventricle during systole (greater inotropy), e.g. by sympathetic stimulation. Oxygen demand of myocardium is increased by both an increase in preload as well as afterload. The importance of this fact lies in the treatment of a patient with congestive heart failure.

Regulation of Cardiac Output

Cardiac output can change from a resting value of 5 L/minute to more than 25 L/minute during exercise. Increase in cardiac output could be because of an increase in one or both of the two variables that determine the cardiac output, i.e. heart rate and stroke volume (since CO = HR × SV). There are basically two regulatory mechanisms which are called upon

to help the increase in cardiac output (CO) in physiological states like exercise or to maintain it in the face of a failing heart:
1. Frank-Starling mechanism (*intrinsic mechanism*) which helps to increase the stroke volume (SV).
2. Sympathetic stimulation of the heart (*extrinsic mechanism*) which helps to increase both heart rate (HR) as well as SV.

Intrinsic Regulation of Cardiac Output(Frank-Starling Mechanism)

Within physiological limits, the stroke volume increases linearly with an increase in end-diastolic volume of the heart (Fig. 11.1). An increase in end diastolic volume results in an increased stretch of ventricular muscle fibers before the contraction (systole) starts resulting in greater force of contraction (greater stroke volume).

The molecular basis of the Frank-Starling law is the sarcomere geometry in the cardiac muscle and skeletal muscle (Fig. 11.2). When a muscle is optimally stretched, there is formation of largest number of cross bridges between the actin and myosin filaments and hence maximum tension is developed during contraction. When the muscle is under-stretched or over-stretched, the cross bridges formed are lesser and hence tension developed is less.

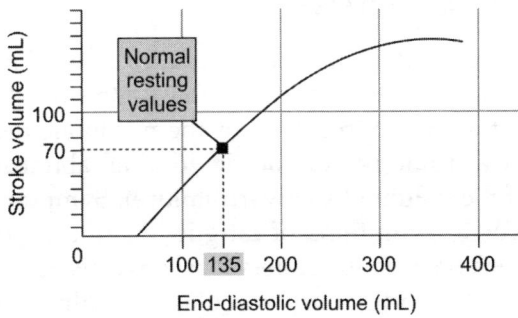

Fig. 11.1: Frank-Starling law of the heart.

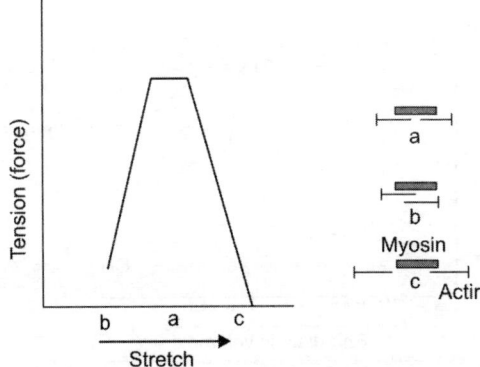

Fig. 11.2: Molecular basis of Frank-Starling law of the heart.

Extrinsic Regulation of Cardiac Output

Both the heart rate and stroke volume of the heart can be altered by an *extrinsic mechanism*. Increased sympathetic discharge to the heart increases the heart rate (chronotropic effect) as well as the stroke volume (force of ventricular contraction, inotropic effect). Thus the cardiac output is increased proportionate to the increase in sympathetic discharge (Fig. 11.3). In the extrinsic regulation, the increase in stroke volume is by a mechanism different from the intrinsic mechanism. In the extrinsic mechanism, the increase in stroke volume is achieved by better emptying as shown be a *decrease in end-systolic volume of the heart.* Under the effect of catecholamines, the cardiac muscle contracts more forcibly. Thus at the end of each systole, only about 30 ml of blood may be left in each ventricle instead of the usual 50 ml.

Even under the effect of extrinsic regulation, the intrinsic regulation, the fundamental property of cardiac muscle, persists. In other words, the heart can utilize both the intrinsic as well as extrinsic mechanism simultaneously. Epinephrine and norepinephrine released from adrenal medulla and circulating in the blood can also reinforce the extrinsic mechanism and increase the cardiac output.

CONGESTIVE HEART FAILURE

Congestive heart failure (CHF**)**, or heart failure is a condition in which an abnormality of cardiac function is responsible for the inability of the heart to pump blood at a rate appropriate for the metabolic requirements of the tissues (forward failure), or can do so at an abnormally elevated ventricular diastolic volume (backward failure). Symptoms of forward heart failure refer to symptoms of fatigue, dizziness, confusion, and asthenia. Backward heart failure refers to a congestive state. Congestion may occur within the pulmonary vasculature (pulmonary edema) or accumulation of fluid within other areas such as the skin (peripheral edema) or abdominal cavity (ascites).

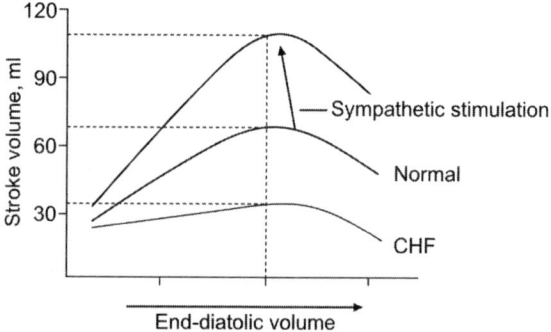

Fig. 11.3: Effect of sympathetic stimulation on Frank-Starling curve.

Heart failure (CHF) should be distinguished from (1) conditions in which there is circulatory congestion consequent to abnormal salt and water retention but in which there is no disturbance of cardiac function per se and (2) non-cardiac causes of inadequate cardiac output, including shock due to hypovolemia and redistribution of blood volume.

Systolic versus Diastolic Failure

This classification relates to whether the principal abnormality is the inability to contract normally and expel sufficient blood (systolic failure) or to relax and fill normally (diastolic failure). The major clinical manifestations of systolic failure relate to an inadequate cardiac output with weakness, fatigue, reduced exercise tolerance and other symptoms of hypoperfusion, while in diastolic failure they relate principally to an elevation of filling pressures. In many patients, particularly those who have both ventricular hypertrophy and dilatation, abnormalities of contraction and relaxation coexist (Fig. 11.4).

Diastolic heart failure may be caused by increased resistance to ventricular inflow and reduced ventricular diastolic capacity (constrictive pericarditis and restrictive, hypertensive, and hypertrophic cardiomyopathy), impaired ventricular relaxation (acute myocardial ischemia, hypertrophic cardiomyopathy), and myocardial fibrosis and infiltration (dilated, chronic ischemic, and restrictive cardiomyopathy). Diastolic failure is manifested by effects of elevated end-diastolic ventricular pressure leading to pulmonary or systemic venous congestion,

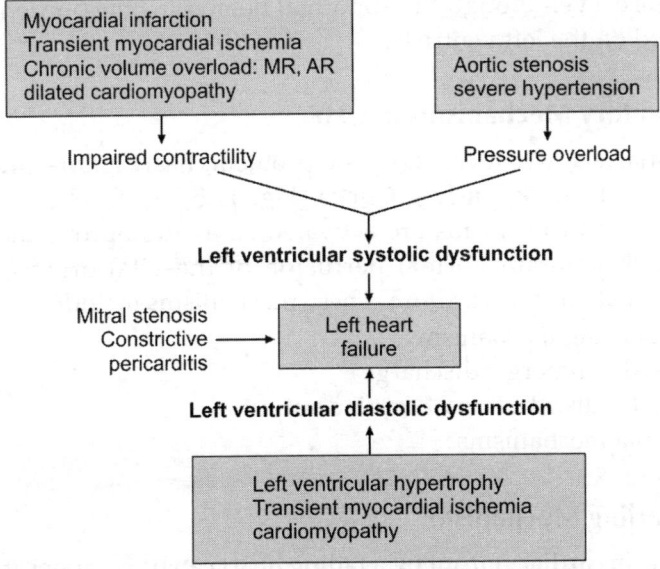

Fig.11.4: Causes of systolic and diastolic heart failure.

e.g. dyspnea, orthopnea, pulmonary edema, edema feet, anorexia, nausea, etc.

High Output versus Low Output Heart Failure

Low output heart failure occurs secondary to ischemic heart disease, hypertension, dilated cardiomyopathy, and valvular and pericardial disease. High output heart failure occurs in hyperthyroidism, anemia, pregnancy, arteriovenous fistulas, beriberi, and Paget's disease. In these conditions, cardiac output is may be more than normal, but it is insufficient for the body's elevated circulatory requirements.

Right Sided versus Left Sided Heart Failure

Patients in whom the left ventricle is mechanically overloaded (e.g., aortic stenosis) or weakened (e.g., post myocardial infarction) develop dyspnea and orthopnea as a result of pulmonary congestion, a condition referred to as left sided heart failure. In contrast, when the underlying abnormality affects the right ventricle primarily (e.g., pulmonic stenosis or pulmonary hypertension), symptoms resulting from pulmonary congestion such as orthopnea and paroxysmal nocturnal dyspnea are less common, and edema, congestive hepatomegaly, and systemic venous distention, i.e., clinical manifestations of right sided heart failure, are more prominent. However, when heart failure has existed for months or years, biventricular failure usually results. For example, patients with long-standing aortic valve disease or systemic hypertension may have ankle edema, congestive hepatomegaly, and systemic venous distention late in the course of their disease, even though the abnormal hemodynamic burden initially was placed on the left ventricle.

Compensatory Mechanisms in CHF

In final analysis, whatever the basic problem, heart failure produces a depression of Frank-Starling Curve (Fig. 11.5). A number of natural compensatory mechanisms are activated so as to improve the cardiac output and maintain normal perfusion of the vital organs, despite depressed state of myocardium. These mechanisms include:
- Frank-Starling mechanism
- Increased adrenergic discharge
- Regional redistribution of cardiac output
- Hormonal mechanisms

Frank-Starling Mechanism

A decrease in cardiac output by a failing heart can be compensated by an increase in end-diastolic volume (Fig. 11.5). However, there is a limit to

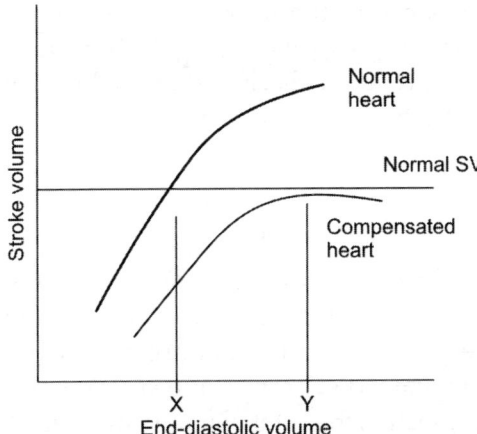

Fig. 11.5: Mechanism of compensation of a failing heart by Frank-Starling mechanism. Failing heart can improve stroke volume by working at greater end-diastolic volume ("Y") instead of normal ("X").

which this mechanism can help. First, the upper part of Frank-Starling curve is flat. That is progressive increase in EDV improves stroke volume only to a limit. Second, a large increase in EDV leads to pulmonary congestion and pulmonary edema. Retention of salt and water through hormonal mechanisms increases the blood volume and therefore helps to increase end-diastolic volume of the ventricle.

Increased Adrenergic Discharge

Increased adrenergic discharge to the heart improves stroke volume at any given EDV (Fig. 11.6). In the failing heart, depressed cardiac output is sensed by high pressure baroreceptors located in the carotid sinus and aortic arch, leading to a reflex increase in adrenergic discharge to the

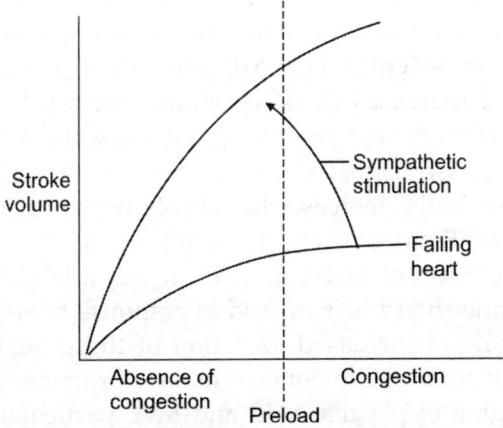

Fig. 11.6: Effect of increased sympathetic discharge on SV in a failing heart.

heart and blood vessels. In the heart, increased adrenergic discharge improves the cardiac output by increasing the heart rate as well as stroke volume. Increased adrenergic discharge to the blood vessels results in selective vasoconstriction, leading to redistribution of cardiac output (discussed next).

Redistribution of Cardiac Output

The redistribution of cardiac output serves as an important compensatory mechanism when cardiac output is reduced. Blood flow is redistributed so that the delivery of oxygen to vital organs, such as the brain and myocardium, is maintained at normal or near-normal levels, while flow to less critical areas, such as the cutaneous and muscular beds and viscera, is reduced. Vasoconstriction mediated by the adrenergic nervous system is largely responsible for this redistribution, which in turn may be responsible for many of the clinical manifestations of heart failure, such as fluid accumulation (reduction of renal flow), low grade fever (redistribution of cutaneous flow), and fatigue (reduction of muscle flow).

Excessive adrenergic stimulation, however, is counter-productive. Excessive arteriolar constriction increases total peripheral resistance and therefore increases afterload. Excessive venular constriction increases venous return to the heart which increases preload to a range where pulmonary congestion occurs. Moreover, prolonged and excessive increase in the sympathetic neural and adrenal medullary discharge results in down regulation of adrenergic receptors in the heart, i.e. heart becomes less responsive to sympathetic stimulation.

Hormonal Mechanisms

Besides increase in adrenergic discharge discussed above, decreased cardiac output (decreased effective circulating volume) activates renin-angiotensin II mechanism. Plasma renin and angiotensin levels are elevated in patients with CHF. Angiotensin II produces arteriolar constriction and increases thirst (↑ water intake). It also increases aldosterone secretion thereby producing salt and water retention. In CHF, ADH secretion is also increased causing renal water retention. All the hormonal changes lead to increased blood volume, which helps to increase cardiac output by Frank-Starling mechanism. As a counter-regulatory mechanism, secretion of atrial natriuretic peptide (ANP) and brain natriuretic peptide (BNP) is increased in response to volume overload. However, in spite of increased secretion of these peptides from the myocardium, salt and water retention remains a prominent clinical feature of CHF. Estimation of plasma ANP and BNP particularly the latter is now considered an important marker of CHF (Fig. 11.7).

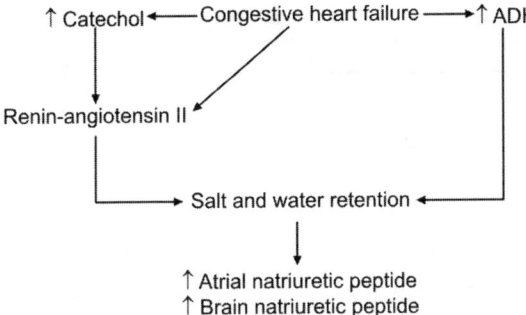

Fig. 11.7: Hormonal changes in congestive heart failure.

Decompensated Congestive Heart Failure

The compensatory mechanisms discussed above may help to maintain cardiac output near normal in the initial stages of the disorder. Gradual progression of the basic disease process or excessive compensatory mechanisms ultimately produce frank heart failure characterized by pulmonary congestion, hypoxia, edema, limitation of physical activity. The precipitating event may be one or more of the following:

- **Increased metabolic demand**
  - Fever
  - Infection
  - Anemia
  - Pregnancy
  - Hyperthyroidism
- **Increased circulatory volume**
  - Excessive sodium or water intake
  - Excessive I/V fluid administration (e.g. following surgery)
  - by renal failure
- **Increased afterload**
  - Severe hypertension
  - Pulmonary embolism
- **Decreased contractility**
  - β-blockers
  - Alcohol abuse
- **Arrhythmias**

Pathophysiological Basis of Various Symptoms and Signs of CHF

Various signs and symptoms of congestive heart failure can be correlated with the effects of primary decrease in cardiac output and various compensatory mechanisms activated in the body have discussed (Fig. 11.8).

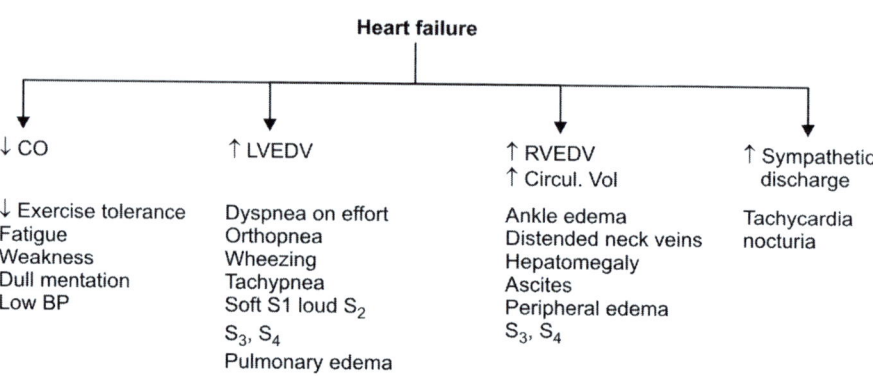

Fig. 11.8: Pathophysiological basis of symptoms and signs of congestive heart failure.

Physiological Principals of Therapeutics in CHF

The rational treatment of congestive heart failure would involve:
- Treatment of underlying cause, e.g. hypertension, valvular heart disease
- Treatment of precipitating cause
- Elimination of pulmonary and systemic vascular congestion
- Improved cardiac contractility

ROLE OF SALT RESTRICTION AND DIURETICS

Salt restriction and diuretics decrease the preload on the heart by decreasing blood volume and therefore venous return to the heart. It helps to bring left ventricular end-diastolic volume (LVEDV) to a value less than that produces pulmonary congestion. However it does not improve stroke volume/cardiac output (action "A" in Fig. 11.9). Vigorous diuretic therapy is to be avoided since may decrease to preload to such an extent that stroke volume decreases. Over-use of diuretics, in addition, is liable to produce hypokalemia and hypomagnesemia which may precipitate dangerous arrhythmias.

Patients with diastolic failure maintain cardiac output only by increasing LVEDV. Such patients are more difficult to treat than systolic dysfunction. If there is pulmonary edema, diuretics are given; however, they are given cautiously because removing too much volume can significantly reduce end-diastolic volume and therefore stroke volume in the stiff ventricles.

Vasodilators (ACE Inhibitors)

ACE inhibitors are especially useful in a patient of systolic heart failure. As mentioned earlier, excessive neuro-humoral compensatory mechanisms are counter-productive. Excessive arteriolar constriction increases

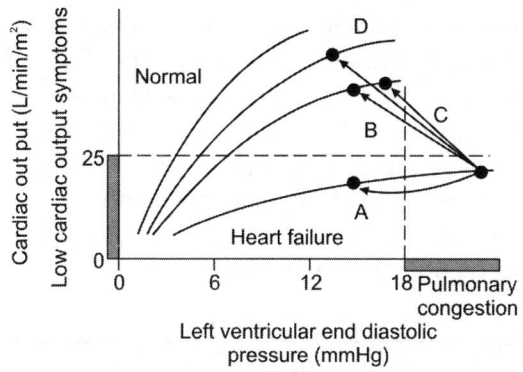

Fig. 11.9: Effect of various drugs used in treatment of CHF.

afterload which impairs cardiac function. Vasodilator drugs tend to reverse this trend. ACE inhibitor drugs are particularly useful since they produce both arteriolar and venous dilatation ("balance vasodilators").

The decrease in plasma angiotensin level as well as aldosterone level reduces intravascular volume also. Thus ACE inhibitors decrease preload as well as afterload (action "B" in Fig. 11.9).

Sympathomimetics

Sympathomimetic drugs increase the stroke volume (action "C" in Fig. 11.9), but they also increase oxygen demand. Moreover, they increase the risk of arrhythmias. Therefore, they are mainly used in acute heart failure or end-stage heart failure.

Digitalis

Digitalis has been used in the treatment of CHF for over one hundred years. The most important effect of digitalis is that, in a failing heart, it increases cardiac contractility and hence it shifts Frank-Starling curve upwards at any EDV. In addition, digitalis has a diuretic effect also. These effects of digitalis are observed only when administered in a patient with

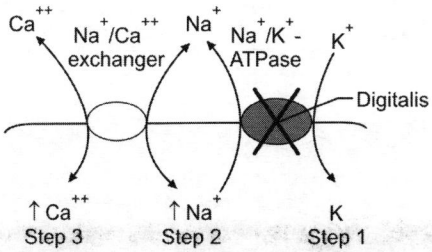

Fig. 11.10: Mode of action of digitalis.

failing heart; not in a person with normal heart. Digitalis acts by inhibiting Na^+/K^+ ATPase activity on the sarcolemma of cardiac muscle fibers. The resulting increase in intracellular Na^+ causes decreased extrusion of Ca^{++} out of the cardiac muscle by Na^+/Ca^{++} exchanger (Fig.11.10). Increased Ca^{++} concentration of sarcoplasm improves the mechanical contractility of the heart by enhancing actin-myosin interaction.

Best results are obtained by use of digitalis along with a diuretic and an ACE inhibitor (action "D" in Fig. 11.9).

Further Reading

Al-Mohammad A, Mant J. **The diagnosis and management of chronic heart failure**. Heart 2011; **97**:411–416.

Klabunde, RE. **Cardiovascular physiology concepts**. 2nd Edi. *2005 Lippincott, Philadelphia.*

Mehta, PA; Dubrey, SW. **High output heart failure**. *QJM 2009; 102:235–241.*

12

Hypertension

DETERMINANTS OF ARTERIAL BLOOD PRESSURE

Following are the important determinants of arterial blood pressure:
- Cardiac output.
- Peripheral resistance.
- Elasticity of the aorta and large arteries (windkessel vessels).
- Blood volume.

Arterioles are the major site of resistance to the flow of blood in the vascular system. Arteriolar smooth muscle tone is most important determinant of vascular resistance, which can show physiological variation. Arteriolar smooth muscle tone is primarily maintained by a tonic vasomotor discharge in the adrenergic postganglionic sympathetic fibers from the thoracolumbar sympathetic outflow (Fig. 12.1). In turn, the preganglionic thoracolumbar fibers are controlled by neurons of medullary cardiovascular centers (popularly known as vasomotor center—VMC). Vasomotor center is under a tonic inhibitory discharge from the high pressure (sino-aortic) baroreceptors.

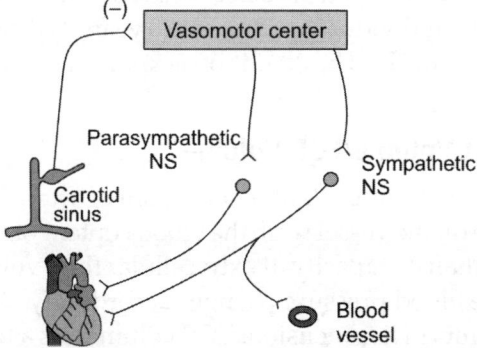

Fig. 12.1: Innervation of the heart and blood vessels. Carotid sinus has a tonic inhibitory discharge on the vasomotor center.

A. Role of Cardiac Output, Peripheral Resistance and Elasticity of the Windkessel Vessels

These factors are of fundamental importance in the creation of arterial pressure. To exert pressure on the vessel wall, first of all, blood needs to be pumped into the arterial system. To be under pressure, the amount of blood entering the arterial system has to be slightly greater than the amount leaving it. Such a situation is created by pumping of blood by the heart into the aorta with each beat and the resistance exerted by the arterioles in its exit out of the arterial system. The importance of these two factors is shown by the equation:

$$\text{Blood pressure} = \text{Cardiac output} \times \text{Peripheral resistance}$$
$$= CO \times PR$$

Since ejection of blood occurs only during ventricular systole (0.3 seconds), the arterial pressure is likely to fall to very low levels during diastole (0.5 seconds). The maintenance of fairly high arterial pressure during diastole (80 mm Hg) is achieved by elasticity of the aorta and its immediate branches (windkessel vessels) and the action of arterioles. The heart ejects about 70 ml of blood during each systole. As a result, the aortic pressure rises to a peak value of approximately 120 mm Hg and stretches the elastic wall of the aorta and its immediate branches. During diastole, the arterial, pressure begins to decline, but does not fall below approximately 80 mm Hg because of (a) elastic recoil of the windkessel (elastic) vessels and (b) resistance offered to the outflow of blood by the arterioles. Elasticity of the windkessel vessels prevents the excessive rise of blood pressure during ventricular systole. The recoil of the elastic fibers helps to maintain fairly high pressure during diastole, when there is no ejection of blood from the heart into the arterial system (Fig. 12.2).

In old age, there is a gradual decrease in the elasticity of the windkessel vessels (due to age-related degeneration of the elastic fibers). As a result, the normal cardiac output produces a greater rise in systolic blood pressure, but the diastolic pressure declines to a value lower than normal. In a normal healthy individual aged about 70 years, typical blood pressure reading is 160/70 mm Hg. The condition is known as *systolic hypertension*.

B. Role of Blood Volume/ECF Volume

The blood volume is an important determinant of arterial blood pressure. To exert pressure on the vessel wall, the blood content of the vessel should be slightly more than its capacity. If extracellular fluid volume is increased or decreased, the blood pressure changes accordingly. Acute blood loss, if significant, results in hypotension. ECF volume has a fundamental role in the long term regulation of blood pressure as well as in therapeutic measures in hypertension.

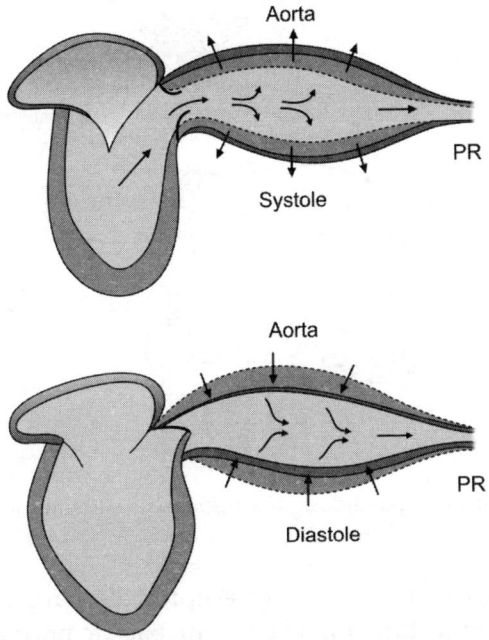

Fig. 12.2: Role of elastic vessels and peripheral resistance (PR) in the maintenance of blood pressure in diastole. Elastic fibers are stretched during systole and recoil during diastole.

REGULATION OF ARTERIAL BLOOD PRESSURE

Adequate blood flow through the vital organs such as the brain and the heart must be maintained all the time. The brain, for example, is irreversibly damaged within three minutes of ischemia. In contrast, many other tissues such as the skin, skeletal muscle or the GI tract can tolerate reduction of bloodflow for a longer duration. The excretory function of the kidney is also critically dependent on normal arterial blood pressure (which provides driving force for the glomerular filtration). It would be obvious that the maintenance of blood pressure within the physiological range is of fundamental importance for the survival of an individual. Besides this, the circulatory system is subjected to various types of stress which may vary from simple change of posture (from supine to upright) to severe hemorrhage. For such eventualities, multiple cardiovascular regulatory systems have evolved in the mammals. Of these, the *neural regulatory mechanism* is most important, since it responds within a few seconds. Some *slow-reacting hormonal mechanisms* provide a second line of defense against a disturbance in blood pressure.

Neural Regulatory Mechanisms

Arterial blood pressure and high pressure sinoaortic baroreceptors are linked in a negative feedback loop (Fig. 12.1). Any increase in blood

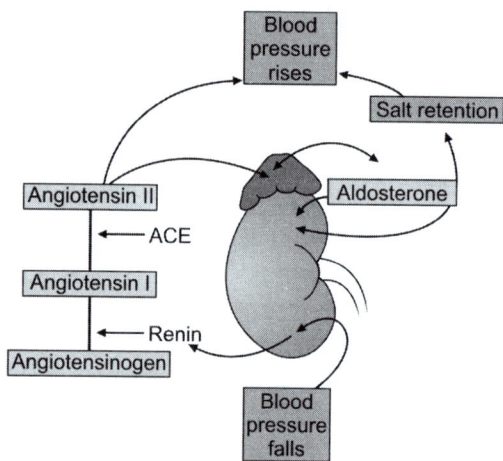

Fig. 12.3: Renin-angiotensin II-aldosterone response to sustained fall in blood pressure.

pressure increases sinoaortic baroreceptor discharge, which, in turn, inhibits VMC and restores blood pressure back to normal. The reverse is also true. The neural regulation of blood pressure is very sensitive and has reflex time of only a few seconds. This mechanism helps to maintain normal arterial blood pressure. During pathological states such as hemorrhage, strong vasomotor discharge is the first line of defense against fall of blood pressure. If neural mechanism is inadequate for the maintenance of blood pressure, activation of renin-angiotensin II system and increased secretion of antidiuretic hormone provides further help to maintain cardiovascular homeostasis (Fig. 12.3).

Long-term Arterial Blood Pressure Regulation

When the blood pressure change is slow; over a period of many days, the neural mechanism loses almost all of its ability to react to the change. Therefore, there has to be a long term regulatory mechanism which maintains the arterial blood pressure in the normal range, week-after-week and month-after-month. The kidneys play a dominant role in this long term regulation of blood pressure. The long term regulation of blood pressure is achieved by changes in the blood volume (actually ECF volume). The kidneys have an ability to regulate the ECF volume by regulation of salt (NaCl) and water excretion. In addition, the rennin-angiotensin-aldosterone system helps in the regulation of salt and water excretion by the kidneys. In normal individuals, any persistent increase in arterial blood pressure leads to increased urinary salt and water excretion resulting in a decrease in ECF volume and arterial blood pressure. Any persistent decrease in arterial blood pressure leads to decreased urinary salt and water excretion. The resultant increase in ECF volume restores the blood pressure to normal. A failure of this long-term regulatory mechanism is believed to be fundamental problem in the pathogenesis of essential hypertension.

WHAT IS HYPERTENSION?

Although hypertension must have existed since ancient times, its recognition as a disease started only in mid-1940s when blood pressure recording became a routine with the physicians in the USA. In the normal population, the distribution of normal blood pressure shows typical "bell-shaped" normal curve (Fig. 12.4). Moreover, blood pressure values, both systolic and diastolic, increase gradually with age. In such a situation, only an arbitrary cut off point can be used to separate those with high blood pressure from those normal blood pressure values. This cutoff point is 140/90 mmHg—systolic blood pressure above 140 mmHg **or** diastolic blood pressure above 90 mmHg is considered abnormal and labeled as hypertension (Fig. 12.4). The basis of this definition was the observation that people with blood pressure values greater than 140/90 showed increased incidence of cardiovascular and renal disorders.

American Heart Association (JNC7, 2003) uses the term **prehypertension** for blood pressure in the range 120–139 mmHg systolic and/or 80–89 mmHg diastolic (Table 12.1). People with prehypertension are at a higher risk for developing hypertension, compared to people with "normal" blood pressure. Prehypertension is believed to increase the risk for heart attacks, strokes, congestive heart failure, and renal failure.

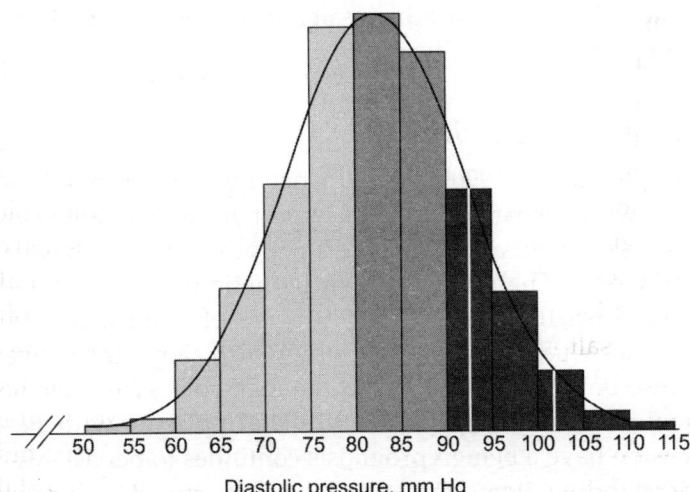

Fig. 12.4: Distribution of diastolic blood pressure in 20–70 years age group. (shaded black: hypertensives; shaded gray: prehypertensives).

Table 12.1: Definitions of disorders of arterial blood pressure

Category	Systolic (mmHg)		Diastolic (mmHg)
Normal	Less than 120	and	Less than 80
Prehypertension	120–139	or	80–89
High blood pressure			
Stage 1	140–159	or	90–99
Stage 2	160 or higher	or	100 or higher
Hypertensive crisis	≥ 180	or	≥ 120
Hypotension	< 90	or	< 60

Since arterial blood pressure fluctuates in most of the individuals, especially on exertion, emotional excitement and psychological stress, it is advisable to confirm elevation of blood pressure on two or more separate occasions.

Pathogenesis of Essential Hypertension

1. *Genetic Predisposition*

In a vast majority of cases of hypertension, no definite cause can be detected. Such patients are said to suffer from "essential hypertension." Epidemiological studies have shown the importance of genetic predisposition in the development of essential hypertension. If family history of hypertension is present, the subject has 3–4 fold greater chance of developing hypertension, at an age earlier than general population. Although genetics appears to contribute to essential hypertension, the exact mechanism has not been established. Genetic factors interact with environmental factors such as high salt intake, male sex, smoking, obesity, stress and physical inactivity, etc.

2. *Sympathetic Overactivity*

According to Julius (1996), the evidence for a widespread autonomic abnormality in the early phases of hypertension is overwhelming and excessive sympathetic activity is consistently present in such patients since their childhood. The enhanced sympathetic tone in hypertension is associated with the metabolic syndrome of insulin resistance and dyslipidemia. Multiple mechanisms by which sympathetic overactivity could cause both hypertension and the metabolic syndrome have been documented. Surprisingly, the myth that patients with neurogenic hypertension have a benign prognosis continues to persist. Much of the misunderstanding stems from the idea that patients with neurogenic hypertension, commonly called "white coat" or borderline hypertension, do not develop established hypertension. There is no support for such an assertion; in fact, patients with neurogenic hypertension are at a high risk of future accelerated hypertension. The evidence is particularly strong for younger patients with early, so-called "borderline" hypertension. The hallmark of the sympathetic overactivity in these patients is the so-called hyperkinetic state that is best characterized by a fast heart rate and an increased cardiac output.

Both the hyperkinetic state and sympathetic overactivity are less readily recognizable later in the course of hypertension. A large proportion of previously hyperkinetic patients later develop established hypertension. Questions arise as to the mechanisms involved in the hemodynamic transition from a fast heart rate/high cardiac output form of borderline hypertension to the later normal cardiac output/high vascular resistance profile that is characteristic of established hypertension.

3. Role of Sodium Intake

Essential hypertension is seen primarily in societies with average sodium intake above 100 mEq/day (2.3 g sodium); it is rare in societies with average sodium intakes of less than 50 mEq/day (1.2 g sodium). These epidemiological observations led to the suggestion that the development of hypertension requires a threshold level of sodium intake. This effect appears to be independent of other risk factors for hypertension, such as obesity. Those in support of salt restriction as a part of prevention and treatment quote the report that reducing salt intake from 170 to 100 mEq/day lowers the blood pressure (BP), on the average, in normotensive adultsby approximately 2/1 mmHg and in hypertensive adults by 5/3 mmHg.

Dietary salt restriction as a measure of prevention/treatment of essential hypertension was initially advocated by Dahl. Dahl demonstrated salt induced hypertension in animals, especially rats, and the cited studies support the notion that chronic excess salt feeding induces hypertension in a considerable fraction of these animals. However later it was pointed out that the amount of salt given to the rats in these studies would correspond to about 560 grams per day in a human, i.e. 50 times more than the average intake in the western world. Therefore, now is considered that these experimental results probably have no physiological relevance for humans.

At the moment,with the availability of efficient drug treatments the place of sodium reduction in the treatment of hypertension is probably rather marginal. Today, we even have a dietary measure that is more efficient and more acceptable for the patients than sodium reduction, namely the intake of fruits and vegetables. In short, the concept of excessive salt intake as a causative factor in essential hypertension is being questioned nowadays.

4. Vascular Hyper-reactivity

Hypertensive patients manifest greater vasoconstrictive response to infused norepinephrine or cold pressor test than normal individuals. Greater vasoconstrictive response to norepinephrine has also been demonstrated in normotensive offspring of hypertensive patients as compared to controls with no family history of hypertension. It suggests that vascular hyper-reactivity may be genetic in origin.

5. Renin-angiotensin-aldosterone-system (RAAS)

In patients of essential hypertension, about 15% have mildly elevated plasma renin activity. In another 60% of hypertensives, plasma renin activity is "within the normal range" but it may inappropriate in presence of elevated blood pressure. Less than 25% patients of essential hypertension have subnormal plasma renin activity. Moreover, favorable therapeutic response to RAAS blockers suggests that renin-dependent mechanism may be involved in the pathogenesis in about 70% cases of essential hypertension. The fundamental cause of elevated renin activity in such cases is not yet clear. It could be due to a chronic sympathetic overactivity. This possibility is supported by the reports that administration of β-blockers in cases with essential hypertension leads to a decrease in plasma renin activity paralleled by a decrease in arterial blood pressure.

6. Endothelial Dysfunction

Due to its position between blood stream and vascular smooth muscle, endothelial dysfunction could either be a consequence or a causative factor in essential hypertension. In recent years, considerable evidence has suggested that changes in vascular endothelial function may cause the increase in vascular tone. For example, in hypertensive patients, the vascular endothelium produces less nitric oxide and the vascular smooth muscle is less sensitive to the actions of this powerful vasodilator. There may also be an increase in endothelin production, which can enhance vasoconstrictor tone.

Complications of Untreated Essential Hypertension

1. Atherosclerosis

Many of the complications of hypertension are related the effects of sustained elevations of blood pressure on vasculature and heart. Atherosclerosis is commonly associated with and is accelerated by long-standing hypertension. Most of the adverse outcomes in hypertension are associated with thrombosis rather than bleeding, and there is evidence that increased vascular shear stress converts the normally anticoagulant endothelium to a prothrombotic state. Atherosclerosis predisposes the hypertensive patient to coronary thrombosis and cerebral stroke. Cerebral strokes are more often due to thrombosis rather than hemorrhage in the cerebral vessels. The excess morbidity and mortality related to hypertension are progressive over the whole range of systolic and diastolic blood pressures. However, target-organ damage varies markedly between individuals with similar levels of hypertension. Atherosclerosis may also result in aortic aneurysm or peripheral arterial disease.

- **Hypertensive cardiomyopathy:** Sustained increase in blood pressure (afterload) results in hypertrophy and subsequent dilatation of left ventricle. Electrocardiographic evidence of left ventricular hypertrophy is found up to 15% of persons with chronic hypertension. Echocardiographic left ventricular hypertrophy is a powerful predictor of prognosis. Left ventricular hypertrophy may cause or facilitate many cardiac complications of hypertension, including congestive heart failure, ventricular arrhythmias, and myocardial ischemia. Left ventricular diastolic dysfunction, which may present with all of the symptoms and signs of congestive heart failure, is common in patients with long-standing hypertension.

- **Cerebral complications:** Hypertension is an important risk factor for cerebral stroke. Approximately 85% of strokes are due to thrombosis and the remainder are due to hemorrhage. Hypertension is also associated with impaired cognition in an aging population. Hypertension-related cognitive impairment and dementia may be a consequence of a single infarct due to occlusion of a "strategic" larger vessel or multiple lacunar infarcts due to occlusive small vessel disease resulting in subcortical white matter ischemia. The term hypertensive encephalopathy is used to describe a group of symptoms and signs that *sometimes* follow a sudden and sustained rise of blood pressure. The symptoms are characterized by a severe headache, restlessness, impaired judgment and memory, confusion, somnolence and stupor. If the condition is not treated, these neurological symptoms may worsen and ultimately turn into a coma. Cerebral encephalopathy seems to result from a failure of autoregulation of cerebral blood flow. The autoregulation falters when hypertension becomes excessive. According to the *over-regulation* concept, brain vessels undergo spasm in response to acute hypertension, which results in cerebral ischemia and cytotoxic edema. According to the *autoregulation breakthrough* conception, cerebral arterioles are forced to dilate, leading to vasogenic cerebral edema.

- **Retinopathy:** The primary response of the retinal arterioles to systemic hypertension is vasoconstriction. Sustained hypertension leads to disruption of the blood-retinal barrier, increased vascular permeability and secondary arteriolosclerosis.

- **Renal complications:** Before effective antihypertensive therapy was available about one-third of patients with essential hypertension developed renal insufficiency. Clinically, macroalbuminuria or microalbuminuria is an early marker of renal injury. Arterial hypertension leads to renal insufficiency via two possible pathways. The traditional view is that arterial hypertension produces renal failure as a consequence of glomerular ischemia induced by damage to preglomerular arteries and arterioles, leading to progressive luminal narrowing and to a fall in glomerular blood flow. Another view is that hypertensive renal damage depends on transmission of the elevated systemic pressure to the glomeruli, inducing glomerular capillary hyperperfusion and hypertension, which in turn causes glomerular structural injury and progressive loss of renal function.
- **Sexual dysfunction:** Sexual dysfunction is more common and more severe in men with hypertension than it is in the general population. Although older drugs used to treat hypertension caused erectile dysfunction as a side effect, more recent evidence suggests that the disease process that causes hypertension is itself the major cause of erectile dysfunction. Experimental studies indicate that essential hypertension results in structural and functional changes in penile vasculature. Cavernous vessels are affected by chronic elevation of arterial blood pressure in the same fashion as other blood vessels. Marked hypertrophy in the smooth muscle of cavernous vessels, increased smooth muscle layer in cavernous space and increased extracellular matrix (collagen) explain the pathophysiological mechanism of erectile dysfunction in essential hypertension.

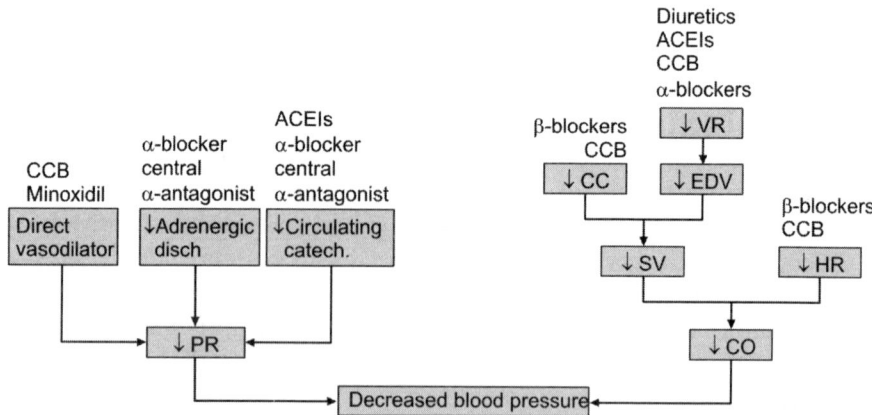

Fig. 12.5: Mechanism of action of anti-hypertensive drugs (CC: Cardiac contractility; VR: venous return; SV: stroke volume; EDV: end-diastolic volume; HR: heart rate; PR: peripheral resistance; CO: cardiac output; CCB: calcium channel blockers; ACEIs: angiotensin converting enzyme inhibitors).

Physiological Basis of Treatment of Essential Hypertension

Non-pharmacological Measures

- Reduction or elimination of factors such as stress, smoking, obesity.
- Regular aerobic exercise.
- Restriction of dietary calories, salt, cholesterol, saturated fats.

Pharmacological Measures

A variety of drugs are being used in the treatment of essential hypertension. They reduce cardiac output, peripheral resistance or both (Fig. 12.5).

Further Reading

Chobanian AV, Bakris GL, Black HR, et al. **The Seventh Report of the Joint National Committee on Prevention, Detection, Evaluation, and Treatment of High Blood Pressure**: the JNC 7 repor. *JAMA. 2003;.289: 2560–72.*

Cowley, AW Jr. **Long-term control of arterial blood pressure**. *Physiol Rev. 1992;72 :231-300.*

Graudal N. Commentary: **Possible role of salt intake in the development of essential hypertension.** *Int. J Epidemiol 2005; 34:972–974.*

Johnson, RJ et al. **Essential hypertension, progressive renal disease, and uric acid: a pathogenetic link?** *JASN. 2005; 16:1909–1919.*

Julius, S; Nesbitt, S. **Sympathetic overactivity in hypertension. A moving target.** *Am J Hypertens 1996; 9: 113S–120S.*

Oparil, S et al. **Pathogenesis of hypertension**. Ann Intern Med 2003; 139: 761–776

Steven, AA. **The renin-angiotensin-aldosterone system: pathophysiological role and pharmacological inhibition.** *J Manag Care Pharm 2007; 13 (suppl S-b): S9–S20*

13 Circulatory Shock

Circulatory shock is a state in which failure of the circulatory system to maintain adequate tissue perfusion results in a reduction of nutrient and oxygen supply to the tissues. Shock produces cellular dysfunction followed by organ dysfunction. Unless treated promptly, it may become irreversible, ending in death.

Circulatory shock is a clinical diagnosis made on the presence of the following signs:
- Pale, cool and moist ("cold and clammy") skin.
- The "thin thready pulse".
- Peripheral cyanosis and mottling
- Hyperventilation.
- Oliguria.
- Restlessness and apprehension.
- Intense thirst.
- Fall in blood pressure.

CLASSIFICATION OF SHOCK

1. Hypovolemic Shock

This is the most common type of shock and based on *insufficient circulating blood volume*. Its primary cause is loss of fluid from the circulation from either an internal or external cause. An internal cause may be hemorrhage into body cavities. External causes may include extensive external bleeding, dehydration, or severe burns.

2. Cardiogenic Shock

This type of shock is caused by the failure of the heart to pump effectively, in spite of normal blood volume. This can be due to damage to the heart muscle, most often from a large myocardial infarction. Other causes of cardiogenic shock include arrhythmias, cardiomyopathy, and end-stage congestive heart failure.

3. Distributive Shock

It is a form of "relative" hypovolemic state caused by dilation of blood vessels due to diminished systemic vascular resistance. Examples of this form of shock are:

a. *Septic shock:* This is caused by an overwhelming infection leading to vasodilatation, such as by gram-negative bacteria or gram-positive cocci.
b. *Anaphylactic shock:* This type of distributive shock results from a severe anaphylactic reaction to an allergen, antigen, drug or foreign protein. The allergic reaction results in the release of histamine which causes widespread vasodilatation, leading to hypotension and increased capillary permeability.
c. *Neurogenic shock:* Neurogenic shock is the rarest form of shock. It is caused by trauma to the spinal cord resulting in the sudden loss of autonomic outflow of impulses below the injury level. Without stimulation by sympathetic nervous system the vessel walls relax, leading to vasodilatation and hypotension.

4. Obstructive Shock

In this situation, the flow of blood into the heart is obstructed which impedes circulation and result in a severe decrease in cardiac output. Several conditions result in this form of shock.

a. *Cardiac tamponade* in which a large volume of fluid in the pericardium prevents inflow of blood into the heart.
b. *Constrictive pericarditis*, in which the pericardium shrinks and hardens, thus interferes with cardiac filling.
c. *Tension pneumothorax*. Through increased intrathoracic pressure, blood flow to the heart is prevented.
d. *Massive pulmonary embolism* resulting in hindrance in the return of blood to the heart.

5. Endocrine Shock

Based on endocrine disturbances. It may be seen both in severe cases of hypo- and hyperthyroidism. These disorders may produce a depression of myocardial function, i.e. the shock resembles cardiogenic type. Acute adrenal insufficiency produces a distributive type of shock. Addison's disease is uncommon. Acute adrenal insufficiency is usually seen when high-dose corticosteroids is discontinued suddenly rather than tapered off. It may also occur in a patient on corticosteroid therapy who undergoes surgery or suffers from an intercurrent illness without appropriate increase in the dose of corticosteroid.

HYPOVOLEMIC SHOCK

This is the commonest type of circulatory shock encountered in clinical practice. Hypovolemia may result from:
- External or internal loss of blood
- Dehydration
- Heavy sweating
- Vomiting
- Severe diarrhea
- Severe burns
- Excessive use of drugs such as diuretics typically used to treat hypertension.

Compensatory Mechanisms

The decrease in blood volume, due any of the reasons listed above, results in a decrease in venous return leading to decreased preload on the heart and hence decreased cardiac output. The decreased cardiac output initially may not be accompanied by a fall in blood pressure. The decreased cardiac output sets into motion a number of compensatory mechanisms, all of which tend to improve the cardiac output and maintain normal blood flow to the vital organs. Neural mechanisms constitute the immediate response. Over time, it is supplemented by slower hormonal and transcapillary fluid shift mechanisms.

1. *Neural Compensatory Mechanisms*

Even when the blood pressure has not fallen, the decreased pulse pressure is sufficient to decrease the impulse discharge from the arterial baroreceptors. The consequent increase in sympathetic vasomotor discharge to the heart, arterioles and veins helps to maintain the blood pressure within the normal range despite decreased blood volume (Fig. 13.1). When the blood pressure begins to fall, adrenal medullary discharge also increases. The increased plasma levels of catecholamines supplement the increased sympathetic neural discharge. The vasoconstriction in the cutaneous, splanchnic, renal and skeletal vessels is proportionate to the degree of hypovolemia and tendency to hypotension. Coronary and cerebral vessels do not participate in the generalized vasoconstriction.

The neural compensatory mechanisms discussed above account for most of the **symptoms and signs of hypovolemic shock.**

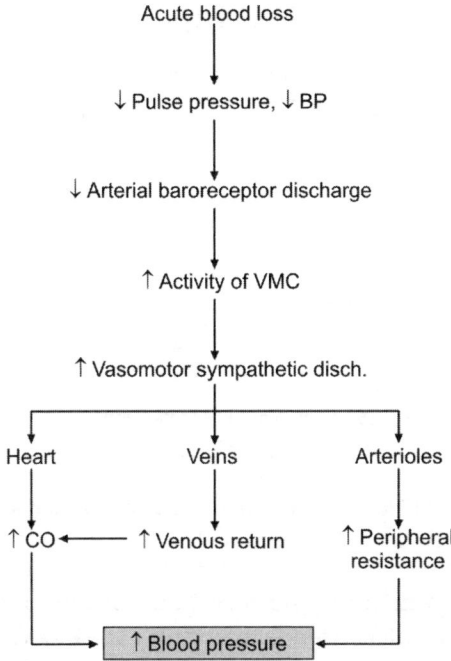

Fig. 13.1: Neural compensatory mechanisms in hypovolemic shock.

- *Pale, cool and moist ("cold and clammy") skin* results from vasoconstriction and sweating because of increased sympathetic discharge to the cutaneous blood vessels and sweat glands.
- *The "thin thready pulse"* results from tachycardia and low pulse pressure.
- *Peripheral cyanosis and mottling* due to tissue hypoxia.
- *Hyperventilation is* due to the presence of metabolic acidosis resulting from poor tissue oxygenation.
- *Oliguria* results from intense renal arterial vasoconstriction.
- *Restlessness and apprehension* are caused by the effects of circulating catecholamines (because of adrenal medullary discharge) on the brainstem reticular formation.
- *Intense thirst* results from fluid shift (*see* below) leading to cellular dehydration. Increased plasma angiotensin II level also promotes thirst by its action on the hypothalamus.
- *Fall of blood pressure* indicates that the neural compensatory mechanisms have not been successful. Gradually, the other two compensatory mechanisms, the hormonal and fluid shift are also recruited.

2. Hormonal Mechanisms

Hypovolemia with or without hypotension increases the secretion of antidiuretic hormone (vasopressin) as well as angiotensin II (Fig. 13.2).

186 Pathophysiology

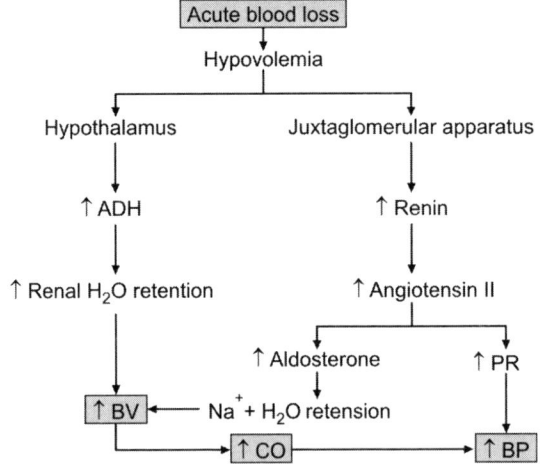

Fig. 13.2: Hormonal mechanisms in hypovolemic shock.

Increased antidiuretic hormone secretion not only increases peripheral vascular resistance but also tends to improve the blood volume by causing renal water retention. Angiotensin II is a powerful vasoconstrictor. In addition, it promotes renal salt and water retention. It is also responsible for the extreme thirst felt by a patient in hypovolemic shock. In short, hormonal mechanisms help to improve blood pressure by increasing peripheral vascular resistance and tend to decrease hypovolemia as well.

3. Fluid Shift Mechanism

Arteriolar vasoconstriction caused by increased adrenergic discharge decreases the capillary hydrostatic pressure. Therefore, the Starling forces governing the transcapillary tissue fluid exchange are shifted towards fluid reabsorption in greater part of the capillary length. The extracellular fluid shift from the interstitial compartment to the intravascular compartment improves intravascular fluid volume but it secondarily leads to cellular dehydration. The cellular dehydration and elevated plasma angiotensin II levels account for the intense thirst and dryness of the mouth felt by the patient.

Symptoms of Hypovolemic Shock in Relation to the Stages of Shock

Stage 1: The Initial Stage

[Up to 15% blood volume loss (750 ml): Compensated by constriction of vascular bed].
- Blood pressure maintained.
- Normal respiratory rate.

- Pallor of the skin.
- Slight anxiety.

Stage 2: The Compensatory Stage

[15–30% blood volume loss (750–1500 ml): Cardiac output cannot be maintained by arterial constriction].
- Tachycardia.
- Increased respiratory rate.
- Blood pressure maintained.
- Increased diastolic pressure.
- Narrow pulse pressure.
- Sweating from sympathetic stimulation. Mildly anxious/restless.

Stage 3: The Progressive Stage

[30–40% blood volume loss (1500–2000 ml): Systolic BP falls to 100 mmHg or less].
- Classic signs of hypovolemic shock.
- Marked tachycardia >120 bpm.
- Marked tachypnea >30 per minute.
- Decreased systolic pressure.
- Alteration in mental status (anxiety, agitation).
- Sweating with cool, pale skin.

Stage 4: The Refractory Stage

[Loss greater than 40% (>2000 ml)]
- Extreme tachycardia with weak pulse.
- Pronounced tachypnea.
- Significantly decreased systolic blood pressure (70 mmHg or less).
- Decreased level of consciousness.
- Skin is sweaty, cool, and extremely pale (moribund).

If the cause of the crisis cannot not be successfully treated, the shock will proceed to the progressive stage and the compensatory mechanisms begin to fail. Increased sympathetic discharge in the blood vessels is a key feature in the compensatory response to hypovolemia. When the hypovolemia is too severe, and the replacement therapy is delayed, the extreme vasoconstriction leads to severe hypoperfusion and tissue damage in the liver and splanchnic area. Hepatic dysfunction includes impairment of both synthetic and detoxification function. The intestinal ischemia is believed to compromise the integrity of mucosal barrier leading to translocation of intestinal bacterial toxins and vasodilator metabolites. The anaerobic metabolism results in release of lactate leading to metabolic acidosis and consequent generalized cellular dysfunction. These metabolites make the arterioles refractory to the vasomotor discharge. The blood pressure can no more be maintained and a permanent downhill course begins. Intense renal vasoconstriction may lead to acute tubular necrosis and renal failure. All this abnormalities produce the stage known as refractory stage (irreversible shock).

Cardiogenic Shock

Cardiogenic shock is a condition in which inadequate tissue perfusion results from cardiac dysfunction, most commonly following *acute myocardial infarction*. Other causes of cardiogenic shock include arrhythmias, cardiomyopathy, and end-stage congestive heart failure. The clinical definition of cardiogenic shock is decreased cardiac output and evidence of tissue hypoxia in the presence of adequate intravascular volume. Hemodynamic criteria for cardiogenic shock are sustained hypotension (systolic blood pressure <90 mm Hg for at least 30 min) and a reduced cardiac index (<2.2 L/min/m^2) in the presence of elevated pulmonary capillary occlusion pressure (>15 mm Hg).

The most common initiating event in cardiogenic shock is acute myocardial infarction. Necrotic myocardium cannot contract. When more than 40% of the myocardium is irreversibly damaged, cardiogenic shock may result. On a mechanical level, a marked decrease in contractility reduces the ejection fraction and cardiac output. These lead to increased ventricular filling pressures, cardiac chamber dilatation, and ultimately ventricular failure that result in systemic hypotension and/or pulmonary edema.

The decreased cardiac output sets up compensatory mechanisms similar to hypovolemic shock. However, the compensatory responses themselves become detrimental to the cardiac function. Tachycardia reduces cardiac filling. Increased peripheral vascular resistance in cutaneous, renal and splanchnic vessels increases the afterload on the heart, whose function is primarily compromised. Fluid retention initially improves the cardiac output, but the increased preload puts an extra burden on the failing heart, resulting in pulmonary congestion and edema.

Symptoms of *cardiogenic shock* are similar to those of hypovolemic shock but in addition: *distended jugular veins* due to increased jugular venous pressure.

Septic Shock

Septic shock is a serious condition caused by decreased tissue perfusion and oxygen delivery *as a result of infection and sepsis*, though the microbes may be systemic or localized to a particular site. It can cause multiple organ dysfunction syndrome (MODS) leading to death. Its most common victims are children, immunocompromised individuals, and the elderly, as their immune systems cannot deal with the infection as effectively as those of healthy adults. The mortality rate from septic shock is approximately 50%.

Septic shock can be broken down into two different phases: (i) warm (or hyperdynamic) shock, and , (ii) cold (or hypodynamic) shock.

Warm Shock

Warm shock characterized by *high cardiac output* and *low peripheral vascular resistance* occurs first. Vasodilation from the effects of histamine, bradykinin, serotonin, and endorphins dramatically decrease total peripheral vascular resistance. It also makes capillaries more permeable causing leakage and fluid shifting into tissues and physiologic third spaces.

Cold Shock—Ominous Late Stage

Most patients will remain in warm shock for 6 to 72 hours before entering cold shock (also known as *low-output or high-resistance shock*). This late and nearly irreversible phase of septic shock is usually indistinguishable from terminal hypovolemic shock.

Two ominous signs of cold shock are a subnormal temperature and a low white blood cell count (with many immature cells). By the time the patient gets to this stage, his hypotension and hypoperfusion are profound. His skin will be cold and mottled in a more generalized fashion-not just below the knees, as in warm shock. Pulse and respirations will still be rapid because of the continued firing of sympathetic nerves and increased catecholamine levels.

The pathophysiology of septic shock is quite different from the other three types of circulatory shock (Table 13.1). In general, septic shock is associated with 3 major pathophysiological effects within the cardiovascular system: vasodilatation, maldistribution of blood flow, and myocardial depression.

1. Vasodilatation

In septic shock, the absolute intravascular volume may be normal. However, because of acute vasodilatation, *relative hypovolemia* occurs. The

Table 13.1: Cardiovascular characteristics of distributive shock as compared to other types of shock

	Hypovolemic	Cardiogenic	Obstructive	Distributive
Cardiac output	low	low	low	high
Vascular resistance	high	high	high	low

physiologic response to infection includes the activation of host defense mechanisms that result in the influx of activated neutrophils and monocytes, the release of inflammatory mediators, local vasodilatation and increased endothelial permeability. Sepsis is characterized by a *similar response to infection, although on a systemic level*, resulting in diffuse endothelial dysfunction. In the case of bacterial infection, the inflammatory response causes release of cytokine and noncytokine mediators, the most notorious of which are tumor necrosis factor-alpha (TNF-α), interleukin 1 (IL-1), and interleukin 6 (IL-6). These factors are implicated in the diffuse activation of a systemic inflammatory response. As a result, mediators with vasodilatory and endotoxic properties are released systemically, including prostaglandins, thromboxane A_2, and nitric oxide. This results in vasodilation and endothelial damage, which leads to hypoperfusion and capillary leak.

2. Maldistribution of Blood Flow

The most characteristic feature of septic shock is the maldistribution of blood flow in the microcirculation. Inadequate tissue perfusion occurs partly because of vascular occlusion. Polymorphonuclear leukocytes may bind abnormally to the endothelium because of endotoxin and inflammatory mediators. These leukocytes and erythrocytes also plug the microvasculature because of the decreased deformability of the cells. In septic shock, endothelial cells are stimulated by proinflammatory mediators [tumor necrosis factor and interleukin-1 (IL-1)] and endotoxin, causing activation of the coagulation cascade, creation of microvascular plugs, and, subsequently, maldistribution of blood flow. The maldistribution contributes to tissue hypoxia.

Even in the stage of increased cardiac output ("warm shock"), vasoactive mediators cause blood flow to bypass capillary exchange vessels (a distributive defect). Poor capillary flow from this shunting along with capillary obstruction by microthrombi decreases delivery of O_2 and impairs removal of CO_2 and waste products. Decreased perfusion causes dysfunction and sometimes failure of one or more organs, including the kidneys, lungs, liver, brain, and heart.

Cardiac output, however, decreases during cold shock. The catecholamines cause selective vasoconstriction of the renal, pulmonary, and splanchnic circulations. This effect coupled with coagulopathy in the microcirculations releases myocardial depressant factor from pancreatic cells. Eventually, cold shock brings multisystem failure—pulmonary edema, adult respiratory distress syndrome, liver and kidney failure, even hemorrhaging from disseminated intravascular coagulation. The patient's mental status and reflexes deteriorate because of hypoperfusion and cerebral microemboli.

3. Myocardial Depression

With adequate fluid resuscitation, patients with septic shock typically have a hyperdynamic state characterized by increased cardiac output and decreased systemic vascular resistance (with or without a decrease in mean arterial pressure). Compared with similarly resuscitated trauma patients, patients with septic shock, despite the hyperdynamic state, have myocardial depression, which is often manifested as decreased ejection fraction, ventricular dilatation, and a flattening of the Frank-Starling curve after fluid resuscitation. Cardiac function usually recovers within 7–10 days in survivors. Myocardial dysfunction does not appear to be due to myocardial hypoperfusion but due to circulating depressant factors, including the cytokines, tumor necrosis factor alpha and IL-1β.

MULTIPLE ORGAN DYSFUNCTION SYNDROMES—MODS (MULTIPLE ORGAN FAILURE SYNDROMES)

This term describes the final clinical picture of a patient in the terminal stages of refractory (irreversible shock). It consists of failure of one or more of the vital organs such as heart, brain, lungs, kidneys, liver and in hematological system.

1. Acute Renal Failure

In all types of shock, the neural response consists of increased vasomotor discharge in blood vessels in the splanchnic area, including renal vessels. Severe renal vasoconstriction results in decreased renal vascular perfusion and a tendency to a decrease in GFR. The compensatory renal responses include autoregulatory renal mechanisms, activation of renin-angiotensin-aldosterone mechanism and increased synthesis of renal prostaglandins. These mechanisms may maintain normal GFR despite decreased renal blood flow. When the renal hypoperfusion is severe, the renal compensatory mechanisms fail resulting in a severe reduction in GFR. The consequent accumulation of nitrogenous waste products (urea, creatinine, etc.) in the plasma and an increase in plasma K^+ and ECF volume is known as prerenal azotemia (Fig. 13.3). This type of acute renal failure is reversible with appropriate therapy to eliminate the basic cause of circulatory shock. If the shock persists, the patient may go into acute tubular necrosis (renal azotemia or intrinsic acute renal injury, intrinsic ATI).

Life threatening complications associated with ARF are:
a. **Hyperkalemia** can be associated with life-threatening **cardiac arrhythmias**.
b. **Salt and water retention often leads to hypertension** and **congestive heart failure (CHF)**.

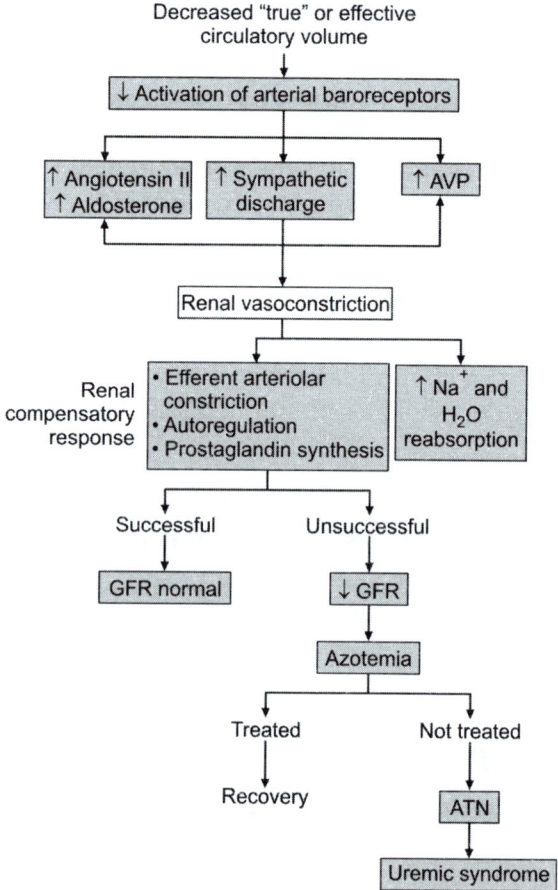

Fig. 13.3: Pathophysiology of prerenal azotemia.

    c. **Hyponatremia** causes concern because of its effects on the central nervous system.

    d. Metabolic acidosis

2. Shock lung [acute lung injury (ALI); adult respiratory distress syndrome (ARDS), non-cardiogenic pulmonary edema]

Acute lung injury/ARDS is one of the important components of multiple organ failure syndromes. The characteristic abnormality of the lung in MODS is a failure of normal gas exchange, reflected predominantly in arterial hypoxemia. ALI is thought to develop when pulmonary or systemic inflammation leads to systemic release of cytokines and other proinflammatory molecules. *It can occur in decompensated stage of all forms of circulatory shock, but occurs more often in septic shock.* Septic shock is more proinflammatory than other forms of circulatory shock because of the actions of bacterial toxins, especially endotoxins. Blood flow to microvessels including capillaries is reduced even though large-vessel blood flow is preserved in settings of septic shock. Mechanical microvascular obstruction is caused by leukocytes and platelets adherence to the endothelium, activation of the clotting system and formation of microthrombi.

Inflammation alone, as in sepsis, causes endothelial dysfunction, fluid extravasation from the capillaries and impaired drainage of fluid from the lungs. Dysfunction of type II pulmonary epithelial cells may also be present, with a concomitant reduction in surfactant production. The cytokines activate alveolar macrophages and recruit neutrophils to the lungs, which in turn release leukotrienes, oxidants, platelet-activating factor, and proteases. These substances damage capillary endothelium and alveolar epithelium, disrupting the barriers between capillaries and airspaces. Protein-rich edema fluid and cellular debris flood the airspaces and interstitium, causing disruption of surfactant membrane which causes collapse of alveoli. In such alveoli, the ventilation is curtailed but blood flow continues, creating physiological shunts and hence severe hypoxia. Stiffening of the lungs parenchyma because of edema and deficiency of surfactant decrease the pulmonary compliance leading to a marked increase in work of breathing. Hypoxia causes pulmonary hypertension.

3. *Myocardial Depression*

In cardiogenic shock, cardiac dysfunction is the primary event. Even in other forms of circulatory shock, severe and persistent hypotension causes further myocardial ischemia and myocardial dysfunction, setting up a vicious circle. Even the neural and hormonal compensatory mechanisms activated in response to fall in blood pressure prove detrimental to the cardiac function by increasing the preload and the afterload.

Among non-cardiogenic types of shock, myocardial depression is seen early in cases with septic shock. In such cases, myocardium dysfunction is because of circulating myocardial depressants such as endotoxins, cytokines and tumor necrosis factor released from the bacteria and immunological response to sepsis.

4. *Disseminated Intravascular Coagulation (DIC)*

Abnormalities of coagulation are frequently observed in shock, especially in septic and traumatic shock. Activation of coagulation cascade within the microvasculature may results from many factors including endotoxins, cell surface components of bacteria, or inflammatory cytokines. The resulting microthrombi in the microvasculature of vital organs may themselves result organ failure.

In addition, the thrombotic phase leads to consumption of circulating coagulant factors. Moreover, many factors that initiate intravascular thrombosis in shock also activate plasminogen activator leading to fibrinolysis of microthrombi. Thus a continuous cycle of fibrin formation and fibrinolysis not only depletes circulating coagulant factors and platelets but also pushes into circulation fibrin degradation products (FDPs), which have a strong anti-haemostatic effect. Diffuse bleeding may be a terminal event.

5. *Cerebral Dysfunction*

Most patients with circulatory failure have abnormal mentation as manifested by mental confusion. Cerebral dysfunction may be multifactorial: cerebral hypoperfusion, hypoxia, acidosis and electrolyte imbalance; all contribute to the failure of autoregulatory mechanisms of cerebral blood flow. When the mean arterial blood pressure falls below 60 mmHg, the cerebral hypoperfusion is severe enough to cause ischemic injury.

6. *Gastrointestinal/Hepatic Dysfunction*

The gut hypothesis is advocated by Deitch to explain MODS in critically ill patient. Due to splanchnic hypoperfusion and the subsequent mucosal ischemia, there are structural changes and alterations in cellular function in the gut. This results in increased gut permeability, changed immune function of the gut and increased translocation of bacteria. Hepatic dysfunction leads to toxins escaping into the systemic circulation and activating an immune response. Under normal circumstances, the tissue macrophage system of the liver acts as a first line of defense in clearing bacteria and their products. Liver dysfunction leads to a spillover of these products into systemic circulation. "Shock liver" can manifest by elevation of liver enzymes and bilirubin, coagulation defects, and failure to excrete toxins such as ammonia, which lead to worsening encephalopathy.

7. *Endocrine/Metabolic*

Multiple metabolic and endocrine abnormalities are evident during MODS; although they are less well-characterized, hyperglycemia and relative insulin resistance is both common and readily detected. Less accessible abnormalities include the sick euthyroid syndrome, and relative adrenal insufficiency. Recognition of the latter has recently gained prominence as a promising therapeutic target for the patient with prolonged inflammation and organ dysfunction.

Further Reading

Kumar, V et al. **"Robbins Basic Pathology"** (8th ed.). *2007 Saunders Elsevier. pp. 102–3.*

Levi M. **Pathogenesis and treatment of disseminated intravascular coagulation in the septic patient.** *J Crit Care. Dec 2001; 16: 167–77.*

Luce JM. **Pathogenesis and management of septic shock.** Chest. 1987; 91:883–8.

Nieuwenhuijzen GA, Deitch EA, Goris RJ. **Infection, the gut and the development of the multiple organ dysfunction syndrome.** *Eur J Surg. 1996; 162:259–73.*

Parrillo JE. **Pathogenetic mechanisms of septic shock.** *N Engl J Med. May 20 1993; 328:1471–7.*

Sethi AK, et al. **Shock: A short Review.** *Indian J Anaesth .2003, 47:345–59.*

14 Obstructive and Restrictive Lung Diseases

NORMAL DEFENSE MECHANISMS OF LUNGS

Since many thousand liters of air enter the respiratory passages each day, lungs are likely to be exposed to a wide variety of assaults by air pollutants such as dust, automobile gases, bacteria, viruses, pollens, etc. In addition, secretions from the mouth and pharynx, rich in bacterial flora of the oral cavity are often aspirated even in normal individuals, especially during sleep. The respiratory passages are supplied with a complex system of protective mechanisms:

- Physical and anatomic factors, especially mucociliary clearance
- Phagocytic and inflammatory cells
- Immune responses

Physical and Anatomic Factors

The anatomic structure of upper respiratory passages (repeated branching) effectively prevents large particles from reaching the alveoli. Particles of $\geq 10\ \mu$ size are likely to settle in the nose. Particles of 5–$10\ \mu$ size are likely to settle in trachea and bronchi. Only particles smaller than $5\ \mu$ size, that include bacteria and viruses are likely to reach the alveoli. Whereas irritant gases provoke cough, large particles in the tracheobronchial tree provoke mucociliary clearance.

Mucociliary Clearance

From trachea down to the terminal bronchioles, the respiratory mucosa is characterized by the presence of cilia, goblet cells, and submucosal mucous glands. The cilia are covered with a blanket of mucus, which traps any incoming particle greater than $5\ \mu$ size. The ciliary movement of adjacent cells is so coordinated that it produces waves of ciliary motions from distal to the proximal parts of tracheobronchial tree (Fig. 14.1). As a result, mucus blanket on the top of cilia laden with dust particles or

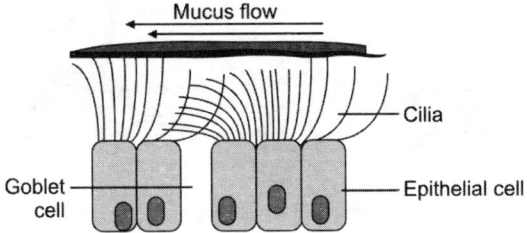

Fig. 14.1: Mucociliary clearance.

bacteria is propelled upwards till it reaches the oropharynx, where it is swallowed or expectorated.

A rare congenital defect in ciliary action, called immobile cilia syndrome results in chronic sinusitis, chronic bronchitis, bronchiectasis, as well as infertility in males (due to poor sperm motility).

Respiratory viral infections produce temporary impairment of tracheobronchial ciliary function. Probably, the most important cause of a defect in mucociliary clearance is cigarette smoking. Pure oxygen, when inhaled for several hours, also impairs ciliary function.

Phagocytic and Inflammatory Cells

Pulmonary alveolar macrophages (PAM, 15–50 µ diameter) constitute the most important defense mechanism in pulmonary parenchyma. Alveolar macrophages are irregular in shape and extend long processes as they move about the alveolar surface. These cells remove all the particles that escape the upper respiratory defenses and reach the alveoli. Bacteria are engulfed by phagocytosis and destroyed by lysosomal digestion. By digestion and processing bacterial antigens, PAM help in cellular and humoral immunity. Some bacteria and viruses, notably *Mycobacterium tuberculosis* and HIV are able to resist the destructive action of PAM (Fig. 14.2).

Viral infections, cigarette smoking, alcoholism, starvation, cold exposure, hypoxia and HIV impair the function of PAM. That explains why bacterial respiratory tract infections are more commonly superimposed in viral respiratory infections or why chronic bronchitis is more common in cigarette smokers.

Polymorphonuclear neutrophils (PMNs) are scarce in normal pulmonary parenchyma. Their number increases remarkably in response to a bacterial infection, e.g. pneumococcal pneumonia. In such cases, PMNs are found not only in the alveolar interstitium but also in the alveolar spaces, engulfing and killing the bacteria. PMN is a defensive phagocyte which is often necessary to clear bacteria from the lung. However, through the release of toxic derivatives of oxygen and of proteolytic enzymes, the PMNs are capable of producing lesions within the pulmonary

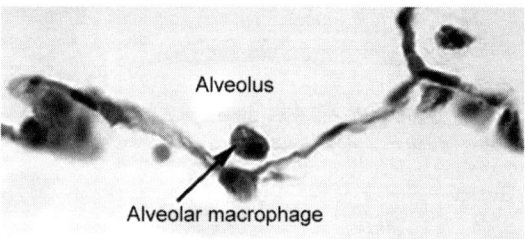

Fig. 14.2: A pulmonary alveolar macrophage.

parenchyma. This double role of defense and aggression makes the PMN an effector cell, which is certainly important, but can be harmful also.

Immune Responses

Both humoral and cellular types of immune responses constitute a strong defense system in the lungs. Secretory form of immunoglobulins (IgA) are present throughout upper tract and lower respiratory tract. Immunoglobulins defend the lungs against many bacteria and a few viruses. T-lymphocyte mediated cellular immunity protects against many viruses, fungi and protozoa.

Defective humoral immune system (e.g. hypogammaglobulinemia) is associated with recurrent bacterial respiratory infections, often leading to bronchiectasis. Cellular immunity is impaired in high-dose corticosteroid therapy and in AIDS. Defective cellular immunity is associated with a different subset of infections, e.g. mycobacteria, fungi, etc.

AIRWAY RESISTANCE

Resistance in the airways (R_{aw}) is basically determined by same factors that determine vascular resistance:

$$Raw = \frac{8nL}{\pi r^4}$$

n = gas viscosity;
L = airway length;
r = radius

In the airways, the variable factor is radius of the airways. Even 4% reduction in airway diameter doubles the airway resistance (Fig. 14.3).

In addition, pattern of airflow is another important factor that determines R_{aw}. Resistance is low when the airflow is laminar, e.g. in bronchi < 2 mm diameter. Airflow resistance is high when the airflow is turbulent. Therefore, 50% of R_{aw} resides *in upper airways*, i.e. nose and pharynx; 40% in trachea and bronchi > 2 mm. Bronchi < 2 mm diameter account for only 10% of total airway resistance (Fig. 14.4).

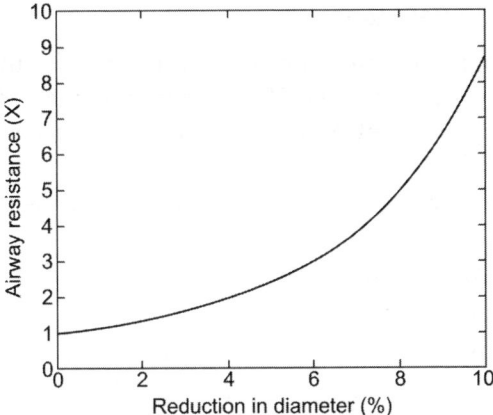

Fig. 14.3: Effect of reduction in airway diameter on airway resistance.

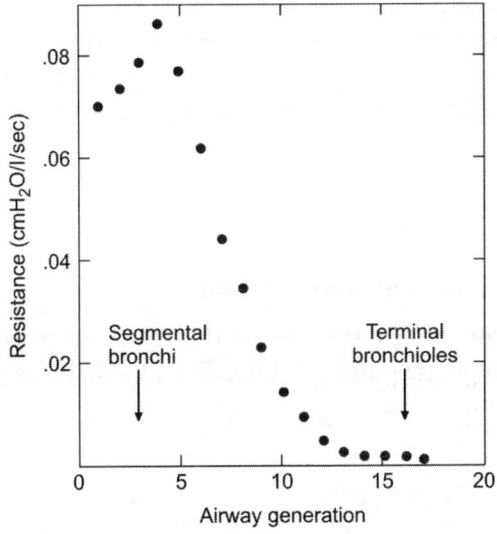

Fig. 14.4: Upper airways are the major site of airway resistance.

The upper airways resistance is not subjected to any physiological variation except that it can be significantly reduced by mouth breathing. During exercise, rapid airflow is likely to markedly increase the air turbulence and hence upper airway resistance. However, it does not happen because, by some unknown mechanism, we shift to mouth breathing during exercise.

Nasal congestion, deviated nasal septum or enlarged adenoids increase upper airway resistance. Mouth breathing is common in these conditions also.

Lower Airway Resistance

The physiological control of airway resistance lies in the medium sized bronchi (2–4 mm diameter). These airways contain, besides supporting cartilage, large amount of smooth muscle. Smooth muscle contraction can substantially increase airway resistance by reducing airway radius. The diameter of these bronchi can be altered by the following factors:
- Bronchomotor muscle tone
- Radial traction by lung parenchyma
- Transmural pressure
- Luminal mucus

Bronchomotor Muscle Tone

Bronchomotor muscle tone is chiefly regulated by parasympathetic neural discharge. It may be reflexly decreased by stretch receptors in the pulmonary parenchyma. Thus, during exercise, deep breathing is helped by bronchodilatation. Circulating epinephrine can also produce bronchodilatation by acting on β_2 receptors present on the bronchial smooth muscle. In allergic asthma, a large number of local chemical mediators, such as histamine, prostaglandins, leukotrienes, kinins, etc. are released. All these mediators produce varying degree of bronchoconstriction.

Radial Traction by Lung Parenchyma

Bronchi and bronchioles are surrounded by lung parenchyma, whose constant pull helps the patency of the airways. This supportive action is

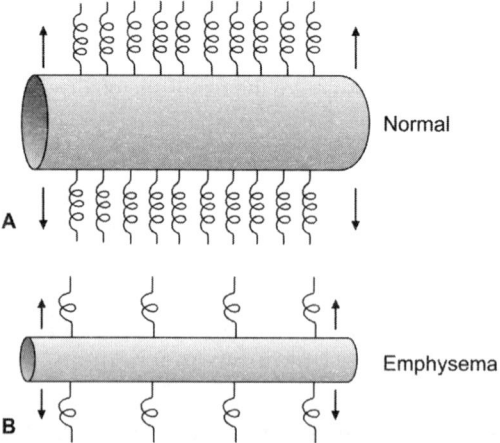

Fig. 14.5: Effect of loss of radial traction in an emphymatous patient on bronchiolar lumen.

called radial traction. Parenchymal destructive diseases such as emphysema cause loss of radial traction. As a result, small airways collapse during expiration (Fig. 14.5). That is why, in emphysema, despite increased pulmonary compliance, the work of breathing is markedly increased by increased airway resistance, especially during expiration.

Transmural Pressure

During inspiration, intrapleural pressure is negative with respect to intrapulmonary pressure which helps to keep airways open. Similar situation exists during tidal expiration also. However, during forced expiration, intrapleural pressure becomes strongly positive, which tends to cause dynamic airway collapse (Fig.14.6). The dynamic airway collapse causes expiratory flow limitations, i.e. beyond a point, increased expiratory effort does not produce further increase in air outflow. The problem is worsened in emphysema due to loss of radial traction, as well.

Mucus in Airways

The presence of mucus or other extraneous material in the airway lumen increases airway resistance (Fig.14.7). Cigarette smoking or respiratory infections enhance the secretion of submucosal mucous glands as well as mucosal goblet cells in the respiratory tract.

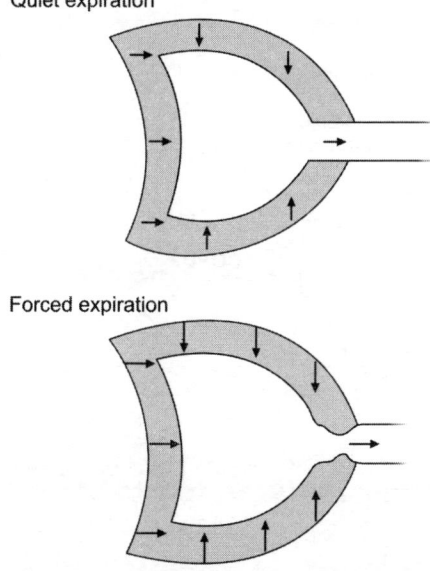

Fig. 14.6: Effect of positive transmural pressure on airway lumen (dynamic collapse of bronchiole in lower picture).

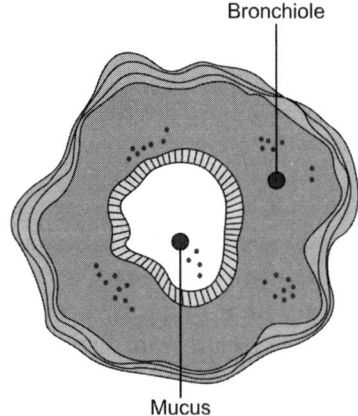

Fig. 14.7: A mucus plug may produce critical narrowing of airways.

OBSTRUCTIVE LUNG DISEASE

Obstructive lung disease refers to a group of diseases that share a common feature—*difficulty in expelling air from the lungs.*
- Asthma
- Chronic bronchitis
- Emphysema

All the three disorders have an increased airway resistance but caused by a different mechanism in each case. However, often there is an overlap (Fig. 14.8). In old cases of bronchial asthma, some element of emphysema

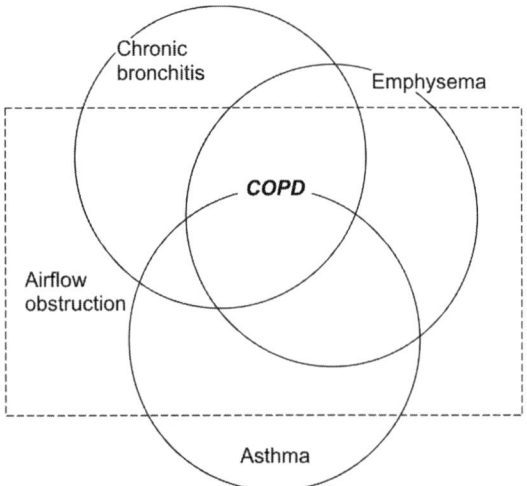

Fig. 14.8: Airway obstruction is a feature common to bronchial asthma, chronic bronchitis and emphysema, through the primary mechanism is different in each.

develops. In chronic bronchitis, some element of bronchospasm is commonly present. Chronic bronchitis and emphysema are considered a spectrum of a chronic obstructive pulmonary disease (COPD) with some patients showing dominantly bronchitis, while others show dominantly emphysema.

Bronchial Asthma

Bronchial asthma is characterized by reversible airway narrowing associated with spasm of smooth muscle in the wall of airways. The airway hyper-responsiveness is the fundamental disorder. The airway smooth muscle shows an exaggerated response to a variety of triggers such as seasonal outdoor allergens (pollens) or allergens derived from house dust, mites present in carpets, beds or domestic animals or cockroaches. In some individuals, even exercise may produce an attack of asthma.

The pathophysiology of asthma is complex and involves the following components:
- Airway inflammation
- Bronchial hyper-responsiveness
- Intermittent airflow obstruction

There is a genetic predisposition to bronchial asthma. A substantial percentage of asthma have elevated IgE levels and history of additional allergic disorders.

All cases of bronchial asthma, provoked by whatever the trigger, have common histological features of underlying inflammatory process. It is characterized by epithelial damage, hypertrophy and hyperplasia of bronchial smooth muscle, enlargement of mucous glands, increased number of goblet cells and infiltration of bronchial wall with eosinophils and lymphocytes (Fig. 14.9). The inflamed tissues responds to any of the triggers by release of mediators such as histamine, leukotrienes and brady-

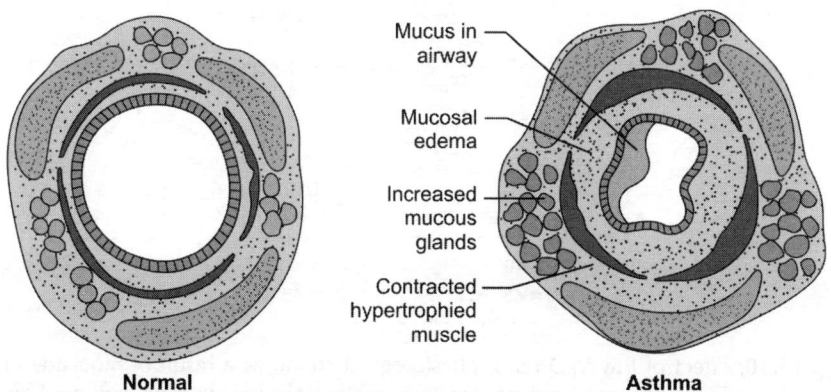

Fig. 14.9: Histological changes in the bronchiole in bronchial asthma.

kinin by the mast cells and eosinophils. These mediators not only alter the extracellular milieu of bronchial smooth muscle causing their hyper-responsiveness (bronchospasm) and increased mucus secretion but also perpetuate local inflammatory reaction. The epithelial damage disrupts the normal mucosal barrier so that antigens or irritants can penetrate the mucosal wall easily.

The combined effect of bronchoconstriction and increased mucus secretion produces a critical narrowing of airways and increased airway resistance, especially during expiratory phase. Even normally, intrathoracic airways are subjected to greater negative transmural pressure during inspiration than expiration. Hence, even normally, airway lumen size tends to be smaller during expiration than inspiration. That why during asthmatic attack, though breathing difficulty is felt during inspiratory phases, it becomes worse during expiratory phases of respiratory cycles. Greatest difficulty occurs when the subject is asked to perform forced expiration. In such a manouver, the highly positive intrapleural pressure may result in almost closure of airways and air traping in the alveoli.

The above mentioned pathophysiological changes are reflected in the followiong laboratory indices *during the attack:*
- Decreased FVC (< 50% of normal) and FEV_1 (<30% of normal)
- Decreased FEV_1/FVC ratio
- Increased residual volume (RV) (up to 400% of normal)
- Increased functional residual capacity (FRC) (up to 200% of normal)

After the attack, FEV_1 improves but usually remains subnormal. FEV1/FVC ratio may be normal in some patients. In such patients, the diagnosis can be confirmed by provoking the attack by a pharmacologic or physical challenge.

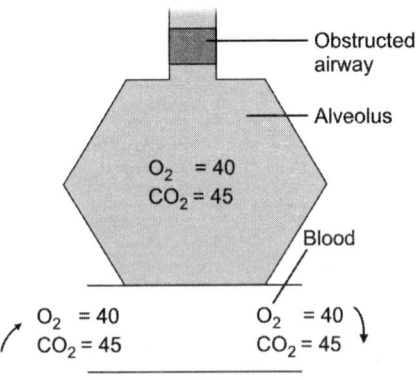

Fig. 14.10: Effect of low V/Q ratio (physiological shunt) as a result of blockade of a bronchus. The venous blood passes to the arterial side without gas exchange (oxygenation). Values shown represent partial pressure in mmHg.

Varying degree of hypoxia occurs during an asthmatic attack. It is caused only partly by the reduction in pulmonary ventilation. Another important factor is *ventilation perfusion mismatch*. During the attack, airway resistance is not increased uniformly in the airways. Some areas are affected more than others and some become blocked by mucus. The blood flow through these hypoventilated areas remains relatively unaffected. Thus in these areas, venous blood is transferred to the arterial side without proper oxygenation (physiological shunt, Fig. 14.10), reducing arterial pO_2 and O_2 content. In the early stages, when ventilation-perfusion mismatch results in hypoxia, hypercarbia is prevented by easy diffusion of carbon dioxide across alveolar capillary membranes. Thus, patients with asthma who are in the early stages of an acute episode have hypoxemia in the absence of carbon dioxide retention. Hyperventilation triggered by the hypoxic drive also causes a decrease in $PaCO_2$. In the early stages of an acute episode, respiratory alkalosis results from hyperventilation. Later, tissue hypoxia worsens because of the increased work of breathing and increased cardiac output. At this stage, a mixed acid-base disturbance, respiratory alkalosis + metabolic acidosis (lactacidosis) is commonly observed. Prolonged and severe attack of asthma may lead to respiratory muscle fatigue and respiratory failure ($\uparrow pCO_2$; $\downarrow pO_2$).

Chronic Obstructive Pulmonary Disease (COPD); Chronic Obstructive Lung Disease (COLD)

COPD is defined as a chronic, slowly progressive disorder characterized by airflow obstruction *which does not change markedly over several months*. Bronchial asthma, though involves airflow obstruction, is excluded by this definition.

The term COPD represents a spectrum of chronic respiratory disorders with predominant bronchitis at one end of spectrum and predominant emphysema at the other. Most patients have characteristics of both the disorders in different proportions. Both disorders cause airway obstruction, though by different mechanisms.

Chronic bronchitis is defined as cough and sputum on most of the days for at least three consecutive months for more than two successive years. In the airways of the lung, the hallmark of chronic bronchitis is hyperplasia and hypertrophy of the goblet cells and mucous glands of the airway. As a result, there is more mucus than usual in the airways, contributing to narrowing of the airways and causing a cough with sputum. Emphysema refers to a permanent destructive enlargement of airways distal to the terminal bronchioles.

Cigarette smoking is considered to be the most important cause of COPD. Some other congenital or acquired factors also seem to be involved, since only about 15% of heavy smokers suffer from clinically diagnosed COPD.

Cigarette Smoke

Cigarette smoke contributes to the development of COPD through a number of mechanisms:
- Inhibits ciliary clearance function
- Inhibits function of alveolar macrophages
- Causes hypertrophy of goblet cells and mucous glands
- Provokes release of elastase from polymorphonuclear neutrophils
- Causes destruction of alveolar parenchyma by inhibiting α_1-antitrypsin
- Increases airway resistance by stimulating irritant receptors.

Genetic Factors

Genetic factors may predispose to COPD possibly by producing deficiency of antitrypsin activity normally present in the lungs to nullify the action of elastase and other proteolytic enzymes produced by leukocytes during acute respiratory infections. However, such deficiency has been detected in only 1–2% of patients of COPD.

Air pollutants may not initiate COPD, but certainly can cause exacerbation of pre-existing disease. Similarly, *respiratory infections* do not initiate COPD, but cause transient worsening of pulmonary function in a patient with pre-existing disease. *Childhood respiratory infections* may predispose to COPD in adult life, if the subject starts smoking.

COPD with Predominant Bronchitis

In such patients, the major pathology is increased activity of hypertrophic and hyperplastic mucus secreting apparatus (goblet cells and mucous glands) throughout large and small airways (Fig. 14.11). Excessive production of thick and viscid mucus results in characteristic cough and copious purulent sputum. The airway obstruction is primarily due to these

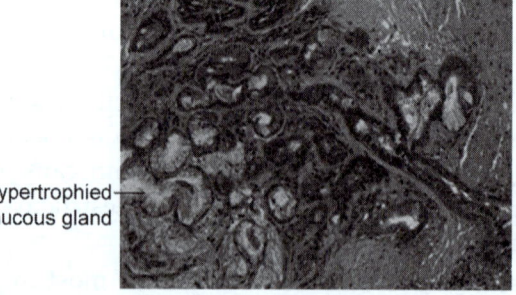

Fig. 14.11: Histological picture of a bronchus in chronic bronchitis.

changes in the terminal bronchioles. Besides intraluminal secretions, some degree of bronchospasm, or thickening of airway wall by edema, inflammation or fibrosis contribute to the increased airway resistance. A component of airway hyper-responsiveness may further aggravate bronchial obstruction resulting in what is called asthmatic bronchitis (Fig. 14.8).

Small airway obstruction is reflected in decreased FEV1, FEV1/FVC ratio and maximum mid-expiratory flow rate. Residual volume (RV) is somewhat increased by air-trapping beyond the obstruction, but total lung capacity (TLC) is normal.

In relatively "pure" chronic bronchitis, pulmonary parenchyma is mostly intact and oxygen diffusion capacity is near normal. However, the patient shows more marked decrease in arterial pO_2 (45–50 mmHg) as well as moderately elevated pCO_2 (50–60 mmHg) and marked polycythemia. The abnormalities in blood gases arise chiefly from uneven ventilation/perfusion in different parts of the lungs. Some bronchioles are obstructed by mucus/inflammation/edema causing marked decrease in ventilation, but fairly well maintained perfusion. The physiological shunts lead to hypoxia and polycythemia. Increased pCO_2 may be due to increased ventilation/perfusion ratio (high V/Q ratio, increased dead space) in many parts of the lungs or hypoventilation due to increased work of breathing resulting from airway obstruction.

Increased pulmonary vascular resistance is important feature of chronic bronchitis. It mainly results from chronic hypoxia. Other contributory factors include increased polycythemia, increased pCO_2 and acidosis. Patients with advanced COPD that have primarily chronic bronchitis rather than emphysema were commonly referred to as "blue bloaters" because of the bluish color of the skin and lips (cyanosis) coupled with congestive heart failure (cor pulmonale).

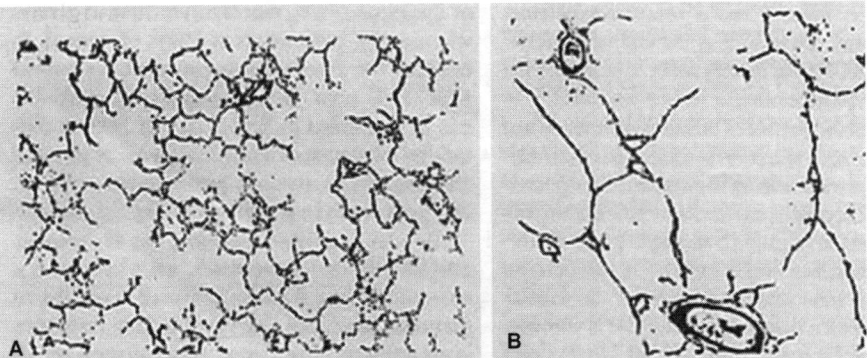

Fig. 14.12: Microscopic appearance of lungs in emphysema (B) as compared to normal (A).

COPD with Prominent Emphysema

In such a patient, the primary problem is degeneration of alveolar tissue. The destruction of airspace walls reduces the surface area available for the exchange of oxygen and carbon dioxide during breathing. It also reduces the elasticity of the lung itself, which results in a loss of support for the airways that are embedded in the lung (Fig. 14.12), leading to a *decrease in elastic recoil of the lungs*. Therefore, the force that normally drives air out of lungs during expiration decreases. Due to disruption of the alveolar septa, the support that keeps the small airways open due to transmural pressure is lost. The difficulty in expiration is further aggravated by *dynamic collapse* (*see* above) of the bronchioles during forced expiration.

Due to loss of elastic fibers, compliance of the lungs increases, the lungs are inflated to a larger volume for a given degree of increase in intrapulmonary pressure. The total lung capacity increases and lungs remain permanently inflated. Residual volume and functional residual capacity are both increased. The chest becomes barrel-shaped. The diaphragm remains permanently flattened (Fig. 14.13).

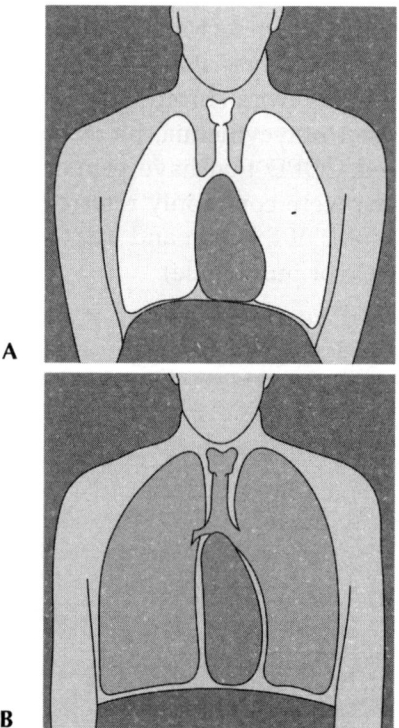

Fig.14. 13: Effect of hyperinflation of lungs on the position of diaphragm during expiration (B). Compare with normal (A).

In a patient with severe emphysema, in spite of the increase in pulmonary compliance, the work of breathing is markedly increased because:
- The diaphragm is ineffective as a muscle of inspiration
- The external intercostals have to contract at an abnormal muscle length
- Additional muscles of inspiration have to be used
- Due to loss of elastic fibers in the alveolar parenchyma, expiration is no more a passive process. Energy is utilized both during inspiration and expiration.
- Airway narrowing due to loss of radial traction of airways adds to difficulty in breathing during expiration

The loss of alveolar tissues markedly decreases the diffusion capacity of lungs. High ventilation/perfusion ratio leads to moderate decrease in arterial pO_2 and as well as mild increase in arterial pCO_2. Severe hypoxia, cyanosis, polycythemia, pulmonary hypertension and cor pulmonale are not seen in patients of COPD with predominant emphysema. Pathophysiological features of the two types of COPD are shown in Table 14.1.

RESTRICTIVE LUNG DISEASE

Restrictive lung diseases are characterized by reduced lung volume, either because of an alteration in lung parenchyma or because of a disease of the pleura, chest wall, or neuromuscular apparatus. In physiological terms, restrictive lung diseases are characterized by reduced total lung capacity (TLC), vital capacity, and resting lung capacity (functional residual capacity—FRC).

Table 14.1: Comparison of pathophysiological features of COPD with predominant bronchitis or emphysema

	COPD Predominant bronchitis	COPD Predominant emphysema
Dyspnea	+	+++
Cough	+++	+
Sputum	+++	±
Bronchial infections	Frequent	Less frequent
Arterial pO_2	↓↓	↓
Arterial pCO_2	↑↑	↑
Acute resp. insuff. episodes	Frequent	Usually at terminal stage
Hematocrit	↑↑	→
Pulmonary hypertension	++ to +++	±
Cor pulmonale	Common	Rare
Elastic recoil	→	↓↓↓
Airway resistance	↑↑↑	±
Diffusion capacity	N	↓↓

There are many disorders that cause restriction of lung volumes but can be divided into 2 groups based on anatomical structures causing the disorder.

1. *Extrinsic disorders or extra-parenchymal diseases:* The chest wall, pleura, and respiratory muscles are the components of the respiratory pump, and they need to function normally for effective ventilation. Diseases of these structures result in lung restriction, impaired ventilatory function, and respiratory failure (e.g., non-muscular diseases of the chest wall and neuromuscular disorders).
2. *Interstitial lung diseases (ILDs):* A large number of disorders involving alveolar walls. The pathology involves all components of alveolar wall and not merely alveolar interstitium. The etiology is diverse and not clear in many types. However, all such diseases have some common features. All of them are chronic disorders with inflammation and fibrosis of alveolar septa. The etiological agents may include:
   - Inorganic dust (silicosis, coal-worker's pneumoconiosis, asbestosis, etc.
   - Immunological assaults (hypersensitive pneumonitis)
   - Dug toxicity
   - Radiation
   - Idiopathic (idiopathic pulmonary fibrosis, sarcoidosis).

Parenchymal fibrosis is the common denominator in all ILDs (Fig. 14.14). Parenchymal fibrosis results in the following pathophysiological features:

Reduced Lung Volumes

A reduction in vital capacity, residual volume, functional residual volume and total lung capacity can be demonstrated. FEV_1/FVC ratio is normal.

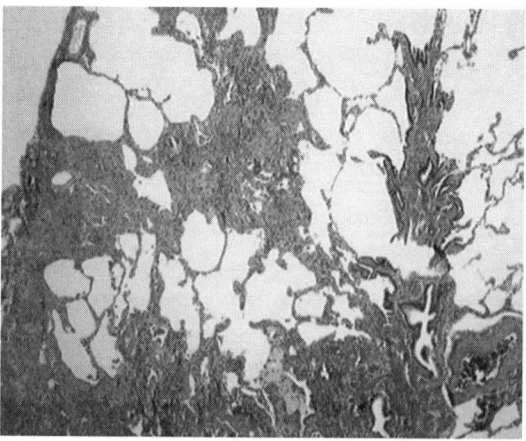

Fig. 14.14: Interstitial lung disease.

Decreased Lung Compliance

The replacement of parenchymal elastic tissue by collagen fibrous tissue decreases the expansibility lungs (pulmonary compliance). Greater inspiratory effort is required to achieve a given tidal volume. Work of breathing is markedly increased. Therefore, the patient tends to breathe with smaller tidal volume in order to decrease the work of breathing. Respiratory rate is increased to maintain adequate alveolar ventilation.

Hypoxia

Arterial hypoxia is a prominent feature of ILDs. Arterial hypoxemia in these disorders is primarily caused by ventilation-perfusion mismatching, with further contribution from an intrapulmonary shunt. The diffusion capacity is impaired, which contributes a little towards hypoxemia at rest but it is primarily the mechanism of exercise-induced oxygen desaturation of blood (the alveolar-arterial pO_2 gradient is elevated, particularly during exercise).

Pulmonary Hypertension

Hypoxia causes pulmonary vasoconstriction. Further, obliteration of pulmonary capillaries by fibrotic process contributes to pulmonary hypertension and development of cor pulmonale.

> ### Further Reading
>
> Rabe KF, Hurd S, Anzueto A, et al. "**Global Strategy for the Diagnosis, Management, and Prevention of Chronic Obstructive Pulmonary Disease: GOLD Executive Summary**". *Am. J. Respir. Crit. Care Med.* 2007; 176: 532–55.
>
> Hogg, JC; Timens, W. The **Pathology of Chronic Obstructive Pulmonary Disease.** *Ann Rev Path.* 2009; 4:435–459.
>
> Hogg JC. **Pathophysiology of airflow limitation in chronic obstructive pulmonary disease.** *Lancet.* 2004; 364:709–21.

15
Ventilatory Disorders

Respiration, though an automatic process, is under two control systems: neural control and chemical control. Neural control is primarily concerned with production of rhythmic alternate inspiration and expiration. Neural control also allows certain reflex responses, e.g. cough reflex. Chemical control is concerned with the regulation of pulmonary ventilation. Chemical control produces changes in alveolar ventilation that are ideal for the metabolic demands of oxygen intake and removal of carbon dioxide from the body.

NEURAL CONTROL OF RESPIRATION

Quiet breathing results from periodic discharge in spinal neurons supplying the inspiratory muscles (diaphragm and external intercostal muscles). Expiration is a passive process. It occurs when the inspiratory muscles cease contraction. The elastic recoil of the lungs expels air out of the lungs. Deep inspiration is brought about by stronger contraction of inspiratory muscles and contraction of accessory muscles of inspiration (scaleni and sternomastoids). Deep expiration is an active process. It is produced by contraction of expiratory muscles—internal intercostals and abdominal muscles. Rhythmic inspiratory and expiratory pattern of breathing is controlled by respiratory centers located in the brainstem.

i. Brain-Stem Respiratory Centers

The medullary inspiratory neurons control the activity of spinal neurons supplying the inspiratory muscles. The medullary expiratory neurons control the activity of spinal neurons supplying the expiratory muscles. There is an inherent pacemaker in the medullary inspiratory neurons. Periodically, these neurons become active and discharge impulses, and then become silent. Thus, the inspiratory neurons have cycles of activity and silence, each lasting 2–3 seconds. This causes periodic contraction and relaxation of inspiratory muscles of the thorax. The switching off point of inspiratory

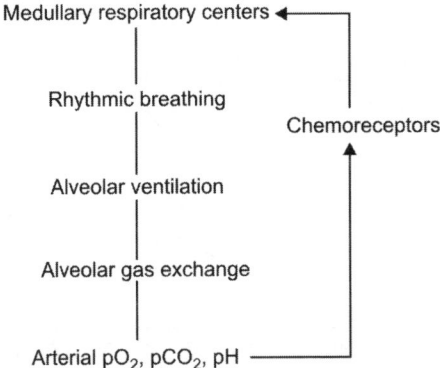

Fig. 15.1: Neural and chemical control of breathing.

neurons is not fully automatic. It is controlled at least partly by the feedback signals from the pontine respiratory center (pneumotaxic center) and vagal receptors located in the thoracic walls and airways. The medullary expiratory neurons remain silent throughout normal tidal breathing. The medullary expiratory neurons and therefore spinal neurons to the expiratory muscle become active only during deep or forced respiration. Thus, activity of various neural mechanisms helps to *control* the rate and depth of breathing (Fig. 15.1).

ii. Chemical Control

The ultimate goal of pulmonary ventilation is to maintain the arterial gases, (oxygen and carbon dioxide), and hydrogen ion concentration within the normal range. Two types of chemoreceptors are sensitive to these chemicals: the central and peripheral chemoreceptors. The central chemoreceptors, located on the ventrolateral surface of medulla oblongata, are very sensitive to changes in the arterial pCO_2. The peripheral chemoreceptors located in carotid and aortic bodies, respond primarily to changes in arterial pO_2 and pH of blood. Chemoreceptors act in a feedback fashion on the activity of brainstem respiratory centers (Fig. 15.1).

The respiratory centers are far more sensitive to hypercapnia (increased arterial pCO_2) than hypoxia. An increase in arterial pCO_2 from 40 to 42 mmHg produces a prominent increase in pulmonary ventilation. However, only an acute increase in arterial pCO_2 sharply increases pulmonary ventilation. Chronic elevation of arterial pCO_2 results in blunting of ventilatory response (Fig 15.2). In cases of COPD, often hypoxia is the chief stimulus for breathing, even though arterial pCO_2 is above 50 mmHg. In such cases, oxygen therapy can result in acute respiratory failure.

Hypoxia increases pulmonary ventilation only when arterial pO_2 decreases below 60 mmHg (normal 100 mmHg). However, ventilatory

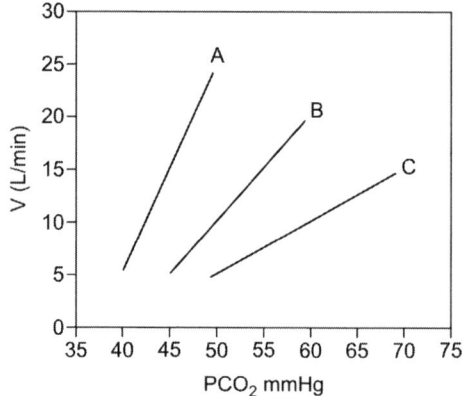

Fig. 15.2: Ventilatory response to an acute increase in arterial pCO_2 (A). Responses (B) and (C) are with increasing chronicity of hypercapnia.

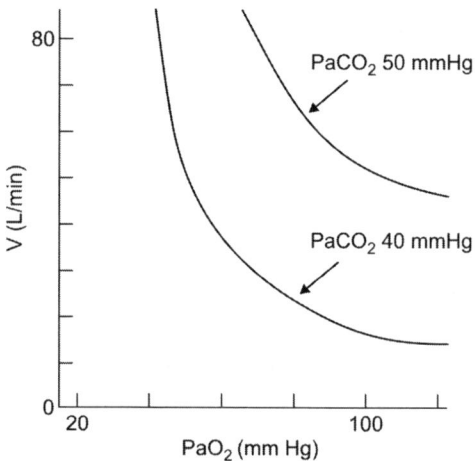

Fig. 15.3: At normal pCO_2, hypoxia increases pulmonary ventilation only when arterial pO_2 falls below 60 mmHg. A combination of hypoxia and hypercapnia dramatically increases pulmonary ventilation.

response to combined hypoxia and hypercapnia is greater than the sum of responses to two stimuli individually (Fig. 15.3).

ANATOMIC AND PHYSIOLOGIC DEAD SPACE

Volume of respiratory conducting passages above the level of respiratory bronchioles is called the *anatomic dead space,* because this volume of air does not participate in gas exchange. *Physiologic dead space* includes anatomic dead space plus the volume of air present in the alveoli where gas exchange does not occur because of insufficient blood supply. Hence, practically these alveoli must also be considered a dead space. Normally the number of such alveoli is very small and physiologic dead space nearly equals the anatomic dead space. However, in certain respiratory disorders (e.g., COPD) physiologic dead space may be as much as ten times the anatomic dead space. Obviously, such patients would have very little effective alveolar ventilation, which results in respiratory distress.

Alveolar Ventilation versus Pulmonary Ventilation

Normal volume of dead space is equal to approximately 150 ml (V_D). Thus, when tidal volume of 500 ml leaves the lungs, the last 150 ml of expiratory alveolar air remains in the conducting passages. Therefore, of 500 ml of air entering the lower respiratory passages during next inspiration (tidal volume, V_T), 150 ml is not fresh atmospheric air but only the alveolar air left behind earlier. Only 350 ml of fresh atmospheric air, reach the alveoli during each inspiration and mix with the alveolar air.

$$\text{Pulmonary ventilation } (V_P) = \text{Tidal volume } (V_T) \times \text{Respiratory rate (RR)}$$
$$= V_T \times RR$$
$$= 500 \times 12 = 6 \text{ L/min}$$
$$\text{Alveolar ventilation } (V_A) = (V_T - V_D) \times RR$$
$$(500-150) \times 12 = 4.2 \text{ L/min}$$

The importance of alveolar ventilation versus pulmonary ventilation can be understood if we calculate alveolar ventilation of two subjects, one with normal breathing (V_T = 500 ml; respiratory rate = 12/min) and the other with rapid shallow breathing (V_T = 200 ml; respiratory rate = 30/min).

Subject A	Subject B
V_P = 500 × 12 = 6 L/min	V_P = 200 × 30 = 6 L/min
V_A = (500–150) × 12	V_A = (200 –150) × 30
= 4.2 L/min	= 1.5 L/min

Hypoventilatory Syndromes

Hypoventilation is said to be present when arterial pCO_2 is above the normal range (37–44 mmHg). Clinically important hypoventilation usually produces arterial pCO_2 in the range of 50–80 mmHg. Acute disorders leading to severe hypoventilation are discussed under the heading of acute respiratory syndrome in Chapter 16. In this chapter, pathophysiology of chronic hypoventilatory syndromes is discussed. Various causes of chronic hypoventilation are listed in Table 15.1.

In most of the cases mentioned in Table 15.1, pCO_2 is elevated because of a decrease in both pulmonary and alveolar ventilation. However, in patients with high ventilation/perfusion ratio (increased physiological

Table 15.1: Causes of chronic hypoventilation

Decreased central respiratory drive
- Narcotic poisoning
- Metabolic alkalosis
- Prolonged severe hypoxia
- Prolonged severe hypercapnia (COPD)
- Bulbar polio
- Head injury

Decreased respiratory neuromuscular activity
- High cervical cord trauma
- Polio
- Myasthenia gravis
- Guillain-Barré syndrome
- Severe hypothyroidism
- Myopathies

Impaired mechanical ventilatory apparatus
- Kyphoscoliosis
- Obesity
- COPD
- Obstructive sleep apnea syndrome

dead space) arterial pCO_2 may be increased despite normal or even increased pulmonary ventilation.

The hallmark of alveolar hypoventilatory syndromes is an increased alveolar pCO_2 (P_ACO_2) and therefore increased arterial pCO_2 (P_aCO_2) leading to respiratory acidosis and cerebral vasodilatation (headache). Simultaneous decrease in P_AO_2 and PaO_2 results in a number of effects: cerebral vasodilatation (headache), mental confusion, polycythemia, pulmonary hypertension and cor pulmonale (Fig. 15.4). The blood gas abnormalities become worse during sleep because of a further reduction in central respiratory drive (Fig. 15.5).

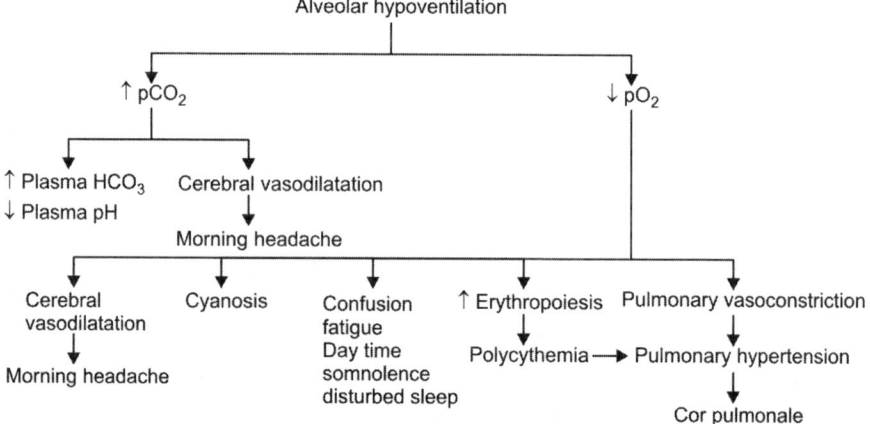

Fig. 15.4: Pathophysiological basis of clinical features of alveolar hypoventilation.

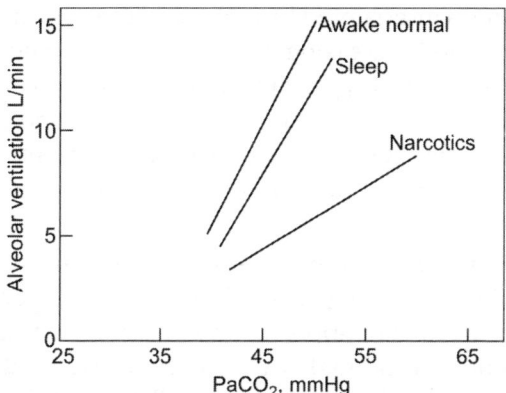

Fig. 15.5: Decreased sensitivity of respiratory centers in sleep and narcotic poisoning.

Sleep Apnea Syndrome

Sleep apnea is defined as an intermittent cessation of airflow at the nose and mouth, for at least 15 seconds each time, during sleep. Commonly apnea lasts 20–30 seconds, but sometimes even 2–3 minutes. The disorder seems to be fairly common. Its prevalence is said to be 2–4% of all middle-aged adults. During each apneic episode, arterial pO_2 drops markedly (Fig. 15.6). When sleep apnea occurs 10–15 times per hour, many clinical problems manifest. Most common is day time somnolence, fatigue and impaired alertness which are dangerous for automobile users. Other consequences include neuropsychiatric and behavioral disturbances caused by sleep fragmentation and loss of slow wave sleep, because of repeated arousals. Nocturnal cerebral hypoxia may play an important role in these manifestations. Polycythemia and pulmonary hypertension may develop.

Two types of sleep apnea syndrome are recognized. The rare central sleep apnea is characterized by breathing interruption due to lack of central respiratory neural drive. In such cases, absence of respiratory movements of the chest is observed during each period of apnea. The other far more common type is known as obstructive sleep apnea (OSA).

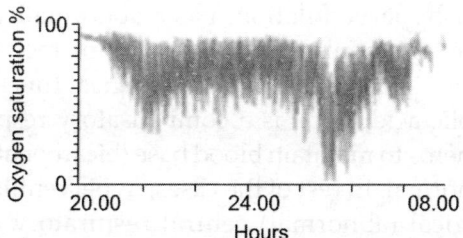

Fig. 15.6: Continuous overnight blood oxygen saturation record in a patient with sleep apnea syndrome.

In OSA, breathing is interrupted by a physical block to airflow. Therefore apnea is accompanied increasing respiratory effort. Snoring is common in OSA. In adults, the most typical individual with OSA syndrome suffers from obesity, with particular heaviness at the face and neck. Obesity is not always present with OSA; in fact, a significant number of adults with normal body mass indices (BMIs) have decreased muscle tone causing airway collapse and sleep apnea.

During normal inspiration, pressure in the throat becomes subatmospheric, which tends to cause collapse of the upper airway. This is prevented by contraction of upper airway dilators which keeps the airway patent. Contraction of genioglossus muscle prevents the tongue from falling against the posterior pharyngeal wall. During sleep, muscle tones declines in general, especially during REM sleep. In those with airways already narrowed by obesity or enlarged adenoids or tonsils, there is a risk of upper airway obstruction during sleep. The result is a gradual progression from initial snoring to OSA. Alcohol and sedatives predispose to OSA by relaxing the upper airway dilators.

During the episode of apnea, the increasing respiratory muscular effort transiently awakens the patient. The patient awakens so briefly that he has no recollection, but long enough for the upper airway dilators to open the airways. Then a series of deep breaths are taken before the patient returns to sleep, snores and apnea. The recurrent cycle of apnea—awakening may be repeated 100 times each night.

Hyperventilation

Alveolar hyperventilation is said to exist when increased rate and depth of breathing result in arterial pCO_2 ($PaCO_2$) below the normal range (37–44 mmHg). Otherwise, increased rate and depth of breathing are referred to as hyperpnea. For example, muscular exercise results in hyperpnea whereas metabolic acidosis results in hyperventilation. In short, hyperpnea is the body's response to increased metabolic requirement, and therefore $PaCO_2$ is maintained within the normal range. Hyperventilation may or may not be associated with dyspnea (a feeling of discomfort in breathing).

In all cases of hyperventilation, basic abnormality is an increased respiratory drive commonly due to hypoxia or metabolic acidosis. In hypoxia, hyperventilation serves a physiological function of improving PaO_2. In metabolic acidosis, it is a compensatory response to depleted buffer base that helps to maintain blood base (bicarbonate)/acid (carbonic acid) ratio near normal. In rest of the cases, hyperventilation results from a non-physiological (abnormal) central respiratory drive (Fig. 15.7). Hyperventilation commonly results in respiratory alkalosis. Therefore, the patient may develop neurological symptoms due to:

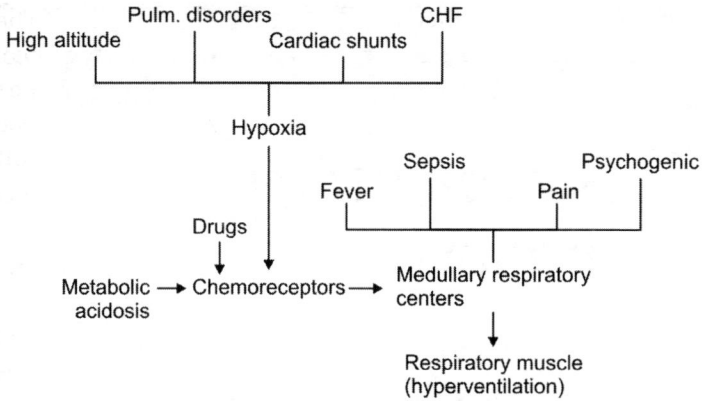

Fig. 15.7: Causes of pulmonary hyperventilation.

- *Hypocalcemic tetany:* Paresthesias, carpopedal spasm sand facial grimacing.
- *Cerebral vasoconstriction:* Light headedness, dizziness, visual impairment, syncope, seizures, etc.

Further Reading

Sean, M, et al. **Obstructive sleep apnea**. *Ann Intern Med. 2005;142:187–197.*

Eckert, DJ and Malhotra, A. **Pathophysiology of adult obstructive sleep apnea.** *Proc Am ThoracSoc 2008;15:144–153.*

16
Respiratory Failure

PHYSIOLOGICAL ASPECTS OF DIFFUSION OF GASES

The Respiratory Parenchyma

The exchange of gases between the blood and the air in the lungs occurs in the terminal region of the air passages. Each respiratory unit consists of a respiratory bronchiole which opens into a number of alveolar ducts. Each alveolar duct opens into a number of sac-like alveoli. The walls of the respiratory units are extremely thin and contain an extremely extensive network of capillaries. The alveoli are lined by two types of epithelial cells (pneumocytes). Type I cells, very thin flat cells with many cytoplasmic extensions, constitute approximately 95% of the surface area of the alveoli. These cells contain only a few cytoplasmic organelles. Type II cells, though similar in number as Type I cells, constitute only 5% of the alveolar surface area. These cells are cuboidal in shape with many microvilli on their apical border. Type II pneumocytes synthesize pulmonary surfactant... the surface tension lowering agent present on the surface of alveolar epithelium. Besides blood capillaries, the alveolar walls contain a few elastic and collagen connective tissue fibers, a few mast cells and tissue macrophages called *pulmonary alveolar macrophages* (PAMs) (Fig. 16.1).

The respiratory membrane is the name given to the tissues which separate the capillary blood from the alveolar air. It consists of cytoplasm of type I epithelial cells, capillary endothelial cells and a very thin interstitial space between the two (Fig. 16.1). Normal respiratory membrane is not more than 0.2–1 μm thick. Hence, under normal circumstances, gases can diffuse across the respiratory membrane with great ease. Pathologically, the thickness of the respiratory membrane may increase due to exudation of fluid from the capillaries (pulmonary edema) or interstitial fibrosis. Under these conditions, the diffusion of gases, particularly O_2, is seriously hampered.

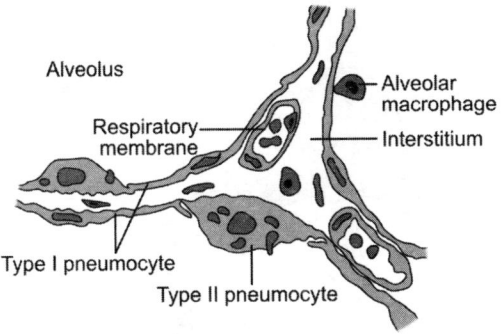

Fig. 16.1: The respiratory membrane

Diffusion Capacity of Lungs

The overall ability of the respiratory membrane to transfer a gas between the alveolar air and the pulmonary blood is expressed in terms of diffusion capacity or transfer factor. Diffusion capacity is defined as a volume of a gas that diffuses through the respiratory membrane each minute for a pressure difference of one millimeter mercury. In young adult males, the diffusion capacity for O_2 under resting conditions is about 25 ml/min/mm Hg. During strenuous exercise, the diffusion capacity of O_2 may increase up to 90 ml/min/mm Hg.

The mechanism of increase is not exactly clear. It may be related to the increased surface area of the respiratory membrane caused by opening up of many dormant pulmonary capillarie. Diffusion capacity for CO_2 is about 400–450 ml/min/mm Hg under resting condition and 1200–1300 ml/min/mm Hg during strenuous exercise. Due to a vast difference in the diffusion capacities for O_2 and CO_2, damage to the respiratory membrane may produce serious impairment of diffusion of O_2 while that of CO_2 may remain normal.

Effect of Ventilation–Perfusion Ratio on Pulmonary Gas Exchange

The resting alveolar ventilation of 4.2 L/min and pulmonary blood flow of 5 L/min give ventilation–perfusion ratio of 0.84. Although there are some regional differences in the ventilation–perfusion ratio, on the whole, the amount of ventilation of the alveoli perfectly matches the amount of blood flow around it. Thus, optimum conditions are produced for gas exchange. In pathological states, the ventilation–perfusion ratio may become below or above normal:

a. *Physiological Shunt (Low V/Q)*

This term is used when ventilation perfusion ratio is below normal. Such a situation occurs when ventilation of a part of the lung is not adequate

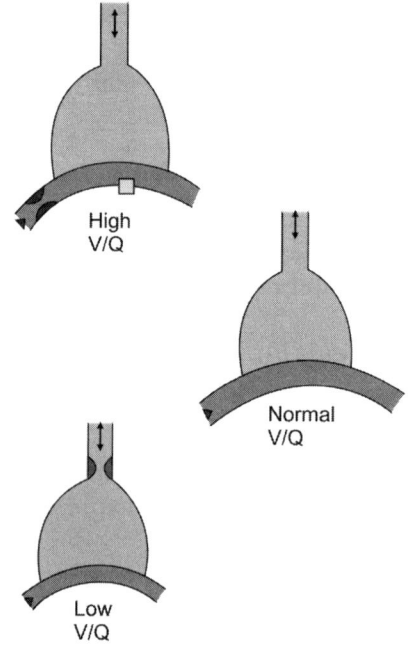

Fig.16.2: Types of ventilation/perfusion mismatch.

enough for the amount of blood flowing through it. Consequently, a certain fraction of the venous blood passes through the area without oxygenation (Fig. 16.2). It seems as if some venous blood has been shunted to the arterial side without oxygenation, and hence the term physiological shunts. In many respiratory disorders like emphysema, and pneumonia, physiological shunts constitute an important cause of fall in the arterial pO_2.

b. Increased Physiological Dead Space (Low V/Q)

In certain lung disorders, blood flow to part of a lung is blocked. Hence, ventilation–perfusion ratio in this region becomes abnormally high (Fig. 16.2). Such alveoli do not take part in gas exchange and therefore constitute a physiological dead space. A large increase in physiological dead space results in severe hypoxia as well as hypercapnia.

RESPIRATORY FAILURE

Respiratory failure is said to exist when the respiratory system fails in one or both of its gas exchange function: oxygenation and elimination of carbon dioxide. In practice, respiratory failure is defined as PaO_2 less than 60 mmHg while breathing air or $PaCO_2$ greater than 50 mmHg. Respiratory failure may be acute or chronic type. The degree of change in the blood gas value cannot help to differentiate an acute from chronic respiratory failure. In patients with chronic respiratory disorders, PaO_2 of 60 mmHg and PCO_2 50–55 mmHg are not unusual. Such a condition is called chronic respiratory failure. In such patients, arterial pH value helps to detect an acute respiratory deterioration superimposed on chronic failure. In chronic respiratory failure, arterial pH is around 7.30–7.35, because of renal compensation (↑ plasma bicarbonate). If it falls to say 7.15 (due to acute rise of $PaCO_2$), or previously stable PaO_2 declines further, an acute upon chronic respiratory failure has set in. Two types of respiratory failure may be recognized: (i) hypoxemic type and (ii) hypercapnic type.

Hypoxemic Type

In this type of respiratory failure, hypoxemia is the chief disorder. $PaCO_2$ is normal or even sub-normal (due to reflex hyperventilation). Such type of acute respiratory failure occurs in patients with acute infections of pulmonary parenchyma (e.g. pneumonia) or a broader group of disorders characterized by increased amount of fluid in the alveolar walls and alveolar spaces, collectively known as *adult respiratory distress syndrome* (ARDS). ARDS is discussed in detail later in this chapter.

In the disorders mentioned above, hypoxia results from decreased ventilation/perfusion ratio (↓ V/Q). Exudation of fluid into alveolar spaces decreases ventilation without matching decrease in blood flow. In pulmonary segments with consolidation P/Q ratio falls to zero and true shunts are said to be present, i.e. pulmonary arterial blood is shunted to the pulmonary veins without any gas exchange. In these types of disorders, elimination of CO_2 remains normal because: (a) diffusion capacity of CO_2 is 20 times greater than that of oxygen; and (b) hyperventilation is induced by hypoxia. Hyperventilation in the non-affected segments is able to produce adequate removal of CO_2. In fact, $PaCO_2$ is often sub-normal, i.e. respiratory alkalosis is present.

Hypercapnic Type

This type is a feature of a large number of chronic respiratory disorders with decreased pulmonary ventilation or decreased alveolar ventilation because of an increase in physiological dead space. Such a problem may arise because of:

a. *Decreased Central Respiratory Drive*
- Narcotic poisoning
- Metabolic alkalosis
- Prolonged severe hypoxia

- Prolonged severe hypercapnia (COPD)
- Bulbar polio
- Head injury

b. Decreased Respiratory Neuromuscular Activity
- High cervical cord trauma
- Polio
- Myasthenia gravis
- Guillain-Barré syndrome
- Severe hypothyroidism
- Myopathies

c. Impaired Mechanical Ventilatory Apparatus
- Kyphoscoliosis
- Obesity
- COPD
- Obstructive sleep apnea

In most of the cases mentioned above, pCO_2 is elevated because of a decrease in both pulmonary as well as alveolar ventilation. Decreased alveolar ventilation results in increased alveolar pCO_2 (P_ACO_2) and hence increased $PaCO_2$. However, in patients with high ventilation/perfusion ratio (increased physiological dead space) arterial pCO_2 may be increased despite normal or even increased pulmonary ventilation.

Adult Respiratory Distress Syndrome (ARDS)

This is the major form of hypoxic respiratory failure. It is being discussed separately because its clinical presentation and pathophysiological features differ markedly from those seen in acute upon chronic respiratory failure.

Causes of ARDS

Rather than a specific disease, ARDS results from acute injury to pulmonary parenchyma from a variety of agents:
- Severe sepsis
- Pneumonia
- Aspiration of gastric contents
- Pregnancy related ARDS
- Multiple trauma
- Shock of any etiology
- Near-drowning

The common denominator in ARDS is a leakage of fluid out of pulmonary capillaries into the interstitium and alveolar spaces. This syndrome is known by a variety of names such as *acute lung injury (ALI), shock lung or non-cardiogenic pulmonary edema.*

Considering the dynamic forces that determine the tissue fluid exchange (Starling forces) would reveal that the pulmonary interstitium and alveolar spaces remain dry because the pulmonary capillary pressure is lower than the plasma protein oncotic pressure. Any little fluid that may be formed in the basal parts of the lungs (due to gravitational effects on capillary hydrostatic pressure) is removed by the pulmonary lymphatics present in the perivascular and peribronchial interstitium. Increased capillary hydrostatic pressure causes pulmonary edema, e.g. left heart failure. In such cases, protein content of edema fluid is low. In ARDS, fluid accumulates in the interstitium and alveoli because of increased capillary permeability. Consequently, protein-rich edema fluid leaks into the interstitial spaces in the alveolar septa and alveoli. In ARDS, capillary hydrostatic pressure is normal. Hence edema of ARDS is also known as non-cardiogenic pulmonary edema.

In terms of pathology, ARDS is characterized by a diffuse alveolar damage of type I pneumocytes. During the initial exudative phase, fluid can be seen in the alveolar septa and alveoli. The inactivation of existing surfactant causes alveolar collapse. Type II pneumocytes are more resistant to damage. One or two weeks later, the exudative phase resolves into the proliferative phase when type II pneumocytes undergo rapid proliferate, differentiate into and replace type I pneumocytes.

Some patients rapidly recover from ARDS, and have no permanent disability. Prolonged inflammation and destruction of pneumocytes leads to fibroblastic proliferation, hyaline membrane formation and lung fibrosis. Subsequent recovery may be characterized by reduced physiologic reserve. It may be clarified that although ARDS is a diffuse process, it is also a heterogeneous process, and not all lung units are affected equally: normal and diseased tissue may exist side-by-side.

Effects on Gas Exchange

In ARDS, the alveoli are flooded with fluid. Hence large parts of the lungs are perfused but not ventilated. Decreased V/Q ratio results in varying degrees of hypoxia. The collapse of alveoli due to deficiency of surfactant adds to the problem of shunts (V/Q = 0). Due to these shunts PaO_2 does not increase to the extent expected from inhalation of pure oxygen, i.e $P_{A-a}O_2$ difference remains substantial.

Hypoxia-induced hyperventilation of the healthy pulmonary segments results in adequate CO_2 removal and often leads to respiratory alkalosis. Only at terminal stage CO_2 retention may occur.

Effect on Work of Breathing

Edema of pulmonary parenchyma as well as deficiency of surfactant reduces the pulmonary compliance. The patient tends to breathe with less tidal volume. To maintain adequate alveolar ventilation, the rate of breathing is substantially increased. The increased energy requirement of such a breathing pattern seems to result in dyspnea, a characteristic clinical feature of ARDS.

Pulmonary Hypertension

Hypoxia, fluid in the interstitial spaces and proliferative changes, all contribute to the increased pulmonary vascular resistance.

Infant Respiratory Distress Syndrome (IRDS)

The surface tension of pure water is so high that every inspiration would require an exhausting muscular effort. However, the presence of a phospholipoprotein complex called *pulmonary surfactant* in the fluid lining the alveoli reduces the surface tension to about one-fourth. Pulmonary surfactant is secreted by type II alveolar epithelial cells, and it mixes with the water molecules on the alveolar surfaces. In the absence of surfactant, the expansion of the lungs becomes extremely difficult. Such a problem occurs in some of the newborn, especially premature babies. The greatest risk factor for respiratory distress syndrome is prematurity, although the syndrome does not occur in all premature newborns. Other risk factors include maternal diabetes, Cesarean delivery, and asphyxia.

The pulmonary system is among the last of the fetal organ systems to mature, both functionally and structurally, since during fetal life, placenta rather than lungs is the site of gas exchange. Fetal lungs consist of only partially opened fluid filled alveoli (Fig. 16.3). The fluid is secreted by pulmonary parenchyma. The lamellar inclusions seen in type II alveolar epithelial cells contain the material that is secreted as surfactant by

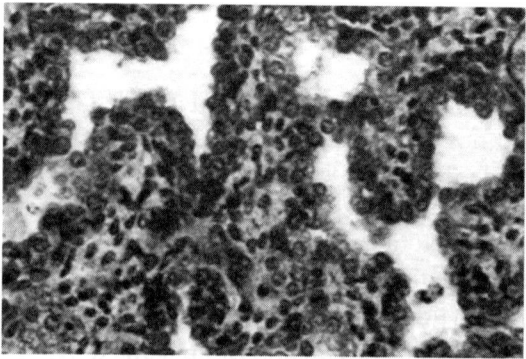

Fig. 16.3: Histological structure of fetal lung.

exocytosis. Glucocorticoids are involved in the maturation of surfactant secretory activity. Normally, there is an increase in the concentrations of cortisol in fetal and maternal blood near term.

Just after birth, a severe inspiratory effort results in expansion of the partially opened fluid-filled alveoli. The presence of surfactant in the alveolar fluid is critically important for the gradual expansion of the alveoli in the next few minutes. Since pulmonary surfactant is mostly synthesized in the last few weeks of gestation, premature infant are more liable to suffer from the pulmonary surfactant deficiency. In such new born babies, high surface tension in the alveolar water-air interface prevents full expansion of the alveoli. Moreover, even the partially opened alveoli tend to collapse gradually. Upon macroscopic evaluation, the lungs of affected newborns appear airless and ruddy (i.e. liver-like).

Atelectasis, low ventilation-perfusion ratio, and hypoventilation result in hypoxemia and hypercarbia. The large V/Q mismatch and right-to-left physiological shunt may involve as much as 80% of the cardiac output. Blood gases show respiratory and metabolic acidosis that cause pulmonary vasoconstriction, resulting in impaired endothelial and epithelial integrity with leakage of proteinaceous exudate and formation of hyaline membranes. That is why; earlier the disorder was known as hyaline membrane disease. Hyaline membranes that line the alveoli may form within half an hour after birth.

Further Reading

Ware LB, Matthay MA. **The acute respiratory distress syndrome**. *N Engl J Med* 2000; 342:1334-1338.

Bernard GR, et al. **The American and European consensus conference on ARDS**. *Am J Resp Crit Care Med* 1994; 149:818-824

Roberts D, Dalziel S. **Antenatal corticosteroids for accelerating fetal lung maturation for women at risk of preterm birth**. *Cochrane Database Syst Rev.* July 2006; 3: CD004454.

17 Physiological Principles of Oxygen Therapy

Oxygen administration is the mainstay of treatment of hypoxemia or respiratory failure. It may produce dramatic improvement in condition of the patient. However, there are several potential hazards associated with its use. These can be avoided if physiological basis of oxygen therapy is clearly understood.

OXYGEN TRANSPORT IN BLOOD

In a subject with normal hemoglobin level, each 100 ml of arterial blood carry about 19.3 ml of oxygen. Oxygen is transported in blood in two forms:
- Physically dissolved form (0.3 ml)
- Combined with hemoglobin (19 ml)

Because of its poor solubility coefficient, very little O_2 is carried in physically dissolved form. However, this amount depends on the partial pressure of O_2 in the blood. For each mm Hg partial pressure, 0.003 ml of O_2 can be dissolved. When fully saturated with oxygen, 1 gram of hemoglobin can take up 1.34 ml oxygen. The relation between partial pressure of oxygen and hemoglobin oxygen saturation is shown by hemoglobin-oxygen dissociation curve (Fig. 17.1). In this curve points of importance are as follows:

Hemoglobin is 100% saturated with oxygen at pO_2 of 100 mmHg (normal pO_2 of alveolar air). An increase in alveolar air pO_2 (e.g. by breathing pure oxygen) does not increase the amount of oxygen carried by hemoglobin. Even at pO_2 of 60 mmHg, hemoglobin is 90% saturated (point B, Fig. 17.1). At pO_2 of 40 mmHg (as that of mixed venous blood), hemoglobin is 75% saturated (point A, Fig.17.1). At lower pO_2 values, there is a steep fall in the amount of oxygen that hemoglobin can hold.

From this discussion, it would be obvious that oxygen delivery to the tissues is dependent on:
- pO_2 of arterial blood

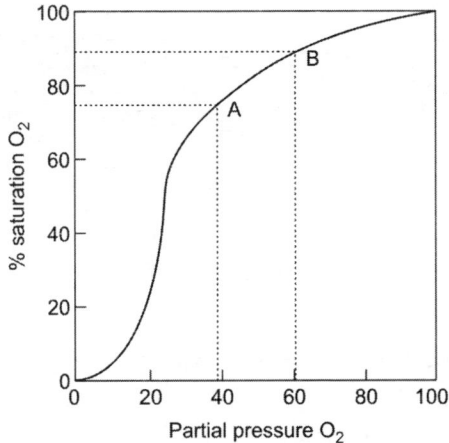

Fig.17.1: Hemoglobin-oxygen dissociation curve.

- Hemoglobin concentration of blood
- Cardiac output and blood flow to the tissues.

A defect in any one of these factors results in tissue hypoxia.

Effects of Inhalation of Pure Oxygen

Fresh air contains 21% O_2 (pO_2 160 mmHg). Alveolar air contains 14% oxygen (pO_2 100 mm Hg). Inhalation of pure O_2 increases PAO_2 and PaO_2 to about 600 mm Hg. At this PaO_2, each 100 ml of blood contains 1.8 ml O_2 in dissolved form (600 × 0.003 ml), but the amount of oxygen combined with hemoglobin does not increase beyond 19 ml% (when hemoglobin concentration is 15 g%). During hyperbaric oxygen therapy, when arterial pO_2 may reach above 2000 mmHg, blood oxygen content increases to 25 ml/dl, purely because of an increase in the amount of oxygen dissolved in plasma (Fig. 17.2).

ROLE OF OXYGEN THERAPY IN HYPOXIA

Oxygen therapy helps to increase P_AO_2 and therefore PaO_2. Thus it would be useful in cases with low PaO_2, i.e. cases with hypoxic hypoxia (Table 17.1). When indicated, aim of oxygen therapy usually is inhalation of air with 25–35% oxygen.

Oxygen therapy in cases with COPD needs special care, because it may lead to acute respiratory failure. Normally, $PaCO_2$ is the driving force for respiration. However, in COPD, chronically elevated $PaCO_2$ acts as a depressor of respiratory centers; hypoxia is the only stimulus for spontaneous breathing. If hypoxia is abolished by oxygen therapy, the patient goes into further hypoventilation and CO_2 retention. That is why patients with COPD are treated by oxygen concentration of about 24%

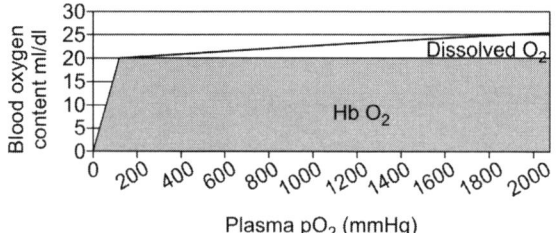

Fig. 17.2: Relation between plasma pO_2 and oxygen content of blood.

Table 17.1: Indications for oxygen therapy

Hypoventilatory Disorders

a. Decreased central respiratory drive
   - Narcotic poisoning
   - Metabolic alkalosis
   - Prolonged severe hypoxia
   - Prolonged severe hypercapnia (COPD)
   - Bulbar polio
   - Head injury
b. Decreased respiratory neuromuscular activity
   - High cervical cord trauma
   - Polio
   - Myasthenia gravis
   - Guillain-Barré syndrome
   - Severe hypothyroidism
   - Myopathies
c. Impaired mechanical ventilatory apparatus
   - Kyphoscoliosis
   - Obesity
   - COPD
   - Obstructive sleep apnea
d. Airway obstruction
   - COPD
   - Severe bronchial asthma

Oxygen therapy is not helpful when hypoxia is due to:
- Anatomical shunts (congenital heart diseases)
- Anemic hypoxia
- Stagnant hypoxia
- Histotoxic hypoxia

and airflow of 1–2 L/min. The aim is to obtain PaO_2 of about 55 mmHg. Ultimate aim is to improve PaO_2 without worsening respiratory acidosis.

Hazards of Oxygen Therapy

Carbon Dioxide Retention

This, a likely complication of oxygen therapy in patients of COPD, has been discussed above.

Oxygen Toxicity

In experimental animals, inhalation of 100% oxygen for two days has led to damage to pulmonary capillary endothelium, alveolar epithelium as well as interstitial and alveolar edema followed by interstitial fibrosis. Therefore, concentrations of O_2 greater than 50% for more than two days are avoided.

Atelectasis: Oxygen therapy may lead to atelectasis by two mechanisms:

i. Following Airway Occlusion

Small airways may be totally obstructed by retained secretions. As a result, slow absorption of gases from the alveoli distal to obstruction may occur. Normally, it is a slow process and takes many hours or even days because 80 of the alveolar air is nitrogen which has very poor solubility coefficient. However, if nitrogen has been replaced by oxygen, atelectasis may occur within minutes.

ii. Respiratory Units with Low V/Q Ratio

Areas of the lungs with low ventilation/perfusion ratio tend to collapse when air containing high concentration of oxygen is inhaled. Hypoxemic blood may rapidly take up oxygen and there is very little nitrogen to keep the alveoli patent.

Retinopathy of Prematurity (Retrolental hyperplasia)

During the 1940s and 1950s, retinopathy of prematurity (ROP) (then known as retrolental fibroplasia), was the leading cause of blindness in children in the United States. In 1951, it was first suggested that ROP was related to the introduction of oxygen therapy into the newborn nursery that was subsequently proved. Nowadays, after oxygen therapy has been studied more extensively, it has been realized that exaggerated oxygenation of retina is not the only causative agent of ROP. Some other factors seem to be at least in part responsible for the disorder.

a. Oxygen-dependent Factors

The development of the human retinal vasculature commences at approximately the 16th week of gestation and concludes at term (i.e., the 40th week of gestation). The exaggerated retinal oxygenation secondary to oxygen supplementation results in exposure of immature tissues to a relative excess of oxygen. This provokes endothelial cell death and thus obliteration of retinal vessels, because infants born prematurely are prone to oxidant injury. On stoppage of oxygen therapy, uncontrolled vasoproliferation begins and spreads into the vitreous, which is devoid

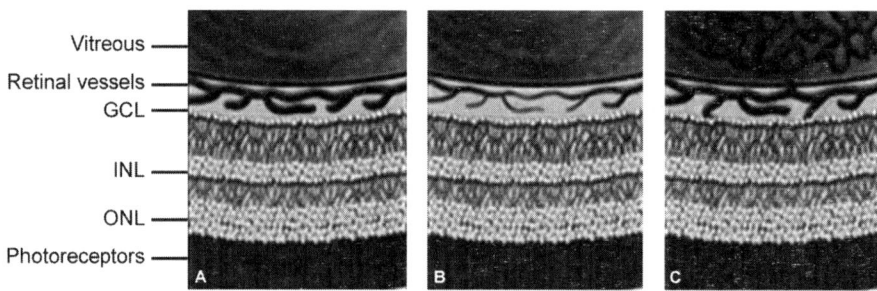

Fig. 17.3: Retinopathy of prematurity. Normal retina (A); vaso-obliteration (B) and neovascularization into vitreous (C). GCL: ganglion cell layer; INL: inner nuclear layer; ONL: outer nuclear layer.

of vessels under physiological conditions (Fig. 17.3). Retinal detachment and blindness follows.

b. *Oxygen-independent Factors*

In light of the major role of high levels of oxygen and their resulting effects in the genesis of ROP, oxygenation protocols limiting hemoglobin saturation with oxygen have been adapted to the clinic and shown to reduce the incidence of ROP. However, these approaches have not eliminated ROP in the industrialized world, suggesting a role for oxygen-independent factors in the development of ROP. Of all these contributors, premature birth remains the greatest risk for ROP, which suggests that perhaps certain factors present in utero required for normal fetal development may be lacking in infants born prematurely.

Further Reading

Sapieha, P, et al. **Retinopathy of prematurity: understanding ischemic retinal vasculopathy at an extreme of age**. *J Clin Invest* 2010; 120: 3022–32.

18 Pulmonary Function Tests

Pulmonary function tests can help to:
- Differentiate between obstructive and restrictive lung disease
- In obstructive disease, differentiate whether obstruction is extrathoracic or intrathoracic
- In obstructive lung disease, whether obstruction is fixed or variable
- Differential diagnosis of dyspnea (cardiac or pulmonary)
- Determine fitness of the patient for major surgery
- Determine the net result of the disorder on blood gases

Pulmonary functions tests can be classified into:
- Tests for lung volumes
- Tests for flow rates and flow volume curve
- Test for diffusion capacity of lungs
- Tests for blood gases (PaO_2 and $PaCO_2$)
- Tests for calculation of $P_{A-a}O_2$ at rest, exercise and after inhalation of pure O_2

1. Tests of Lung Volume

Following lung volumes can be measured:
- Forced ventilatory capacity (FVC)
- Forced expiratory volume 1st second (FEV_1)
- FVC/FEV_1 ratio
- $FEV_{25-75\%}$
- Functional residual capacity (FRC)
- Residual volume (RV)
- Total lung capacity (TLC).

Of these, FVC, FEV_1 and FEV_1/FVC ratio can be easily measured by a spirometer (Fig. 18.1).
- A vital capacity is an important preoperative assessment tool. Significant reductions in vital capacity (less than 20 cc/kg of ideal body

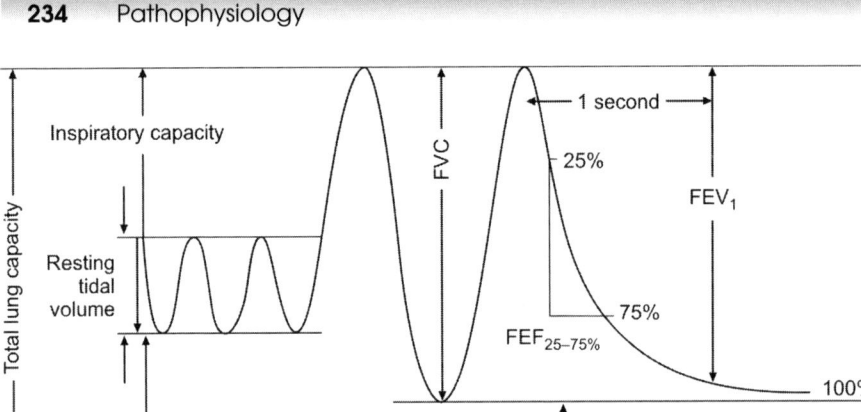

Fig. 18.1: A spirogram.

weight) indicate that the patient is at a higher risk for postoperative respiratory complications. This is because vital capacity reflects the patient's ability to take a deep breath, to cough, and to clear the airways of excess secretions. Estimation of FVC of the patient prior to surgery is important, especially in who:
- Are older than 60–65 years of age
- Are known to have pulmonary disease
- Are obese (as in pathologically obese)
- Have a history of smoking, cough or wheezing
- Will be under anesthesia for a lengthy period of time
- Are undergoing an abdominal or a thoracic operation

Measurement of FVC and FEV_1 and FEV_1/FVC ratio helps in the differential diagnosis of obstructive and restrictive lung disorders. Besides FEV_1, another index of flow rate can also be estimated from a spirogram, i.e., $FEF_{25-75\%}$ (Fig.18.1). This index reflects flow rate in the middle half of the forced expiration. It is a sensitive index of airway obstruction. In some patients of obstructive lung disease, $FEF_{25-75\%}$ is abnormal, even though FEV_1/FVC ratio is normal.

Measurement of Functional Residual Capacity

FRC is the amount of air left in the lungs at the end of tidal expiration. It can be measured by the **helium dilution technique**. This technique is a closed-circuit system where a spirometer is filled with a mixture of helium (He) and oxygen. The amount of He in the spirometer is known at the beginning of the test (Concentration × Volume (V_1), = Amount). A helium meter records the concentration of helium (C1) (Fig. 18.2A). The patient

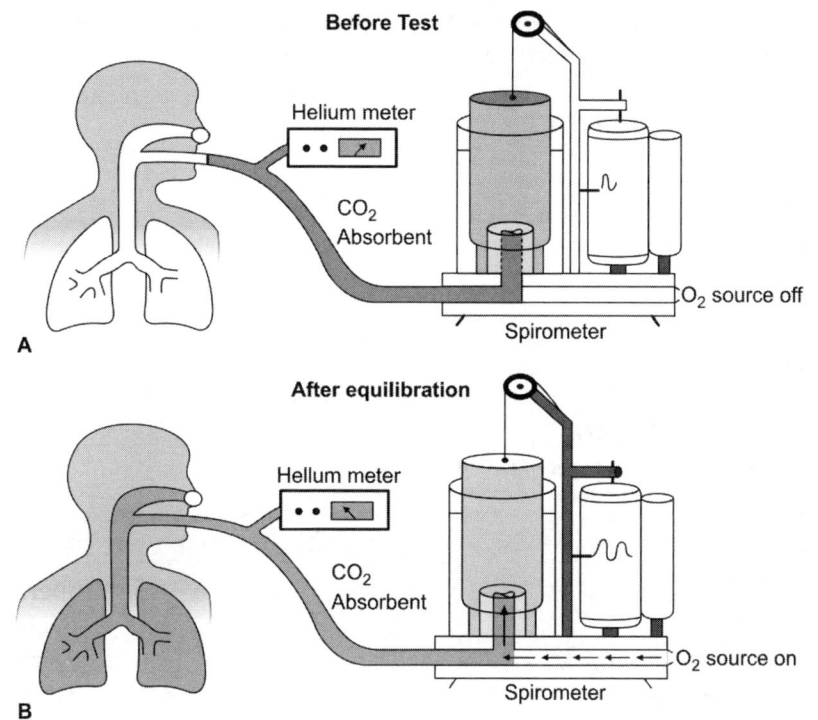

Fig. 18.2: Estimation of functional residual capacity by helium dilution method. Distribution of helium before (A), i.e. V_1 and after equilibrium is achieved (B) V_1 + FRC.

is then asked to breathe the mixture from the spirometer starting from the end of a tidal expiration. The helium spreads into the lungs of the patient, and settles at a new (lower) concentration (C_2) (Fig. 18.2B). Now helium has spread in a new volume, V_2 (= air in spirometer + FRC)

$$C_1 \times V_1 = C_2 \times V_2$$
$$C_1 \times V_1 = C_2 \times (V_1 + FRC)$$
$$FRC = [(C_1 \times V_1)/C_2] - V_1$$

With the knowledge of FRC, values of RV and TLC can be calculated from the spirogram of the patient (Fig. 18.1).

Interpretation

Nowadays, computerized spirometers not only give the observed value of lung function, but also the predicted normal value corrected for the patient's height and age. The results also show the percent deviation from the predicted normal value. Any result that is within ± 20% of the predicted value is considered normal.

From the results of ventilatory function, two major patterns of abnormalities can be detected:

A. *Obstructive Pattern*
- VC ↓
- $FEV_{1\%}$ ↓
- FEV_1/FVC ratio ↓
- FEF 25–75% ↓
- RV ↑
- TLC N or ↑

B. *Restrictive Pattern*
i. *Extra-parenchymal restrictive disorder*
- VC ↓
- RV N
- TLC ↓
- $FEV_{1\%}$ N
- FEV_1/FVC ratio N or ↑
- FEF 25–75% N or ↑

ii. *Pulmonary parenchymal restrictive disorder*
- VC ↓
- *RV* ↓
- TLC ↓
- $FEV_{1\%}$ N
- FEV_1/FVC ratio N or ↑
- FEF 25–75% N or ↑

2. Spirometric Response to Inhaled Bronchodilators

This test helps to determine:
- Whether there is an unsuspected element of reversible airflow obstruction in patients who are thought not to have asthma.
- The degree of reversibility in a known case of asthma

In this test, a forced expirogram is recorded before and 10–20 minutes after inhalation of 2 puffs of salbutamol inhaler separated by 30–60 seconds interval.

3. Diffusion Capacity (Transfer Factor)

Due to technical reasons diffusion capacity for carbon monoxide (or to say more accurately, transfer factor for CO, TF_{CO}) is estimated instead of oxygen diffusion capacity.

In the lungs, diffusion of CO (or oxygen) is limited by:
- The surface area in which diffusion occurs
- Capillary blood volume
- Hemoglobin concentration
- Properties of the lung parenchyma that separate the alveolar gas from the red blood cell within the capillary
    i. alveolar-capillary membrane thickness and/or
    ii. the presence of excess fluid in the alveoli

Important causes of decreased TF_{CO} include:
- Loss of lung parenchyma in diseases like emphysema.
- Interstitial lung diseases, such as idiopathic pulmonary fibrosis, or sarcoidosis.
- Pulmonary edema due to heart failure, or acute interstitial pneumonitis.
- Diseases of the blood vessels in the lung, such as pulmonary vasculitis and pulmonary hypertension.

4. Flow Volume Loops

Most of the modern computerized recorders of ventilatory function also show a graphic record of the relation between volume and flow during maximum inspiratory and expiratory effort. A typical normal pattern is "a triangle sitting on a semicircle". During expiration, the flow during the early part is effort dependent, but later part is effort independent; it is determined by the mechanical properties of the lungs and resistance to airflow. In patients with airflow obstruction, the flow rate at any given volume is decreased, particularly in the later part of expiration, giving a "scooped out" appearance to the expiratory curve (Fig. 18.3). In some

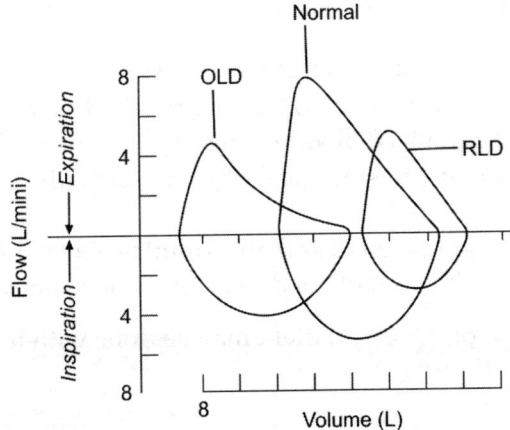

Fig. 18.3: Flow volume loops. OLD: obstructive lung disease. RLD: restrictive lung disease.

cases of obstructive lung disease, such an abnormal flow volume loop may be observed at an earlier stage of the disease than abnormalities in FEV_1 or $FEF_{25-75\%}$.

5. Arterial Blood Gases

Interpreting an arterial blood gas (ABG) report is a crucial skill for physicians, nurses, and respiratory therapists. ABG interpretation is especially important in critically ill patients. Arterial blood gas determinations will indicate two basic body functions:
- Acid-base balance of the blood
- Oxygenation status of the blood

The topic of acid–base status of the body constitutes a separate chapter (Chapter 30) in this book. The interpretation of oxygenation status is discussed below.

Oxygenation Status

The normal PaO_2 (partial pressure of oxygen in arterial blood is) is easily estimated by blood oxygen analyzer. Its normal range is 80–100 mm Hg. Any value below this range reflects hypoxia (usually named as hypoxic hypoxia). The commonest cause hypoxia is hypoventilation due to various pulmonary disorders (*see* Table 15.1). However, a decrease in PaO_2 may result from causes other than hypoventilation:
- Intra-cardiac right to left shunts
- Pulmonary disorders with physiological shunts
- Pulmonary disorders with diffusion block

If diffusion block is suspected estimation of **Alveolar arterial pressure gradient of oxygen ($P_{A-a}O_2$)** is required. PAO_2 is calculated as follows:
$$PAO_2 = 150 - [1.25 \times PaCO_2]$$

Normally, PaO_2 is less than PAO_2 because:
- Mixture of some venous blood from bronchial veins and the besian vessels with arterialized blood.
- Small number of physiological shunts normally present in lung parenchyma.

Normal $P_{A-a}O_2$ gradient is less than 15 mmHg. Greater $P_{A-a}O_2$ gradient is observed in the three set of conditions mentioned above.

Determination of $P_{A-a}O_2$ gradient may be done with inhalation of:
- Room air
- Pure oxygen

This modification of the procedure helps to differentiate hypoxia due to V/Q mismatch from that due to predominant shunts. In case of former,

$P_{A-a}O_2$ gradient is narrowed when tested with pure oxygen. In a case with predominant shunts, the difference persists.

6. Exercise Testing

In most of the patients with respiratory disorders, the pulmonary function tests discussed above are able to give a clear-cut pathophysiological diagnosis. However, in a few patients, all these tests may fail to explain the severity of dyspnea present. In such cases, blood gases, particularly PaO_2 is estimated while (i) breathing room air and (ii) breathing pure oxygen at:

i. At rest

ii. During exercise on a treadmill or a cycle ergometer.

A widened $P_{A-a}O_2$ gradient during exercise suggests a diffusion defect.

Further Reading

Macintyre N, et al. **Standardisation of the single-breath determination of carbon monoxide uptake in the lung.** EurRespir J. 2005; 26:720–35

www.radiometeramerica.com/.../**Blood**% 20gas% 20 hand

19
Disorders of Motor Control

GENERAL CONSIDERATIONS

The motor system generates three types of movements:

1. Reflex responses, e.g. postural reflexes, withdrawal reflex
2. Rhythmic motor pattern, e.g. walking, running, chewing, etc. These movements combine features of (1) and (3). Typically, only initiation and termination of the sequence is voluntary. Once initiated, the relatively stereotyped activity continues almost automatically.
3. Voluntary movements. The movement involved may be as simple as lifting a book off the table or as complex as writing or playing a musical instrument. These are purposeful movements and completely voluntary in nature. Their execution, however, may improve with learning.

It must be appreciated that most of the voluntary movements are executed over the background of reflex postural adjustments. While taking one step forward, one is most likely to fall but for the various postural reflexes which allow the body to be balanced on one foot, while the other is off the ground.

In the central nervous system, there are three hierarchical levels of motor control (Fig. 19.1):

- Motor cortex
- Brain stem
- Spinal cord

Each level is provided with sensory information essential for its motor function. Spinal cord and brain stem generate reflexes so that the motor cortex is left free to give general commands to lower centers to execute movements with appropriate postural adjustments.

The overall planning and programming and execution are complex processes (Fig. 19.2).

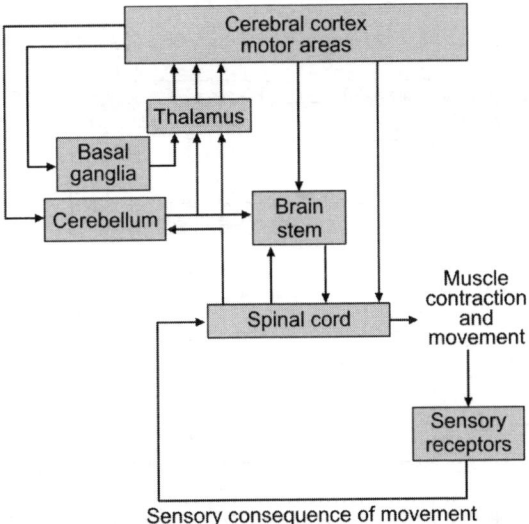

Fig. 19.1: Hierarchy in control of motor activity.

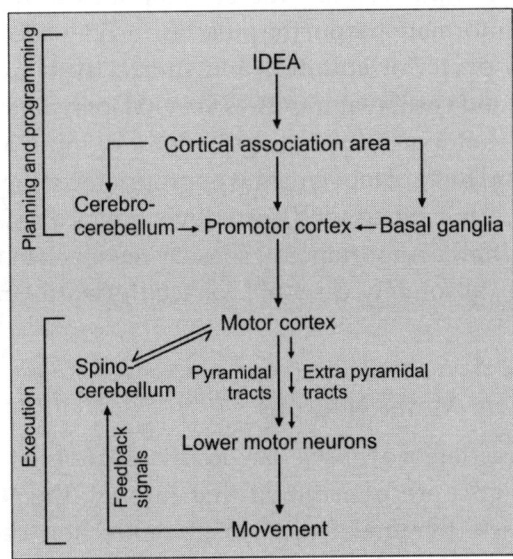

Fig.19.2: Planning, programming and execution of motor activity.

ROLE OF SENSORY INFORMATION IN MOTOR ACTIVITY

Large amount of exteroceptive (visual, auditory, and cutaneous) and proprioceptive impulses (from muscles and joints as well as vestibular apparatus) provide a constant feedback information which is essential

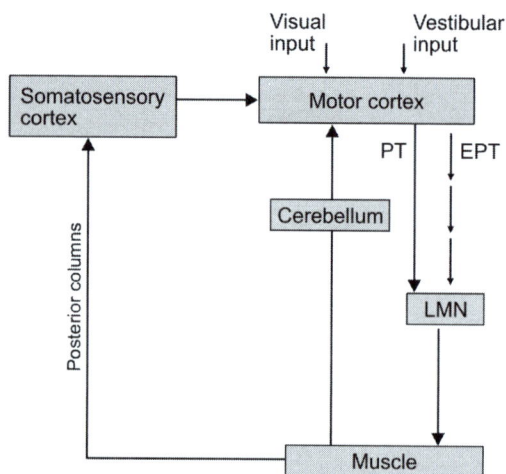

Fig. 19.3: Sensory feedback in motor activity. PT: pyramidal tracts; EPT: extrapyramidal tracts; LMN: lower motor neuron.

not only execution of motor activity with accuracy and precision but also for reflexes and rhythmic motor patterns mentioned above. The feedback proprioceptive information from the muscles and joints reaches the motor cortex through posterior columns and indirectly via cerebellum. In addition, visual and vestibular impulses are vital for maintenance of stable posture during motor activity (Fig. 19.3). Sensory input assures that the rate, direction and force of movement is appropriate for the desired target. The motor defects in patients with posterior columns disease or cerebellar disorder highlight the importance of sensory feedback in motor activity. Sensory input is absolutely essential for feedforward control of motor activity.

Upper and Lower Motor Neurons

Voluntary contraction of a muscle can occur only if signals originating in primary motor area are transmitted first through the corticospinal or corticobulbar tracts (pyramidal tracts) to the ventral horn cells in the spinal cord (or their cranial equivalents in brainstem). Efferent fibers arising from ventral horn cells (α-motor neurons) carry signals to the skeletal muscle (Fig. 19.4). In other words, voluntary control over skeletal muscle is exerted by a two-neuron chain constituted by corticospinal neurons and α-motor neurons. Lesion of either of neurons of this chain results in paralysis of the muscle. The terms upper motor neuron (UPN) type of paralysis and lower motor neurons (LMN) type of paralysis are used to describe paralysis due to a lesion of corticospinal fibers and α-motor spinal neurons (or their cranial equivalents), respectively.

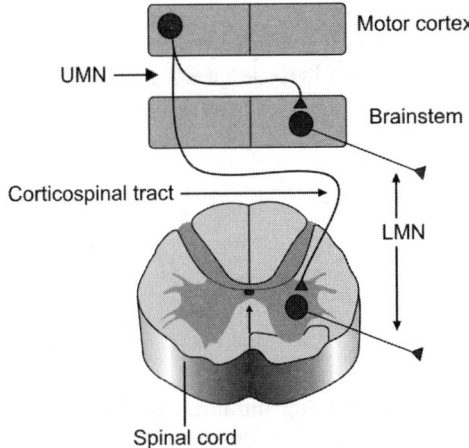

Fig. 19.4: Upper motor neuron (UMN) and lower motor neuron (LMN).

Regulation of Muscle Tone

Normal motor activity involves a controlled contraction of a group of skeletal muscles for the intended aim. It also involves contraction of several other muscles to produce appropriate postural background. All this is made possible by a constant feedback from the muscles regarding their length, velocity of change in length and the degree of force generated by the contracting muscles. This sensory information, called proprioceptive information, is monitored by two types of sensory receptors: (i) muscle spindles, and (ii) Golgi tendon organs. The activity of these sensory receptors is modulated by cortical and brainstem motor areas through gamma (γ) motor neurons.

THE MUSCLE SPINDLES

Muscle spindles are spindle-shaped sensory receptors (1–5 mm long) present in the belly of skeletal muscle. They are located in parallel with skeletal muscle fibers (average length 30 mm). Either end of the spindle is attached to the endomysium of a skeletal muscle fiber. Each spindle contains 2–10 intrafusal muscle fibers in the polar region and a group of nuclei in the non-contractile central region. Central region of the spindle is surrounded by type Ia afferents which carry proprioceptive information generated in the spindle to central nervous system. The intrafusal fibers are innervated by γ-efferents (Fig. 19.5). (Skeletal muscle fibers or extrafusal fibers are innervated by α-motor neurons.) Increased discharge in γ-efferents fibers causes contraction of the intrafusal fibers leading to greater sensitivity of muscle spindles. When skeletal muscle fibers (extrafusal fibers) are stretched, muscle spindles are also stretched which increases the Ia afferent discharge.

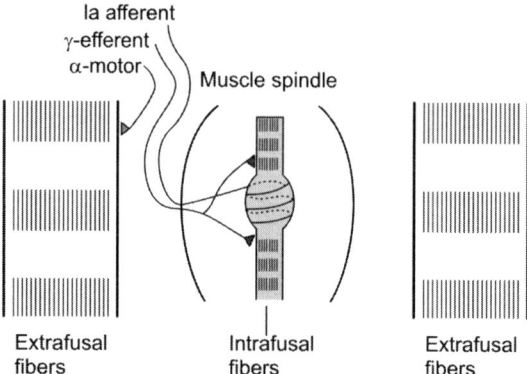

Fig.19.5: Muscle spindle (containing intrafusal fibers) and skeletal muscle fibers (containing "extrafusal" fibers) with their innervation.

Muscle spindles generate proprioceptive information which reaches the CNS both at unconscious and conscious levels. Unconscious proprioceptive information reaches the spinal cord and results in stretch reflex. Further, unconscious proprioceptive information reaches the cerebellum through spinocerebellar tracts. Muscle spindle also generate conscious kinesthetic sensation, which reaches the somatosensory cortex via posterior while columns.

Stretch Reflex

Afferent fibers (Ia type) from the muscle spindles make monosynaptic connection with ventral horn cells (α-motor neurons) of the spinal cord, which innervate the (extrafusal) skeletal muscle fibers close to the respective muscle spindle (Fig. 19.6).

Any passive stretch of the skeletal muscle causes increased discharge in the Ia afferent fibers results in increased discharge in the appropriate α-motor neurons. The reflex contraction of the skeletal muscle brings the

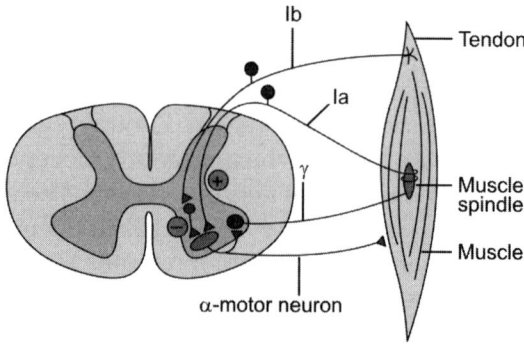

Fig. 19.6: Reflex arcs of stretch reflex (initiated from a muscle spindle) and inverse stretch reflex (initiated from a Golgi tendon organ).

muscle length to the original (pre-stretch) condition. The stretch reflex is of fundamental importance in maintenance of muscle tone and posture.

Inverse Stretch Reflex

Golgi tendon organs are slender encapsulated structures located at the junction of muscle fibers and collagen fibers that constitute the tendon. In contrast to the muscle spindles, Golgi tendon organs are located in series with the muscle fibers. Golgi tendon organs are innervated by type Ib afferents. Golgi tendon organs monitor the tension developed in the muscle during contraction. Excessive muscle tension increases discharge rate in Ib afferents, which through a disynaptic pathway inhibits the appropriate α-motor neurons, leading to a decrease in the force of muscle contraction (Fig. 19.6). Physiologically, inverse stretch reflex operates as a feedback mechanism to control muscle tension by causing muscle relaxation before muscle force becomes so great that tendons might be torn. Clinically, the clasp-knife effect seen in spastic muscles of a patient with UMN lesion results from initial over-activation of stretch reflex followed by activation of inverse stretch reflex.

Withdrawal (Flexor) Reflex

Stimulation of cutaneous pain afferents results in flexion of the affected limb. As a result, the limb is withdrawn away from the noxious stimulus. The reflex is mediated through a polysynaptic pathway (Fig. 19.7).

Clinical Testing of Reflexes

Tendon Jerks

The tendon jerks (deep reflexes) test the integrity of stretch reflexes. When the reflex hammer is suddenly tapped on the patellar tendon of a passively stretched quadriceps muscle, the transient deformity of tendon results in a sudden but transient stretch of quadriceps. The consequent increase in

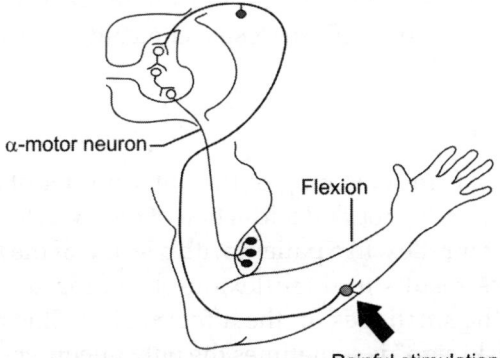

Fig. 19.7: Withdrawal reflex arc.

Table 19.1: Segmental level of various reflexes

CNS level	Reflex
Cranial nerves	
II, III	Pupillary light reflex
V, VII	Corneal
IX, X, XI	Gag
Spinal segments	
C5,6	Biceps
C6	Brachioradialis
C7	Triceps
T7–9	Upper abdominal
T10–12	Lower abdominal
L1	Cremasteric
L3,4	Knee jerk
L5,S1	Ankle jerk
L52S2	Plantar
S3,4,5	Anal

discharge in the muscle spindles located within the muscle activates stretch reflex leading to a brief contraction of quadriceps. All the tendon jerks are based on this principle. A lesion of the afferent limb or efferent limb of the reflex arc abolishes the reflex response. On the other hand, increased γ-motor discharge from the spinal cord (to the muscle spindles) produces exaggerated reflex response. Gamma-motor discharge may be increased physiologically because of mental excitement or deliberately by asking the patient to hook fingers of the two hands and pull the two hands apart. This maneuver, called "reinforcement" is used when a deep tendon jerk seems to be equivocal. In cases with upper motor neuron lesion, tendon jerks are exaggerated because of a pathologically increased γ-motor discharge.

Superficial reflexes (e.g. abdominal, plantar) are clinical equivalents of with drawal reflex. A particular superficial reflex is abolished by lower motor neuron lesion at the spinal segment involved in the reflex. In pyramidal tract lesion, all superficial reflexes are abolished on the affected side because of loss of facilitatory input from the corticospinal tract. The segmental level of various reflexes tested clinically is shown in Table 19.1.

BABINSKI SIGN

In normal adults, firm scratching of the outer border of a foot results in plantar flexion of the big toe and adduction of the small toes. This response constitutes plantar reflex. In a patient with a lesion of the pyramidal tract, similar stimulus results in dorsiflexion of the big toe and abduction ("fanning") of the small toes on the affected side. This response, called "positive Babinski sign" is sometimes the only unequivocal sign of upper motor neuron lesion.

Regulation of Muscle Tone

Muscle tone is the force with which a muscle resists being passively lengthened. It is assessed clinically by quickly extending and flexing a limb alternately and feeling the resistance offered by the muscle. The most commonly used maneuvers for the upper extremities are flexion and extension at the elbow and wrist. The most commonly used maneuvers for the lower extremities are flexion and extension at the knee and ankle. Besides the intrinsic stiffness, there is a neural component of muscle tone, i.e. the stretch reflex resists the passive increase in muscle length.

The sensitivity of spinal stretch reflex mediating the muscle tone is modulated by a number of supraspinal centers, namely, brainstem reticular formation (through descending facilitatory and inhibitory reticulospinal tract), vestibular nuclei, basal ganglia, cerebellum and cerebral cortex (Fig. 19.8).

Inhibitory signals arrive at gamma neurons through the lateral reticulospinal tract from Brodmann area 6, the paleocerebellum and the red nucleus. Facilitatory signals arrive through the ventral reticulospinal tract from Brodmann area 4, the neocerebellum and the vestibular nucleus.

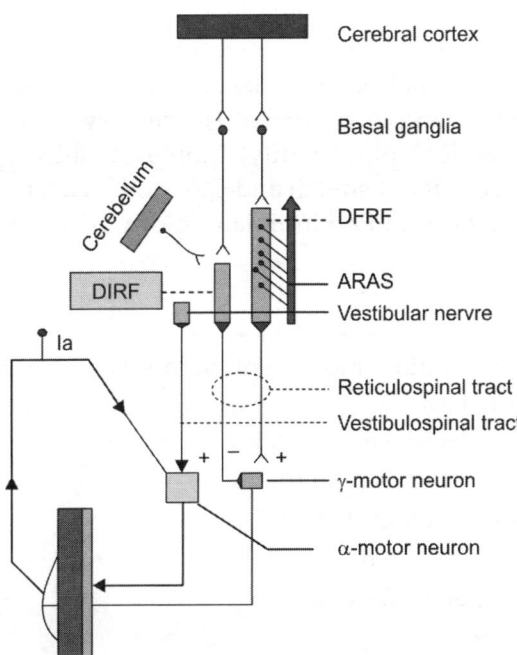

Fig. 19.8: Supraspinal control over stretch reflex. DFRF: descending facilitatory reticular formation; DIRF: descending inhibitory reticular formation; ARAS: ascending reticular activating system.

Disorders of Muscle Tone

Since the stretch reflex is the basis of muscle tone, it would be decreased whenever there is a lesion of any part of its reflex arc. Thus hypotonia is a prominent feature of lesions of ventral horn cells (lower motor neuron paralysis) or a lesion of sensory fibers (polyneuropathy). In cerebellar lesions also hypotonia is a prominent feature since α–β linkage, a prominent function of cerebellum is affected.

Hypertonia may be due to an upper motor neuron lesion, e.g. vascular lesion in the internal capsule (spasticity, or clasp-knife rigidity) or a basal ganglion disorder, e.g. Parkinson disease (lead-pipe rigidity).

Spasticity results from relative overactivity of supraspinal facilitatory control over γ-motor neurons resulting in oversensitivity of stretch reflex. Such response is typical of upper motor neuron type of paralysis. Spasticity is characterized by marked resistance at the beginning of passive flexion but the resistance suddenly disappears when greater force is used to produce flexion (clasp knife effect). In spastic muscles, the resistance varies with the speed of passive movement, i.e. rapidly executed passive movement at the joint meets greater resistance than a slow one. This response is due to strong activation stretch reflex initially and activation of inverse stretch reflex subsequently. Spasticity can be demonstrated especially in extensor muscles of the lower limbs and flexor muscles of the upper limbs (anti-gravity muscles). Spasticity is associated with exaggerated tendon jerks. Tendon jerks are clinical test of stretch reflex.

In *Parkinsonian rigidity* flexor muscles are involved more than extensors, both in upper limbs and lower limbs. The rigidity lasts throughout the passive movement (lead-pipe rigidity). Moreover, unlike spasticity, there is little effect of velocity of stretch and clasp knife effect is not observed. The physiological basis of Parkinsonian rigidity is yet not clear.

TREMOR

The oscillatory involuntary movements across a joint are called a tremor. Tremor is classified as:
- *Tremor at rest:* Parkinsonian tremor.
- *Tremor on movement:* Action tremor
   i. Postural or physiologic tremor
   ii. Essential (familial) tremor
   iii. Cerebellar (intention) tremor

Resting Tremor

Resting tremor is pathognomonic of Parkinson disease. It typically involves *distal muscles of the hands ("pill-rolling movements")*. Parkinsonian tremor are coarse and slow (4–6 Hz). Parkinsonian tremor disappear when the muscle is put to voluntary motor activity. Thus a patient, whose hand is shaking badly, may pick up a cup of tea, take it to the lips and drink with out spilling a drop.

The exact pathophysiology of parkinsonian tremor is not clear. The EMG records an alternating activity in agonists and antagonist muscles. The oscillations seem to be generated centrally, probably involving thalamocortical activity. Parkinsonian tremor is reduced by dopamine replacement therapy. A surgical lesion of ventrolateral thalamic nucleus abolishes tremor on the contralateral side. Besides resting tremor, a patient of Parkinson disease may also suffer from exaggerated physiologic tremor (Fig. 19.9).

Physiologic Tremor

A small degree of tremor is present in normal individuals which may be unmasked by fatigue, hypoglycemia, CNS stimulants, alcohol hangover or hyperthyroidism. Physiologic tremor is fine and relatively rapid oscillations (8–12 Hz), seen when an individual is doing some delicate task or asked to hold an outstretched arm (postural tremor). The tremor disappears when the muscle is relaxed (Fig. 19.9).

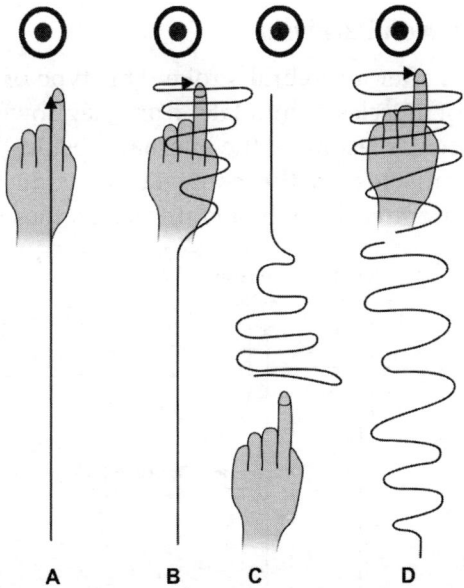

Fig. 19.9: Characteristics of different type of tremor. (A) Normal: Smooth trajectory throughout movement. (B) Cerebellar syndrome: Tremor increase in amplitude as finger approaches target. (C) Parkinsonism: Tremor may be present at initiation of movement, but smoothen out as finger approaches target. (D) Essential tremor: Low-amplitude fast tremor throughout trajectory which may worsen as finger approaches target.

Physiologic tremor seems to be caused by a mechanism at spinal cord level. It can be expected from the basic feedback sensory control over all motor activities. A slight delay in feedback sensory and motor elements of the loop would result in fine tremor, which is unmasked only by factors mentioned above.

Essential (Familial Tremor)

Essential/familial tremor commonly involves the head where it produces nodding or "no-no" effect. Parkinsonian tremor usually spare the head. Essential tremor are usually slower and have greater amplitude than physiology tremor. The exact mechanism of essential tremor is not clear (Fig. 19.9). Due to some unknown reason, essential tremor is suppressed by alcohol.

Cerebellar Tremor

Cerebellar tremor are slower, side-to-side oscillations when a voluntary movement is performed. The term "intention tremor" is a misnomer because there is no tremor on merely having an intention for voluntary movements. The tremor amplitude increases as goal is approached (Fig. 19.9). Cerebellar tremor is caused by a defective cerebellar servo-mechanism (Fig. 19.10).

Upper Motor Neuron Paralysis

It is typically seen after a cerebral stroke. This type of paralysis always involves a group of muscles. Contralateral arm, leg, lower face and tongue are affected in vascular lesions of the internal capsule. Paralysis does not involve all the muscles on the contralateral side to same degree. Movements that are invariably bilateral, such as those of the eyes, jaw,

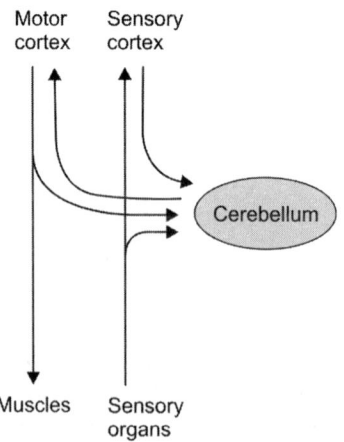

Fig. 19.10: Cerebellar servo mechanism.

pharynx, larynx, neck, thorax and abdomen are usually unaffected because these muscles have bilateral cortical control.

Just after the cerebral stroke, there is a total paralytic flaccidity of muscles and areflexia (stage of spinal shock). After a few days or weeks, flaccidity disappears, motor tone returns, and gradually spasticity becomes a prominent feature. In patients with paresis (not paralysis), spasticity may add to the difficulty in performance of voluntary movements. Drugs that decrease spasticity may be of help in such patients. In hemiplegia, discrete movements of the hands and fingers are lost, but voluntary control over proximal muscles of the limbs is maintained. Synergistic movements ultimately become prominent. For example, in the upper limb, an effort to grasp an object results in flexion of the wrist, pronation and flexion of elbow and elevation and abduction of shoulder. Attempt at pushing with hand results in pronation of the hand, extension of wrist and elbow, adduction of upper arm and lowering of shoulder. Similar synergism is seen in lower limbs. Here extensor synergism is more powerful and facilitates weight bearing and walking. These synergisms indicate that corticospinal lesions diminish voluntary control on anterior horn cells and augment reflex synergistic discharge on the motor neuron pool.

Lower Motor Neuron Paralysis

Damage to the ventral horn cells or a lesion of anterior root or motor nerve produces paresis or paralysis. This type of paralysis is characterized by loss of all movements, voluntary, postural or reflex. The absence of stretch reflex produces hypotonia (or atonia), flaccidity of muscles and absence of tendon jerks in the concerned muscle. The denervated muscle undergoes atrophy (Table 19.2).

Muscle fasciculations. This term is used to describe the twitching of paralyzed muscle. Fasciculation is a spontaneous, isolated contraction (twitch) of individual motor units. The sign is seen only when there is a slow degeneration of the motor neuron, e.g. motor neuron disease.

Table 19.2: Comparison of clinical features of upper motor neuron (UMN) paralysis and lower motor neuron (LMN) paralysis (+ : present; – : absent)

	UMN paralysis	LMN paralysis
Loss of voluntary control	+	+
Lesion	Pyramidal tract	Ventral horn cell or motor nerve
Distribution	Diffuse or patchy	Segmental
Muscle tone	Increased (spasticity)	Decreased (flaccidity)
Tendon jerks	Exaggerated	Absent in concerned muscle
Superficial reflexes	Absent	Absent in concerned muscle
Babinski sign	+	–
Muscle wasting	–	+
Muscle fasciculations	–	+

Fasciculation is more often seen with nerve root compression than it is with more distal peripheral nerve compression.

A lesion in the internal capsule typically produces UMN type of paralysis on the contralateral side of the body. A lesion in the spinal cord produces a combination of LMN paralysis in the muscle innervated by the damaged spinal segment(s), and UMN paralysis in the muscles innervated by spinal segments below the level of the lesion. A lesion in the brainstem would produce LMN paralysis in muscles supplied by the concerned cranial nerve(s) and UMN paralysis of muscles of the upper and lower limb(s).

Further Reading

Muscle tone-spinal reflexeswww.neuro physiology.ws/muscletone.htm
Viktor's Notes—**UMN&LMN Disorders**—www.neurosurgeryresident.net

20. Cerebrovascular Accidents

GENERAL CONSIDERATIONS

The brain receives blood supply from four arteries, the two internal carotids and the two vertebral arteries. Internal carotid artery gives off anterior cerebral artery and the trunk that remains is designated as middle cerebral artery (Fig. 20.1). The two anterior cerebral arteries run along the corpus callosum. They supply blood to the medial aspect of frontal lobe, cingulate gyrus and anterior portion of corpus callosum. Therefore, leg area of primary motor cortex and somatosensory cortex and supplementary motor area are in the territory of anterior cerebral cortex.

The middle cerebral artery runs along the Sylvian fissure and supplies blood to the lateral aspect of cerebral cortex. Therefore, territory of middle

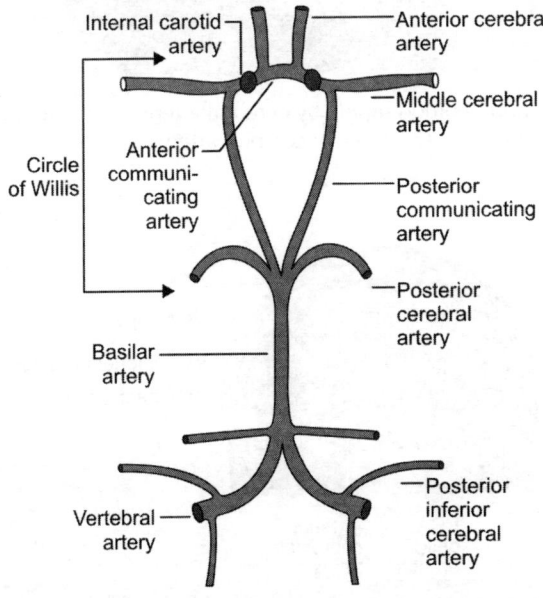

Fig. 20.1: The circle of Willis.

cerebral artery includes face, arm and trunk areas of sensory-motor homunculi, parts of frontal, parietal and temporal lobes adjacent to the Sylvian fissure, including basal ganglia and internal capsule (Figs 20.2 and 20.3).

The two vertebral arteries supply blood to upper spinal cord, medulla and cerebellum. At the lower border of pons, the two vertebral arteries unite to form basilar artery which runs along the middle of pons and supplies to pons and cerebellum. The basilar artery divides into two posterior cerebral arteries which supply blood to midbrain, thalamus, occipital lobe, and inferior temporal lobe.

By anterior communicating artery between two anterior cerebral arteries and the posterior communicating artery between the posterior cerebral arteries, the six cerebral arteries constitute the circle of Willis. Considerable anatomic variation exists in the circle of Willis. The truth is that about two-thirds of the human population does not have a complete "circle"—most have one or more connections missing. No concrete evidence supports the view that a person with an incomplete circle of Willis is at greater risk for strokes.

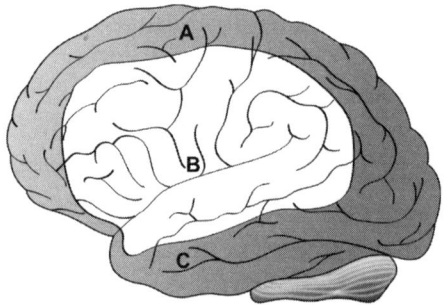

Fig. 20.2: Distribution of blood supply by cerebral arteries. (A) anterior cerebral artery; (B) middle cerebral artery; (C) posterior cerebral artery.

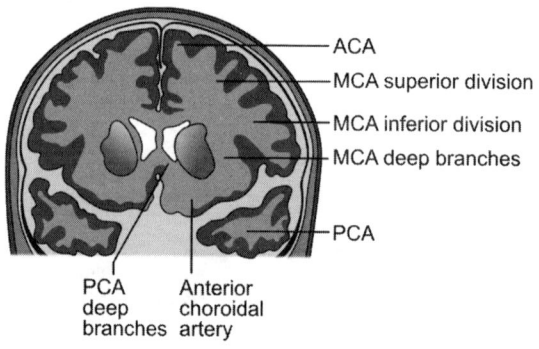

Fig. 20.3: Territories of anterior cerebral artery (ACA), middle cerebral artery (MCA) and posterior cerebral artery (PCA) shown in coronal section of brain.

CEREBRAL BLOOD FLOW

The brain receives approximately 800 ml of blood per minute (50–60 ml/100 gm/min), which reflects fairly high metabolic demand (oxygen consumption) of the brain. The cerebral metabolism, hence cerebral blood flow, does not vary with the mental activity. Only extreme conditions like general anesthesia or a seizure causes a large decrease or increase in cerebral blood flow, respectively. The constant rate of cerebral blood flow is maintained by the autoregulation of blood flow, mediated through vasodilator metabolites, chiefly CO_2. Variations in arterial pCO_2 produce significant variations in cerebral blood flow. Local tissue hypoxia also produces vasodilatation.

The autoregulation of cerebral blood flow normally operates between 60–150 mmHg blood pressure. Outside this range, cerebral blood flow passively and linearly follows the blood pressure. In chronic hypertension, the curve is shifted to the right (Fig. 20.4). As a result, even a mild hypotension may be more damaging than that in normotensive individuals.

Cerebral autoregulation is ineffective in patients with cerebral injury due to trauma, hemorrhage or ischemic stroke. Such patients revert to passive near-linear relationship between the arterial blood pressure and cerebral blood flow. Hence, such patients are not only more prone to hypotensive cerebral damage, but also non-responsive to therapeutic alterations in the cerebral blood flow.

The factor most important to cerebral circulation is cerebral perfusion pressure and not blood pressure as such. Perfusion pressure is the difference between mean arterial pressure (MAP) and venous blood pressure values. Because pressure in the cerebral venous system approximates intracranial pressure (ICP), cerebral perfusion pressure is usually calculated as MAP–ICP. An important consequence is that patients with increased ICP should never undergo deliberate hypotension before the dura is opened unless measurement of ICP is available before the surgical procedure. Higher cerebral perfusion pressure is required for patients with chronic hypertension and altered cerebral autoregulation.

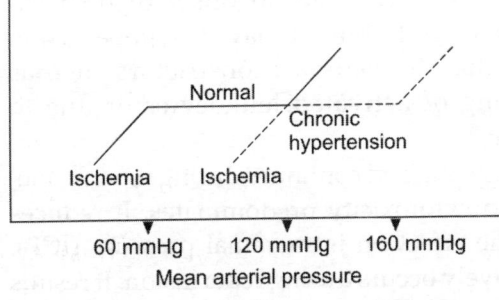

Fig. 20.4: Autoregulation of cerebral blood flow in a normal individual (——) and in a patient of chronic hypertension (-----).

Tissue Level Effects of Cerebral Ischemia

An interruption of blood flow to the brain for more than 10 seconds causes unconsciousness. Interruption of blood flow more than a few minutes may result in irreversible brain damage. In the nervous tissue, neurons are by far more vulnerable to hypoxia than glial cells. Most vulnerable are pyramidal neurons of the hippocampus followed by neurons of cerebellum, striatum and neocortex.

Normal cerebral blood flow has a moderate margin of safety for most of the physiologic variations. When the blood flow drops to 50% of normal, symptoms often begin. A drop below 30% of normal produces profound functional disturbance (electrical failure) but the tissue is still viable. At this stage, there is attenuation of EEG and absence of cerebral evoked potentials. Cerebral blood flow below 15% of normal results in irreversible brain damage as shown by ionic failure caused by deficiency of ATP and hence failure of ATP-driven Na^+–K^+ pump. K^+ leaks out of neurons. Glial mechanisms for glutamate uptake do not function consequently; excess glutamate opens membrane channels leading to intracellular accumulation of Na^+ and Ca^{++}. The entry of Ca^{++} into the cells is destructive. Some degree of intracellular acidosis also occurs due to anaerobic glucose metabolism to lactate, which hastens cellular death.

Effects of Global Cerebral Ischemia

Global cerebral ischemia means diminished blood flow over the entire brain. It is common in patients who have suffered cardiac arrest, shock, asphyxia or during complex cardiac surgery. Neurological symptoms include unconsciousness, coma, seizers, ischemic stroke, and delirium and neurocognitive impairment. Focal cerebral ischemia involves reduction in cerebral blood flow (CBF) in a specific vascular territory and is typically encountered in cerebral strokes due to thromboembolism in cerebral vessels.

Reperfusion injury: Restoration of cerebral blood flow after cardiac arrest allows reperfusion of the ischemic region. Reperfusion itself results in many pathophysiologic responses harmful to the neurons. Immediately after the onset of reperfusion, CBF is greater than normal for several minutes. This stage is followed by a gradual onset of delayed hypoperfusion which may last several hours. Delayed hypoperfusion possibly results from endothelial-derived vasoconstrictors such as endothelin, or due to clumping of activated leukocytes or due to coagulation in microvasculature.

Brain edema begins during ischemia and continues during reperfusion. During ischemia, swelling from cytotoxicity predominates. It reduces intracellular space and has little effect on intracranial pressure (ICP). Vasogenic edema almost exclusively occurs during reperfusion. It results

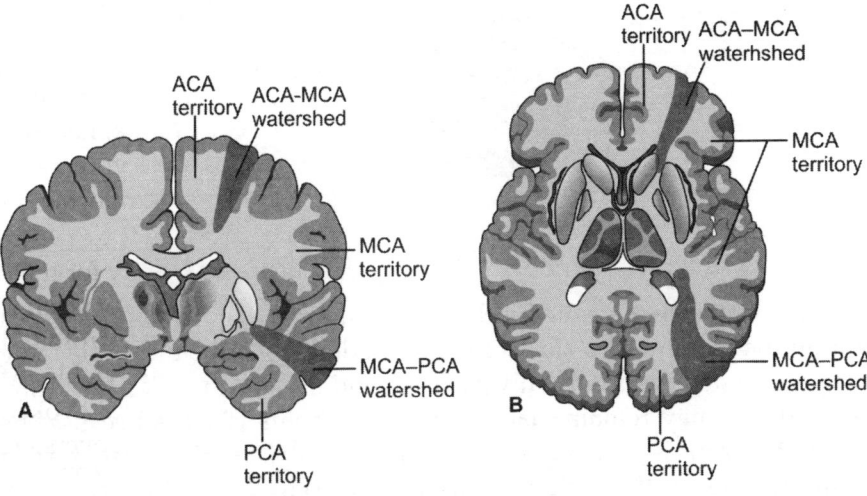

Fig. 20.5: Watershed areas in coronal section (A) and axial section (B) of brain.

from damage to blood–brain barrier during ischemia and reperfusion injury.

Global ischemia causes greatest damage to areas between the territories of major cerebral and cerebellar arteries, known as the watershed areas. The parieto-temporal-occipital triangle at the junction of anterior, middle and posterior cerebral arteries is most commonly affected (Fig. 20.5). Infarction of watershed area causes paralysis and loss of sensation involving arm; face is not affected and speech is spared.

Acute Ischemic Stroke

Cerebral strokes are examples of focal ischemia. The occlusion of a cerebral blood vessel usually because of a thrombosis/embolism initiates a series of events which end up as irreversible neuronal death (cerebral infarction) in the territory of the blood vessel. In the cerebral tissue, a series of changes occur in the neurons, glial cells and other structural components which progress from an initial loss of function to complete structural death and cellular death. In other words, unlike what is generally assumed, cerebral infarction is not an "all or none" episode that produces instantaneous maximum damage. In fact, the effects of thrombosis or embolism progress over time. In clinical practice, efforts are being made to devise a therapeutic approach that may minimize or even reverse the effects of cerebral ischemia. In this context, the concept of ischemic penumbra is important.

Ischemic penumbra: Focal ischemia, as occurs during a cerebral stroke, results in a series zones with varying degree of hypoperfusion. The central core of the affected area consists of area of complete cell death (ischemic necrosis). Outside the core, there is a zone of electrically non-functional,

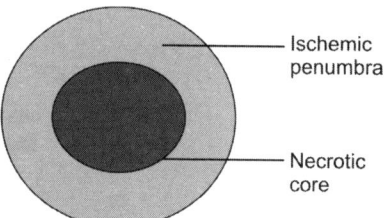

Fig. 20.6: The ischemic penumbra.

but still viable tissue called ischemic penumbra (Fig. 20.6). Brain cells within the penumbra, a rim of mild to moderately ischemic tissue lying between tissue that is normally perfused and the area in which infarction is evolving, may remain viable for several hours. That is because the penumbral zone is supplied with blood by collateral arteries anastomosing with branches of the occluded vascular tree (Fig. 20.7). However, even cells in this region will die if reperfusion is not established during the early hours since collateral circulation is inadequate to maintain the neuronal demand for oxygen and glucose indefinitely.

Stroke therapy is mostly directed at rescue of this zone by increasing oxygen delivery and decreasing tissue acidosis. The neurons of the ischemic penumbra are vulnerable to further assaults that may occur because of hypovolemia secondary to dehydration, medications that lower blood pressure or even standing up quickly. The penumbra area can be saved from becoming a necrotic area by avoiding these assaults. The size and the fate of zone of ischemic penumbra varies in different patients of ischemic strokes and possible explains the large variation in permanent effects of ischemic attack.

Intracerebral Hemorrhage

Intracranial hemorrhage may be a cerebral hemorrhage (an **intra-axial hemorrhage**); that is, it occurs within the brain tissue (intracerebral

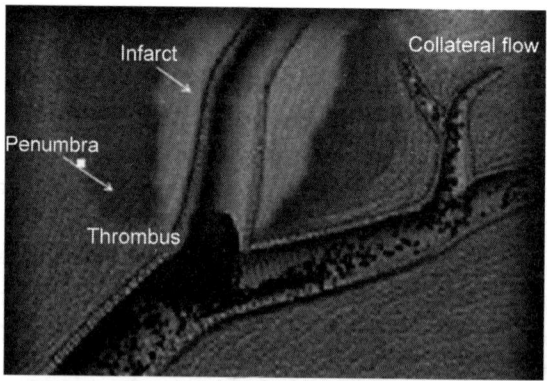

Fig. 20.7: Anatomic basis of ischemic penumbra.

hemorrhage—ICH) or extra-axial hemorrhage, which all occur within the skull but outside of the brain tissue. Predilection sites for intracerebral hemorrhage include the basal ganglia (40–50%), lobar regions (20–50%), thalamus (10–15%), pons (5–12%), cerebellum (5–10%), and other brainstem sites (1–5%).

Unlike the declining mortality with subarachnoid hemorrhage (SAH) due to improvements in surgical and critical care techniques, the morbidity and mortality of ICH have remained relatively unchanged throughout the past several decades.

Hypertension is the most important cause of CH. Risk of ICH appears to be related to the severity and the duration of hypertension. Control of hypertension notably decreases the risk of ICH.

PATHOPHYSIOLOGY

Intracerebral hemorrhage secondary to hypertension occurs in areas of the brain that are perfused by the perforating arteries that arise directly from the large basal cerebral arteries. These perforating arteries are directly exposed to the effects of hypertension because they lack the protection normally afforded by a preceding gradual decrease in vessel caliber. Chronic hypertension induces a series of pathologic changes that lead to segmental constriction of these vessels. This process is called lipohyalinosis.

Lipohyalinosis represents two pathologic processes that include atherosclerosis of the larger perforating arteries and arteriolosclerosis of the smaller perforating vessels. Atherosclerosis occurs most commonly at the branch points of vessels and is characterized by subintimal fibroblast proliferation accompanied by deposition of lipid-filled macrophages. Arteriolosclerosis involves the replacement of smooth muscle cells in the tunica media with collagen. These processes result in the development of noncompliant, narrowed vessels that are susceptible to both sudden closure (lacunar infarction) or rupture (ICH). The mechanism of actual hemorrhage is presumably due to rupture of these fragile vessels, but this has been difficult to prove pathologically. Cerebral microaneurysms, are described in only a small number of patients.

A substantial amount of tissue damage occurs after an initial hemorrhage. CH was once considered to be a simple monophasic event that produced neural damage by mass effect of expanding hematoma. However, animal models have failed to reveal a local pressure effect of an introduced non-hemorrhagic focal mass. Now, with CT scans, ICH has been shown to be a dynamic response that gradually evolves to produce neural damage. Three important phases include:

  a. *Expansion of hematoma:* Most hematomas result from rupture of an artery or an arteriole. Their expansion is most likely to be due to

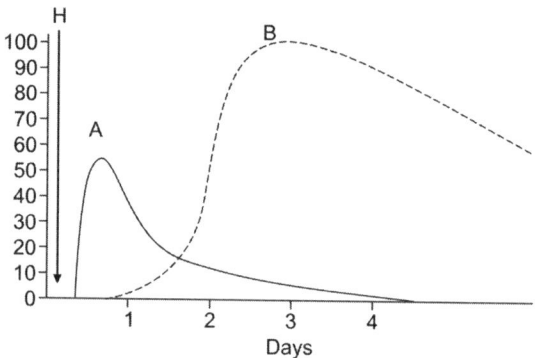

Fig. 20.8: Time-course of different mechanisms of edema after intracerebral hemorrhage (H). (A) Edema due to osmotic effect of clot. (B) Edema due to cytotoxicity because of degradation product of red cell lysis and thrombin.

continuous bleeding from the primary source or due to mechanical rupture of surrounding blood vessels.

b. *Brain edema:* Neurologic deterioration after this point often is attributed to the development of cerebral edema which appears within hours secondary to clot retraction with extrusion of plasma proteins into the underlying white matter..

c. *Cytotoxic products:* Thrombin may contribute directly to neural toxicity or indirectly through damage to the blood–brain barrier with subsequent worsening of vasogenic edema. Peak edema occurs 3 to 7 days after the hemorrhage and correlates with lysis of red blood cells. Both hemoglobin and its degradation products have been implicated in direct and indirect neural toxicity (Fig. 20.8). The importance of the development of cerebral edema in ICH has been supported by retrospective evidence suggesting that patients with a larger amount of cerebral edema relative to the initial hemorrhage volume have worse clinical outcomes.

The recent advances in the pathophysiology of intracerebral hemorrhage discussed above are likely to lead to better therapeutic measures in the management of patients with intracerebral hemorrhage.

Further Reading

Bergman, RA; Afifi, AK; Miyauchi, R; **Circle of Willis. Illustrated Encyclopedia of Human Anatomic Variation**, URL: http://www.anatomyatlases.org/AnatomicVariants/Cardiovascular/Text/Arteries/CircleofWillis.shtml

Harukuni, A; Bhardwaj, A. **Mechanisms of brain injury after global cerebral ischemia**. *NeurolClin* 2006; 24:1–21.

Manno, EM, et al. **Emerging medical and surgical management strategies in the evaluation and treatment of intracerebral hemorrhage**.*Mayo Clin Proc.*, 2005; 80:420–433.

Chakrabarty, A.; Shivane, A. **Pathology of intracerebral hemorrhage.** *ACNR* 2008; 20:20–21.

21. Disorders of Consciousness

RETICULAR ACTIVATING SYSTEM

The mid-ventral core of the brainstem contains a complex network of cells and fibers which extends into diencephalon above and spinal cord below. It contains specific anatomically well-defined collection of neurons, e.g. cranial nerve nuclei. In addition, there are aggregates of neurons, though not having well-defined anatomic entity, have well-defined physiologic functions, e.g. respiratory center, cardiovascular center. Besides these anatomic and physiologic groups of cells, there is a complex network of neurons that constitutes the brainstem reticular formation. Among the cells of reticular formation, a group of neurons form a descending system while others constitute an ascending system. The descending system, known as reticulospinal tract, is a component of extrapyramidal tracts, which is primarily involved in regulation of muscle tone. The ascending system constitutes what is known as reticular activation system (RAS). RAS is a polysynaptic pathway that extends from brainstem reticular formation to non-specific thalamic nuclei and then projects diffusely to all over cerebral cortex (Fig. 21.1). The long ascending

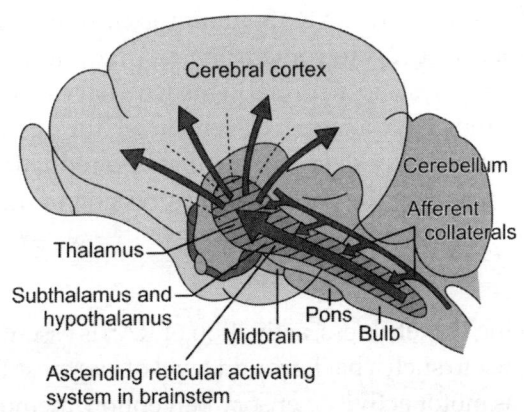

Fig. 21.1: The brainstem reticular activating system.

sensory tracts, as they ascend in the brainstem, give collaterals to RAS. Visual, auditory and olfactory tracts also give collaterals to RAS. Thus, neurons of RAS can be excited non-specifically by any of the sensations, especially pain. Stimulation of RAS causes an immediate and marked activation of cerebral cortex leading to arousal, if the subject is asleep. The cerebral cortical function of control of movement, speech, somatosensory perception, etc. is localized to well-defined areas of cerebral cortex. In contrast, wakefulness is related, in semi-quantitative way to the total mass of cerebral cortex and its connections to RAS. Coma may result from an interruption of RAS pathways or a generalized hemispherical lesion or a cerebral metabolic derangement, e.g. encephalitis, global cerebral ischemia, narcotic poisoning of severe hypoglycemia, etc.

Experimental work in animals suggests that the following structures play key roles in the maintenance and modulation of wakefulness: cholinergic neurons in the upper brainstem and basal forebrain; noradrenergic neurons, in particular the locus ceruleus; a histaminergic projection from the posterior hypothalamus; and probably dopaminergic and serotonergic pathways arising from the brainstem.

Functions of RAS

a. *Sleep–Wakefulness Cycles*

There are distinct differences in the brain's electrical activity during periods of wakefulness and sleep: Low voltage fast burst brain waves (EEG desynchronization) are associated with wakefulness; large voltage slow waves are found during non-REM sleep stimulation of the RAS in a sleeping individual produces EEG desynchronization and arousal.

The physiological change from a state of deep sleep to wakefulness is reversible and mediated by the RAS. Inhibitory influence from the brain, active at sleep onset, seems to come from the preoptic area (POA) of the hypothalamus. During sleep, neurons in the RAS have a much lower firing rate; conversely, they have a higher activity level during the waking state. In order that the brain may sleep, there must be a reduction in ascending afferent activity reaching the cortex by suppression of the RAS.

b. *Alertness*

Besides producing wakefulness, activation of RAS is essential for bringing the cerebral cortex to such a background level of alertness that other brain functions such as motor activity, sensory perception, memory and abstract thinking, etc. are possible.

DISORDERS OF CONSCIOUSNESS

The highest level of altered consciousness is lethargy, in which there is decreased responsiveness, although the patient remains arousable. Stupor is a slightly more diminished level of awareness, there is less meaningful cortical interaction. The eyes remain open in stupor allowing stimulation of the reticular activating system. Coma refers to an even more diminished state of consciousness, in which the patient is unarousable to external stimuli of any kind. Sleep-wake cycles are absent in coma. A hallmark of coma is the lack of eye opening.

- **Coma:** The patient usually cannot be aroused, and the eyes do not open in response to any stimulation.
- **Stupor:** The patient can be awakened only by vigorous physical stimulation.

Coma

Sleep is a state of unconsciousness from which a person can be readily aroused by appropriate sensory stimulation. Coma is defined as a pathological loss of consciousness. Basically, coma may result from two causes: (i) due to diffuse cerebral cortical failure and (ii) due to a failure of brainstem arousal mechanism.

I. *Coma due to Diffuse Cerebral Cortical Failure*

1. Metabolic or toxic encephalopathy
   - Narcotic poisoning
   - Hypoglycemia
   - Ketotic coma
   - Hyperosmolar coma
   - Hepatic coma
   - Uremic com
   - Hypercapnic coma
   - Myxedema coma
   - Severe hyponatremia
2. Seizures
3. Hypothermia
4. Heat stroke
5. Viral encephalitis
6. Meningitis

The above mentioned conditions produce a variety of metabolic derangements in the nervous tissue (both neurons and astrocytes). Although the exact derangement is likely to be different in each case, the

net effect is neuronal failure through one or more of the following mechanisms:
- Impaired supply of energy
- A change in the resting membrane potential
- Impaired release of neurotransmitters
- A morphological change

In all cases of coma mentioned above, brainstem reflexes are normal. CT scan is also normal.

II. Coma due to Failure of Brainstem Arousal Mechanism

a. *Primary brainstem failure:* Basilar artery stroke, pontine hemorrhage or destruction of brainstem by a posterior fossa tumor disrupts the brainstem arousal mechanism. Absence of brainstem reflexes (pupillary light reflex, corneal reflex, oculocephalic reflex and vestibulo-ocular reflex) is indicative of this type of lesion.

b. *Brainstem dysfunction due a space occupying lesion:* An expanding mass in a cerebral hemisphere can cause displacement of vital structures involved in arousal mechanism. The intracranial compartment has a limited capacity to accommodate a space occupying lesion. When a mass in a hemisphere grows to occupy 30–60 ml of space, some other tissue has to get displaced. The displacement of a temporal lobe through the tentorium causes compression of brainstem structures. This mechanism accounts for about 15% of cases of coma. Subdural hemorrhage, intracranial hemorrhage and brain tumor cause coma by this mechanism.

c. *Surgical coma:* Concussion causes transient coma probably from torsion of hemispheres at the brainstem-diencephalon junction leading to a brief interruption of function of RAS. The mechanism of persistent coma after head trauma is more complex.

SYNCOPE

Syncope is the term used to describe an acute temporary loss of consciousness with spontaneous recovery caused by short-term cerebral hypoperfusion. Syncope should be differentiated from other causes of transient loss of consciousness (T-LOC) such as seizures, hypoglycemia, hyperventilation, episodic weakness, concussion or narcolepsy.

In all forms of syncope, cerebral hypoperfusion is the common denominator (Fig. 21.2). Transient cerebral hypoperfusion produces unconsciousness by a brief reduction in oxygen supply to the parts of the brain sub-serving consciousness. The causes of syncope may vary from most benign vasovagal attack to most serious disorders such as a decrease in cardiac output (MI, Stokes-Adams syndrome, tachyarrhythmias), or a

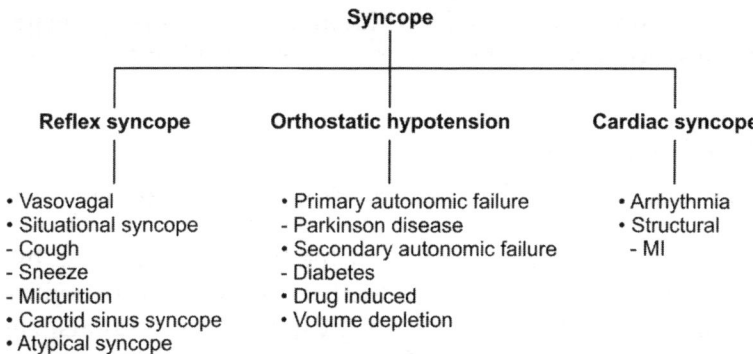

Fig. 21.2: Classification of causes of syncope.

decrease in cerebral blood flow (transient ischemic attack, vertebra-basilar artery insufficiency). In all types of syncope, the loss of consciousness is caused by hypoperfusion of the brain.

Vasovagal syncope is due to a disorder of autonomic control of the cardiovascular system. It commonly occurs in normal people of all ages. Precipitating factors include alcohol consumption, fatigue, pain, hunger, and prolonged standing. It can also be triggered by situations causing anxiety, such as having blood drawn, as well as by hot or crowded situations. The pathophysiology of the hypotension/bradycardia reflex responsible for vasovagal syncope is not completely understood. The main trigger for this reflex loops seems to be a reduction in venous return during upright position. Factors which augment this reflex response include extravascular factors such as a warm environment or psychological stress. In the first moments of a vasovagal syncope an empty heart is seen in echocardiographic investigations because of an acute loss of preload ('empty heart' syndrome). According to one hypothesis, the initial responses appear to be venous pooling and increased activity of the sympathetic nervous system. This causes the heart to contract forcefully while relatively empty, triggering stimulation of ventricular mechanoreceptors leading to Bezold Jarisch reflex response. This reduces sympathetic activity and stimulates parasympathetic activity, resulting in bradycardia and vasodilation, followed by syncope (Fig. 21.3C). This mechanism is probably not the only explanation. Many of inciting factors, such as hunger or anxiety, sight of blood, etc. do not involve venous pooling. Also, patients with transplanted hearts (which are not innervated) also exhibit vasovagal syncope-like episodes. Although presentation of reflex syncope is similar to that of other types of syncope, loss of consciousness in patients with vasovagal syncope may be preceded by prodromata such as nausea, diaphoresis, lightheadedness, blurred vision, headaches, palpitations, paresthesias, and pallor, which usually occur in the upright position and resolve almost immediately when the patient assumes the supine position. In addition, after recovery, patients with vasovagal syncope may complain of a "washed out" and tired feeling.

Orthostatic Hypotension

A change from supine to standing posture results in gravitational pooling of blood in the veins of the lower limb ("venous pooling"). As a result, capacity of veins in the lower half of the body may increase by 300–800 ml. Reduced venous return to the heart leads to decreased cardiac output and fall in blood pressure. In normal individuals, serious hypotension and hypoperfusion of the brain is prevented by baroreceptor-mediated increase in vasomotor increase in sympathetic discharge to the heart and blood vessels (Fig. 21. 3A). A failure of this compensatory mechanism may occur due to primary or secondary autonomic failure leading to a significant fall blood pressure, cerebral hypoperfusion and syncope (Figs 21.3B and 21.4).

Autonomic failure may be primary (earlier called idiopathic orthostatic hypotension) or secondary to some metabolic disease such as diabetes mellitus. Orthostatic hypotension is only one of the numerous manifestations of autonomic failure such as disturbed bowel, bladder, sudomotor, thermoregulatory, and sexual function. Symptoms are slow

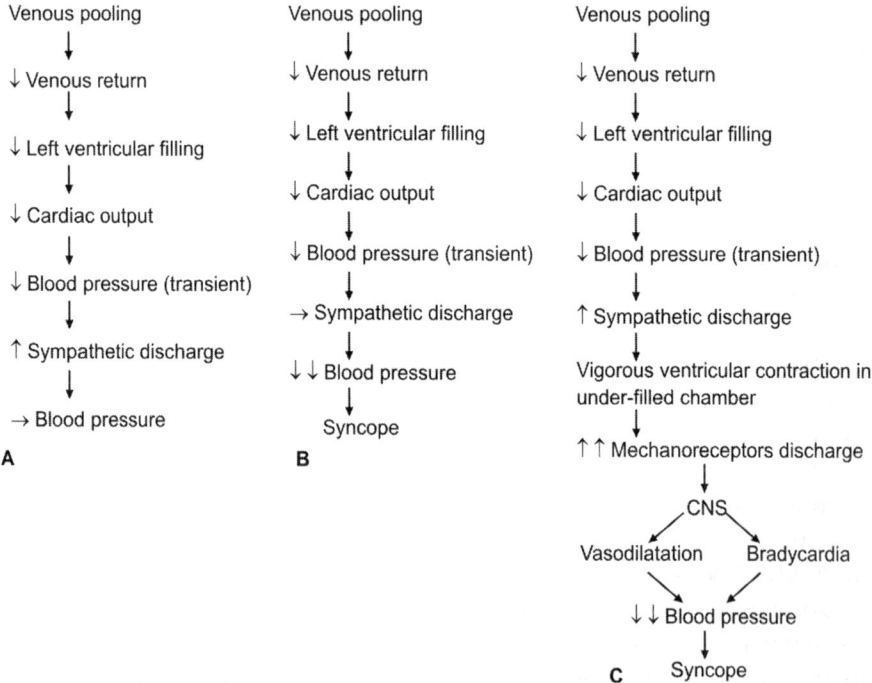

Fig. 21.3: Response to change of posture from supine to standing in a normal individual (A), a patient of orthostatic hypotension (B) and vasovagal syncope (C).

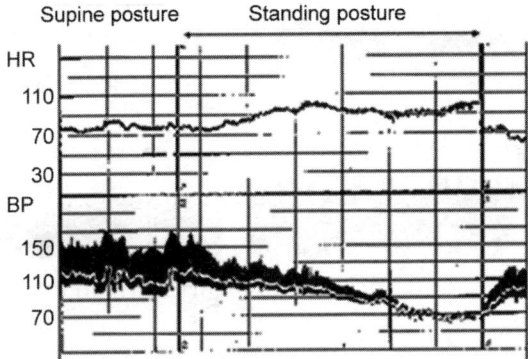

Fig. 21.4: Effect of a change from supine to standing posture on blood pressure and heart rate in a patient of orthostatic hypotension.

and insidious in onset, usually beginning with vague complaints of orthostatic weakness, dizziness, and lightheadedness that are often dismissed by physicians as insignificant. As their orthostatic hypotension worsens, patients experience near syncope or syncope, which often prompts the patient to seek initial medical attention. In men, the earliest symptoms of autonomic failure are impotence and loss of libido, whereas in women, urinary retention and incontinence occur first. Although PAF may lead to severe functional impairment, only rarely is it fatal.

Postural Tachycardia Syndrome (POTS)

Failure of the regulatory mechanism to respond properly to change from supine to standing posture may lead to either *orthostatic hypotension*, as is seen in autonomic failure, or *orthostatic tachycardia*, as is seen in POTS. Orthostatic hypotension is defined as a fall in pressure on standing of more than 20/10 mmHg. However, it is common in patients with autonomic failure for the decline to be much greater than this, which may result in loss of consciousness soon after standing. On the other hand, in POTS, blood pressure is typically maintained on standing or may even increase. Heart rate rises more than 30 bpm and symptoms reminiscent of impaired cerebral perfusion may develop (Fig. 21.5).

POTS is currently defined as the presence of symptoms of orthostatic intolerance associated with a heart rate increase of 30 bpm (or rate that exceeds 120 bpm) that occurs within the first 10 minutes of standing or upright tilt, not associated with other chronic debilitating conditions such as prolonged bed rest or the use of medications known to diminish vascular or autonomic tone. It is important to recognize that this syndrome is typically disabling. Hence, the mere observation of orthostatic tachycardia is not, by itself, sufficient to make the diagnosis of POTS. Symptoms include mental clouding ("brain fog"), blurred or tunneled

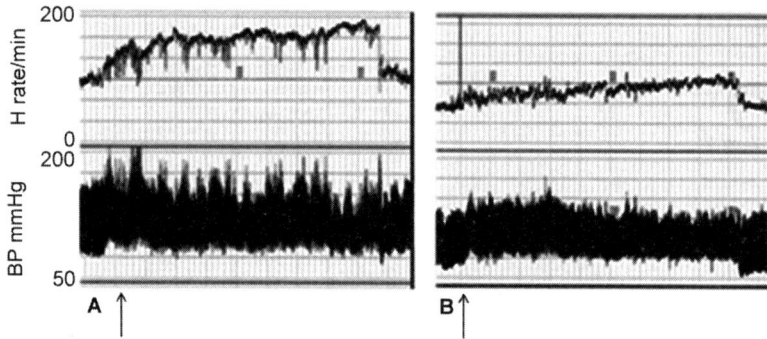

Fig. 21.5: Heart rate and blood pressure record of a patient suffering from POTS (A) and a normal individual (B). Arrow (↑) indicates the change from supine to standing posture.

vision, and shortness of breath, palpitation, tremulousness, chest discomfort, headache, lightheadedness and nausea. While pre-syncope is common in these patients, only a minority (~30%) actually pass out.

> **Further Reading**
>
> Scarabelli, CC; Scarabelli, TM. **Neurocard-iogenic syncope** BMJ. 2004; 32: 336–41.
>
> Aydin, MA, et al. **Management and therapy of vasovagal syncope: A review** *World J Cardiol. 201; 2: 308–15.*
>
> Grubb, BP. **Neurocardiogenic syncope and related disorders of orthostatic intolerance.** *Circulation 2005; 111:2997–3006.*
>
> Raj, SR. **The Postural Tachycardia Syndrome (POTS): Pathophysiology, Diagnosis and Management.** *Indian Pacing Electrophysiol. J. 2006; 6:84–99.*

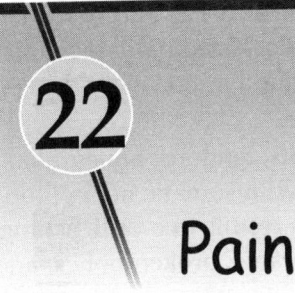

22

Pain

Pain constitutes one of the most important indications of ill-health. Pain occurs whenever tissues are damaged. Hence, pain is basically a protective mechanism of the body. It is meant to produce responses which induce the individual to get rid of the injurious stimulus. The danger of lack of pain sensation is best demonstrated in paraplegics due to spinal cord injury. Within weeks, the patient often develops ulcers on the pressure points of the body.

Nociceptive pain and **neuropathic pain** are the two main kinds of pain when the primary mechanism of production is considered (Fig. 22.1). Nociceptive pain results from stimulation of nociceptors, i.e. sensory receptors that detect tissue damage. It could be due to a chemical, thermal, or mechanical event that has the potential to damage body tissue. Neuropathic pain results from damage to pain pathways in the peripheral nerves or a part of CNS.

NOCICEPTIVE PAIN

Nociceptive pain may be classified further in three types that have distinct organic origins and felt qualities.

A. **Superficial somatic pain** (or cutaneous pain) is caused by injury to the skin or superficial tissues. Cutaneous nociceptors are present just below

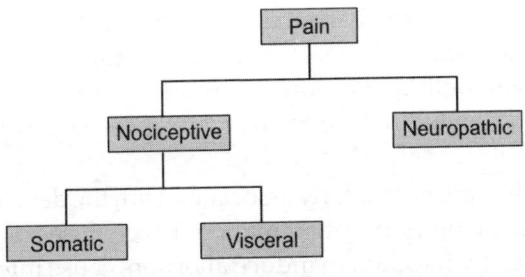

Fig. 22.1: Classification of pain.

the skin, and due to the high concentration of nerve endings, their stimulation results in a sharp, well-defined, localized pain. Examples of injuries that produce cutaneous pain include minor wounds, and minor (first degree) burns.

B. Deep somatic pain originates from ligaments, tendons, bones, blood vessels, fasciae, and muscles. It is detected with somatic nociceptors. The scarcity of pain receptors in these areas results in a dull, aching, poorly-localized pain. Examples include sprains, broken bones, and myofascial pain.

C. Visceral pain originates from body's viscera. The even greater scarcity of nociceptors in these areas produces pain that is usually more aching or cramping than somatic pain. Visceral pain may be well-localized, but more often it is not. Visceral pain may be referred to a superficial structure.

PAIN RECEPTORS

Pain receptors are *free nerve endings* of two types of nerve fibers, A-α and C fibers. High density of pain receptors is present in the superficial layers of the skin and in many deeper tissues such as periosteum, joints, arterial wall, and falx and tentorium in the cranium. Most other deeper tissues have relatively sparse pain nerve endings, but widespread tissue damage always results in pain, even in these areas. Such pain receptors may be stimulated by excessive mechanical stress, mechanical damage, extreme heat or cold or electrical damage.

Visceral pain is often due to excessive tension on nerve endings in the smooth muscle, e.g. pain due to uterine contractions during childbirth or pain due to colics of alimentary, biliary or urinary tracts.

Chemical Mediators of Pain

A number of substances normally present inside the cells, produce pain when released from damaged tissues into extracellular fluid. For example, 5-hydroxy tryptamine (5-HT), prostaglandins; K^+, AMP and ADP and acids stimulate pain nerve endings. In addition, plasma and other extracellular fluids normally contain a protein system, from which very potent pain producing plasma kinins can be formed. Bradykinin and kallidin are two well-known kinins produced from a substrate called kinogen (A = α2-globulin) by certain enzymes formed by tissue injury or inflammation.

Prostaglandins are particularly associated with the development of pain that accompanies injury or inflammation. Large doses of PGE_2 or PGF_2, given to women by injection to induce abortion, cause intense local pain. Prostaglandins can also cause headache and vascular pain when infused intravenously in man. While the doses of prostaglandins required to elicit pain are high in comparison with the concentrations expected *in vivo*, induction of hyperalgesia occurs when minute amounts of PGE_1 are given intradermal to man. Furthermore, in experiments in man where separate infusions of PGE_1, bradykinin, or histamine caused no pain, marked pain was experienced when PGE_1 was added to bradykinin or histamine. The important role of prostaglandins as the chief chemical mediator of pain shown by the fact that main mode of action of non-narcotic analgesic agents is suppression of prostaglandin synthesis.

Transmission of Pain Signals: Fast and Slow Pain

In the peripheral nerves, pain signals are transmitted through two types of fibers: (a) through fast conducting A-δ fibers and (b) through slow conducting C fibers. In the spinal cord A-δ fibers and type C fibers terminate in the dorsal gray horn. The second order neurons give rise to long axons which cross to the opposite side and ascend as lateral spinothalamic tract. Even in the spinal cord and brain stem, there seems to be a fast-acute pain pathway (composed of myelinated fibers and a slow-chronic pain pathway (composed of unmyelinated fibers).

Some of the fast conducting fibers terminate in the reticular formation of the brain stem and the rest terminate in the posterolateral ventral nucleus of the thalamus. From thalamus, some fibers relay to the somatic sensory cortex to help in the localization of pain.

Almost all the slow conducting fibers terminate in the reticular formation of the brain stem. However, sensory signals are further relayed to the nonspecific intralaminar nuclei of the thalamus, which in turn relay activating signals to all parts of the brain (Fig. 22.2).

The transmission of pain signals through two routes explains why a single prick with a sharp needle produces almost immediately sharp localized pain, followed about one second later by slowly increasing painful sensation which lasts many seconds and sometime even minutes. Fast pain plays an important role in making the person react immediately to remove himself from the stimulus. Fast pain sensation is not felt in the deeper tissues in the body. The slow type of pain is usually associated with tissue destruction. Slow pain receptors are located both in the skin and in almost any deep tissue and most of the organs.

Site of Pain Perception

Pain perception occurs at subcortical levels, i.e. in the thalamus and in the reticular formation of the brain stem. However, *cerebral cortex helps to interpret the quality and localization of pain*. Pain not only indicates the existence of tissue damage but also may prevent further damage by

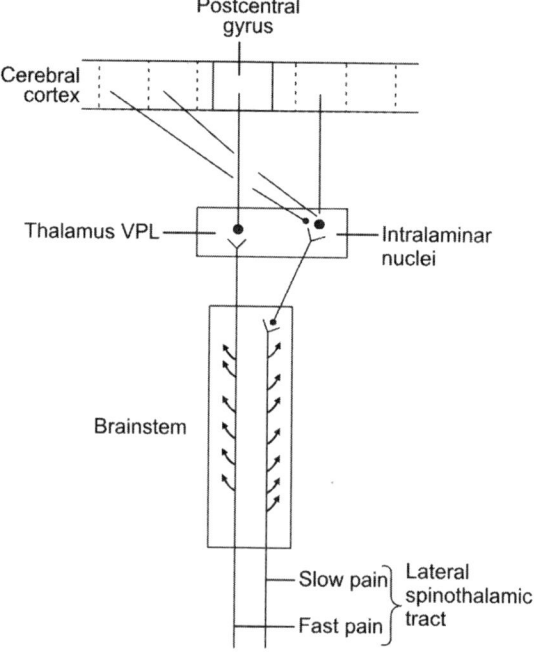

Fig. 22.2: Pathways of slow and fast pain.

initiating a withdrawal reflex or forcing the person to give rest to the affected part.

Visceral Pain

Natural stimuli associated with visceral pain are:
- Ischemia
- Hollow organ distension
- Inflammation
- Muscle spasm
- Traction

Due to high density of pain receptors in the skin, *superficial pain* is accurately localized. On the other hand, *deep somatic pain and visceral pain* are poorly localized, due to sparse distribution of pain receptors. It may also be mentioned that the viscera do not have any other sensation except pain and that is partly the reason why visceral pain is poorly localized. Localized tissue damage in the viscera may not produce any pain at all. If the abdominal wall is infiltrated with a local anesthetic and opened, localized cuts or burns in the gut do not produce any pain. Diffuse visceral inflammation or distension of the hollow viscera produces intense pain.

Visceral pain sensation is carried mostly by unmyelinated type-C afferents in the sympathetic (from all the thoracic and most of the abdominal viscera) and parasympathetic (from many pelvic viscera) nerves. A few A-δ fibers also seem to be involved in the transmission of visceral pain. In the central nervous system, visceral pain fibers accompany somatic pain fibers in the spinothalamic tract and the medial lemniscus.

Characteristics of Visceral Pain

- Diffuse and difficult to localize.
- Very commonly perceived in the midline at the level of lower sternum or upper abdomen.
- May be accompanied by cutaneous or deep tissue hyperalgesia.
- Usually associated with stronger autonomic reflexes than somatic pain.
- Psychologically more disturbing than somatic pain.
- The intensity of visceral pain may not reflect the true extent of visceral damage.
- Often referred to the skin or a superficial somatic structure.

Due to the low density of sensory innervation of viscera and the extensive divergence of visceral input within the central nervous system (CNS), *visceral pain* is a vague, diffuse, and poorly defined sensation.

Regardless of the specific internal organ of origin, it is usually perceived in the midline at the level of the lower sternum or upper abdomen. Whether the origin is from the heart, esophagus, stomach, duodenum, gallbladder, or pancreas, visceral pain in its early phase is perceived in this same general area. Additional stimuli such as local compression applied to this area fail to worsen the pain.

Visceral pain is typically associated with marked autonomic phenomena, such as pallor, profuse sweating, nausea, vomiting, changes in blood pressure and heart rate, gastrointestinal disturbances (e.g., diarrhea), and changes in body temperature. Strong emotional reactions are commonly present that include anxiety, anguish, and sometimes even a sense of impending death.

Sometimes visceral pathology may manifest principally through vegetative and emotional reactions, with minimal pain and discomfort. A typical example is painless myocardial infarction, which may produce a sense of gastric fullness, heaviness, pressure, squeezing, or choking. These deceptive symptoms may lead to an incorrect diagnosis such as gastrointestinal pathology, especially when vegetative signs such as nausea and vomiting are present.

The intensity of visceral pain may bear no relationship to the extent of the internal injury. Again, this is evident in the example of painless myocardial infarction, which involves death of cardiac muscle, versus angina, which reflects only ischemia without permanent tissue damage.

Effect of Age on Visceral Pain Perception

Many studies have revealed an age-related change in pain symptoms and presentation, typically in the direction of reduced or absent pain in older people. In cases of appendicitis, about 45% of older adults with appendicitis do not have lower-right quadrant pain as a presenting symptom, whereas it is the chief complaint in 95% of younger adults. Visceral pain associated with various types of malignancy is also reported to be less intense in adults of advanced age than in younger individuals. The pathophysiology of decreased visceral pain sensitivity with aging is not exactly clear, but possible mechanisms may include an age-related decline in the density of nociceptors. Also worth noting is the higher prevalence in the elderly of medical conditions such as diabetes that are associated with impaired pain perception because of autonomic neuropathy. Thus, elderly patients affected with these conditions may have the highest risk of presenting with painless visceral diseases. These factors should be kept in mind by clinicians, who should be prepared to suspect and pursue the diagnosis of potentially dangerous or life-threatening diagnoses in elderly patients.

Referred Pain

Pain due to a disorder of a deep somatic tissue or a viscus is usually felt in the structure concerned. However, in many tissues, pain may be felt in some other deeper or superficial structure supplied by the same neural (spinal) segments. Such a pain is said to be referred to the second structure. For example, in myocardial ischemia, pain is referred to the left shoulder and arm. Pain due to a stone in the lower part of the ureter is usually referred to the corresponding testis and inner thigh. Similarly, inflammation of the diaphragm due to pleurisy or severe cholecystitis produces pain at the tip of the shoulder. The site where pain can be referred is determined by the dermatomal rule. Pain is usually referred to a structure with common embryonic origin and hence both are innervated by a common neural (spinal) segment. Embryologically, the heart originates from structures in the neck and upper thorax and hence the visceral pain fibers enter the spinal segments from C_3 to C_5. Important sites where visceral pain is referred are shown in Fig. 22.3.

Mechanism of Referred Pain

All the nerve fibers of a given dermatome enter the same spinal segment. Moreover, pain afferents in the peripheral nerves are far more in number than in the lateral spinothalamic tracts. Therefore many primary pain afferents must be converging on each of the second order neurons of the spinothalamic tract. So when somatic and visceral pain afferents converge on the same second order neuron, pain due to a disorder in the viscus is interpreted as coming from the somatic structure (Fig. 22.4). Pain is more

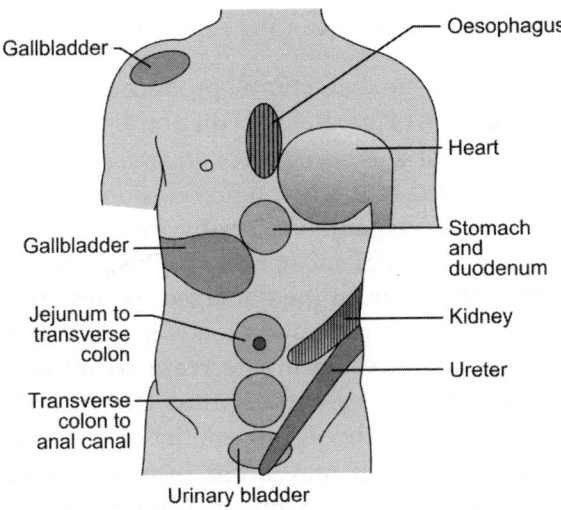

Fig. 22.3: Important sites where visceral pain is referred.

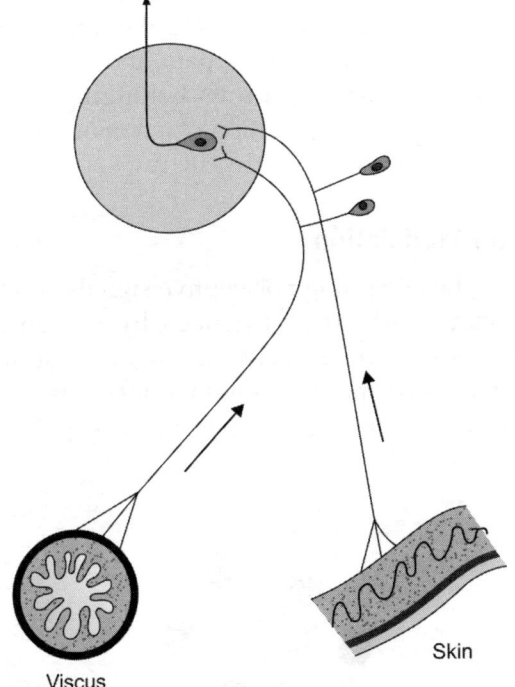

Fig. 22.4: Mechanism of referred pain: Convergence of first order neurons from the viscus and the skin on a common second order neuron.

often referred to the anterior than the posterior half of the body. This is probably because we are more conscious of the front than the back of the body.

HYPERALGESIA

It is a condition in which noxious stimuli produce more severe pain than expected. Two main types of hyperalgesia may be distinguished (Fig. 22.5):

Primary hyperalgesia: This occurs over an area of tissue damage. The pain threshold is lowered so that, even non-noxious mechanical (touch) or thermal stimuli produce pain. Primary hyperalgesia is due to release of algogenic (pain producing) substances like histamine, 5-HT, plasma kinins and prostaglandins from the damaged tissues. Nociceptors and their neurons also display sensitization following repeated stimulation. Sensitization of nociceptors results in a decrease in threshold, an increase in frequency response, a decrease in response latency and spontaneous firing even after cessation of the stimulus (after discharge).

Secondary hyperalgesia: It may occur in a normal healthy tissue surrounding the diseased tissue. In this condition there is no lowering of pain threshold. However, noxious stimuli produce far more severe pain than expected in a normal skin. Secondary hyperalgesia may be due to the phenomenon of subliminal fringe. Primary pain afferents from an area of tissue damage not only stimulate the appropriate 2nd order neurons to threshold level, producing pain and primary hyperalgesia, but also excite the 2nd order neurons belonging to nearby area to subthreshold degree. Hence application of a noxious stimulus produces more intense pain in this area.

Endogenous Pain Modulation

The magnitude of the ascending nociceptive signals and the consequent pain sensation can be greatly influenced by descending pathways originating in the brainstem and terminating in the spinal dorsal horn. The descending pathways may be inhibitory or facilitatory in nature. The descending pain inhibitory system has been investigated more thoroughly.

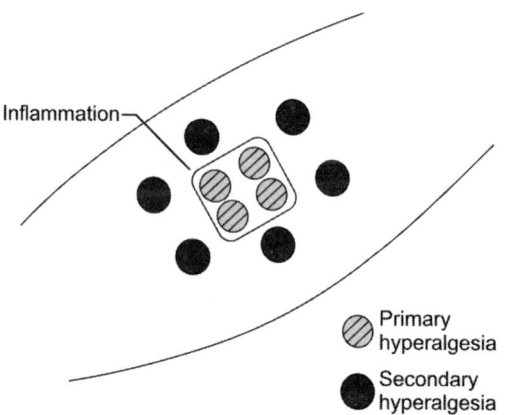

Fig. 22.5: Primary and secondary hyperalgesia.

1. Gate Control Hypothesis

First order neurons carrying the sensation of pain (Aδ and C fibers) terminate in the substantia gelatinosa in the dorsal horn of the spinal cord. The second order neurons situated in the substantia gelatinosa give rise to long axons which cross to the opposite site and ascend as lateral spinothalamic tract. Thus, dorsal horn of the spinal cord may be considered as a gate for the transmission of all the pain signals into the CNS. It has been shown that the gate may be partially or completely closed, i.e. the transmission of pain signals may be partially or completely blocked:

i. *Impulse discharge in the large afferent fibers carrying sensation of touch can partially block pain signals.* It is a common observation that touching the area of inflammation usually gives partial relief from pain. It is believed that touch signals, as they enter the dorsal columns, give off collaterals that synapse with short interneurons that produce opioid peptides and produce presynaptic inhibition of the second order neurons carrying pain signals (Fig. 22.6). Counter-irritants and transcutaneous electrical stimulation is believed to produce partial pain relief through this mechanism.

ii. A more powerful mechanism of gate control is the descending inhibitory pathways arising from the brain stem nuclei and terminating on the second order pain neurons in the dorsal horn. The periaqueductal grey (PAG) matter in the midbrain and Raphe nuclei (RN) in the medulla oblongata receive collaterals from the ascending lateral spinothalamic tract carrying pain signals. When activated by ascending pain signals, pathways descending from the PAG and RN produce inhibition of second order pain neurons in the dorsal horn (Fig. 22.7). Persistent pain signals ascending in the ascending pathways, in a feedback manner, are believed to activate PAG and RN and thereby reduce the intensity of nociceptive signals reaching the brain.

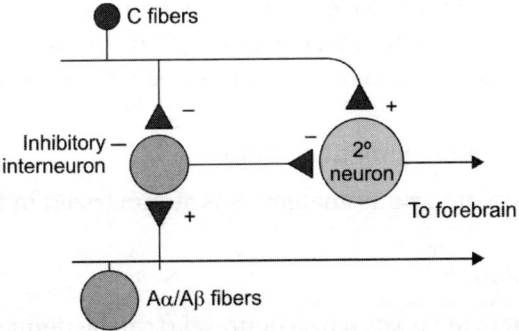

Fig. 22.6: Mechanism of gate control of pain in the dorsal horn of spinal cord.

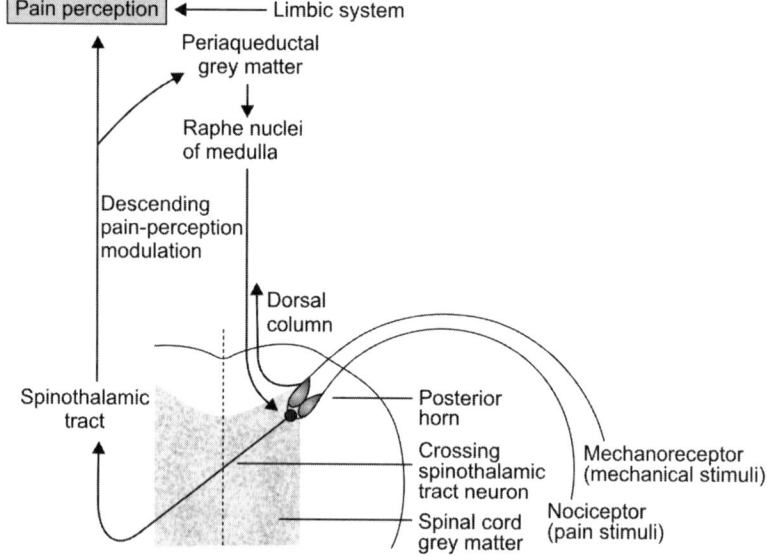

Fig. 22.7: Inhibition of pain sensation in the dorsal horn of spinal cord by (i) mechanoreceptor afferents and (ii) descending pain inhibitory pathway.

2. Role of Endorphins

Morphine, the active ingredient of opium is an extremely potent pain killer. A search was made for the morphine-sensitive receptors in the CNS, acting on which morphine relieves pain. Such receptors, known as *opioid receptors,* were found in various parts of CNS, particularly in hypothalamus, brain stem and dorsal horn of the spinal cord.

A number of peptides have been found in the brain stem and dorsal horn of the spinal cord which have analgesic action like morphine. These opioid polypeptides include α-endorphin, met-endorphin, leu-encephalin and dynorphin. Obviously certain neurons in the CNS secrete these analgesic polypeptides. These opioid polypeptides cause presynaptic inhibition of pain sensation either in the dorsal horn of the spinal cord (Fig. 22.8) or pain signals ascending in the brain stem. It seems the brain possesses its own internal mechanism to limit the intensity of chronic pain. Acupuncture seems to help in relief of pain by releasing endorphins.

Implications in Management of Pain

The site of action of various analgesics is summarized in Fig. 22.9.

Neuropathic Pain

Neuropathic pain (also known as neuralgia) can be defined most simply as non-nociceptive pain, or in other words, pain that is not related to

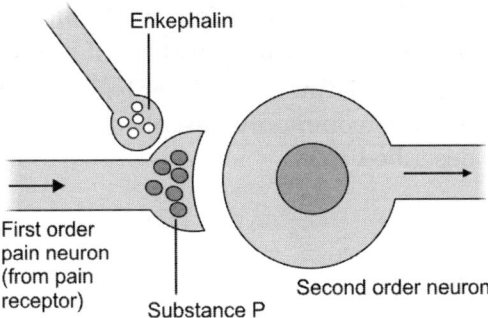

Fig. 22.8: Presynaptic inhibition of pain in the dorsal horn of spinal cord.

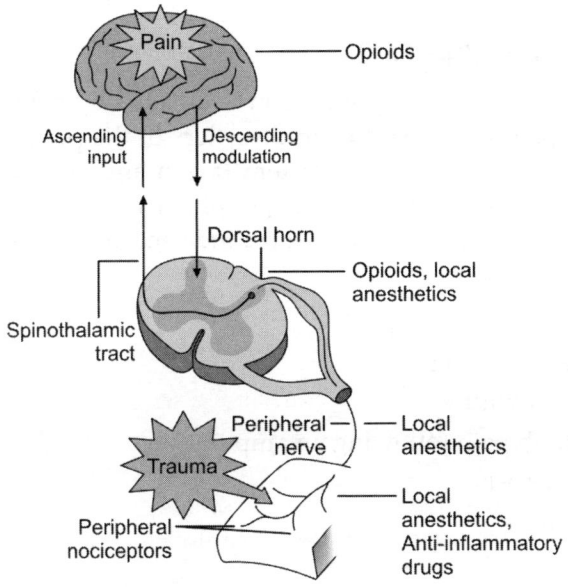

Fig. 22.9: Site of action of various analgesics.

activation of pain receptors in any part of the body. Neuropathic pain results from damage to the peripheral nerves or a part of CNS. Unlike nociceptive pain, neuralgia exists with no continuous nociceptive input. Pain occurs without any apparent tissue injury, because the pain nerve fibers are pathologically stimulated. Peripheral neuropathy (diabetes mellitus, chronic alcohol abuse), prolapsed intervertebral disc (PIVD) or nerve entrapment in a cancerous growth are common causes of neuropathic pain. Neuropathic pain does not respond to ordinary analgesics. Even morphine, the most potent analgesic ingredient of opium may be ineffective. This type of pain is biologically useless, but it produces profound psychological effects. Some important differences between the nociceptive pain and neuropathic pain are shown in Table 22.1.

Neuropathic pain is distinctly different from nociceptive pain. Nociceptive pain is more commonly described as aching. Neuropathic pain is variously described as:
- Burning
- Tingling
- Like an electric shock
- Shooting
- Coldness
- "Pins and needles" sensations
- Numbness
- Itching

Causes of Neuropathic Pain

As much as 7 to 8% of the population is affected by neuropathic pain. Neuropathic pain may result from disorders of the peripheral nervous system or the central nervous system (brain and spinal cord). Thus, neuropathic pain may be divided into peripheral neuropathic pain, central neuropathic pain, or mixed (peripheral and central) neuropathic pain.
- Trigeminal neuralgia
- Intervertebral disc prolapse
- Post-herpetic neuralgia
- Diabetic neuropathy
- Phantom limb pain following an amputation
- Multiple sclerosis
- HIV infection
- Alcoholism
- Cancer

In patients with cancer, peripheral neuropathic pain can be caused directly by infiltration or compression of the nerve by the tumor or

Table 22.1: Differences between nociceptive pain and neuropathic pain

Nociceptive pain	Neuropathic pain
Nociceptive stimulus evident.	No obvious tissue damage.
Well localized.	Poorly localized.
Visceral pain may be referred	Not referred
It is "typical" or "has been experienced before".	It is different from the usual somatic or visceral pain.
It responds to common analgesics.	Only partially relieved by narcotic analgesics.

indirectly by cancer treatments such as radiation therapy and chemotherapy.

PATHOPHYSIOLOGY

The mechanisms involved in neuropathic pain are complex and involve both peripheral and central pathophysiologic phenomenon. The underlying dysfunction may involve deafferentation within the peripheral nervous system (e.g. neuropathy), deafferentation within the central nervous system (e.g. post-thalamic stroke) or an imbalance between the two (e.g. phantom limb pain).

a. Peripheral Mechanisms: Ectopic Discharges and Ephaptic Conduction

In normal primary afferent neurons, it is rare for firing threshold to be reached without the input of a stimulus. However, following a nerve injury, it has been demonstrated that there is a large increase in the level of spontaneous firing in the afferent neurons linked to the injury site. This has been termed ectopic discharge and has also been demonstrated in humans, suffering from neuropathic pain.

Certain investigations in animals suggest that abnormal electrical connections can occur between adjacent demyelinated axons. These are referred to as ephapses. "Ephaptic cross talk" may result in the transfer of nerve impulses from one axon to another. Cross talk between A and C fibers often develops in the dorsal root ganglion.

b. Central Mechanisms

Following a peripheral nerve injury, anatomical and neurochemical changes can occur within the central nervous system (CNS) that can persist long after the injury has healed. This "CNS plasticity" may play an important role in the evolution of chronic, neuropathic pain. As is the case in the periphery, sensitization of neurons can occur within the dorsal horn following peripheral tissue damage. It is characterized by an increased spontaneous activity of the dorsal horn neurons, a decreased threshold and an increased responsivity to afferent input. In the non-injured state, Aβ fibers (large myelinated afferents) penetrate the dorsal horn, travel ventrally, and terminate in lamina III and deeper. C fibers (small unmyelinated afferents) penetrate directly and generally terminate no deeper than lamina II. However, after peripheral nerve injury there is a prominent sprouting of large afferents dorsally from lamina III into laminae I and II. After peripheral nerve injury, these large afferents gain access to spinal regions involved in transmitting high intensity, noxious signals, instead of merely encoding low threshold information. Evidence also suggests that excessive nociceptive input to the dorsal horn can have excitotoxic consequences resulting in the death of inhibitory interneurons. This inhibition may contribute to spinal hyper-excitability.

CHRONIC PAIN SYNDROME

There is no clear definition what constitutes chronic pain. Pain is said to be chronic when it lasts 3 to 6 months. Some argue that any pain that persists longer than the reasonable expected healing time for the involved tissues should be considered as chronic pain.

Most of us have suffered from acute pain some time or the other, e.g. because of physical injury, mild burns, colics, minor or major surgeries. This type of pain is short lived and disappears when the offending agent disappears or healing occurs. Chronic pain is different in that it persists. Pain signals keep firing in the nervous system for weeks, months, even years. There may have been an initial mishap, a sprained back or a serious infection, from which the patient has long recovered. There may be an ongoing cause of pain such as arthritis or cancer. It may occur in patients with neuropathic pain. Whatever the matter may be, chronic pain is real, unrelenting, and demoralizing.

Effects of Pain

Acute Pain Responses

Somatic and visceral pain fibers are fully integrated with the skeletal motor and sympathetic systems in the spinal cord, brain stem and higher centers. These synapses are responsible for reflex muscle activity (muscle spasm, or "guarding") that is associated with pain. In a similar fashion reflex sympathetic activation causes the release of catecholamines, locally and from the adrenal medulla. This increases heart rate and blood pressure with a consequent increase in myocardial work, increased metabolic rate and oxygen consumption. Gastrointestinal tone is decreased leading to delayed gastric emptying. Pain also causes an increase in the secretion of catabolic hormones and decreased secretion of anabolic hormones. The metabolic responses to pain include hyperglycemia due to gluconeogenesis and decreases in insulin secretion or action, increased protein catabolism and increased lipolysis. The respiratory responses could be either hyperventilation due to stimulation of respiratory center or hypoventilation due to splinting and reflex muscle spasm. The cortical responses include anxiety and fear.

Chronic Pain Responses

Chronic pain syndrome results in chronic anxiety and depression, anger, and changed lifestyle, all due to a variable but significant level of genuine neurologically-based chronic pain. Pain of such proportions overwhelms all other symptoms and itself becomes the problem. People may not be able to work. Their appetite falls off. Physical activity of any kind is exhausting and may aggravate the pain.

Soon the person becomes the victim of a vicious circle in which total preoccupation with pain leads to irritability and depression. The sufferer cannot sleep at night and the next day's weariness compounds the problem, leading to more irritability, depression, and pain. Chronic pain syndrome tends to be very difficult to manage because of is its complex natural history, unclear etiology and poor response to therapy.

Pathophysiology of Chronic Pain

The exact mechanisms involved in the pathophysiology of chronic pain are complex and remain unclear. It is believed that following an injury, rapid and long-term changes occur in parts of the CNS that are involved in the transmission and modulation of pain.

Why does local injury resulting from trauma lead to chronic, intractable pain in some patients? What is responsible for the translation of local injury with acute pain into a chronic pain state? Long-term pain is classically known to persist following amputation of an extremity, and is often present following thoracotomy, mastectomy, laparotomy, herniorrhaphy, and orthopedic procedures. Apart from the actual discomfort experienced by the patient, even relatively low levels of persistent pain following surgery have been associated with decreased physical and social function as well as a decreased perception of overall health. Patients already suffering from chronic painful conditions often report a more intense pain following subsequent surgery than normal individuals.

A central mechanism in the spinal cord, called 'wind-up', also referred to as hypersensitivity or hyperexcitability, has been proposed to explain such types of chronic pain. Wind-up occurs when repeated, prolonged, noxious stimulation causes the dorsal horn neurons to transmit progressively increasing numbers of pain impulses. The patient begins feel intense pain in response to a stimulus that is not usually associated with pain, for example, touch. This is called **allodynia**. This abnormal processing of pain within the PNS and CNS may become independent of the original painful event. Such types of chronic pain may result from peripheral or central sensitization of neural pathways concerned in the conduction of pain signals in the peripheral nerves (*peripheral sensitization*) or within the CNS (*central sensitization*). In some cases, for example, amputation, the original injury may have occurred in the peripheral nerves, but the mechanisms that underlie the phantom pain are generated in both the PNS and the CNS.

Implications in Pain Management

When pain occurs as a consequence of injury or surgery, the spinal cord can reach a hyperexcitable state wherein excessive pain responses occur that may persist for days or weeks (or even years).

It is possible to limit sensitization of the pain pathways by initiating appropriate pain therapy before the onset of a noxious stimulus. This approach is often referred to as *preemptive analgesia* or treatment before pain progresses. The acute pain that accompanies surgical procedures represents an ideal setting for a preemptive analgesia therapy, because the timing of the beginning of noxious stimulation is known in advance (Fig. 22.10).

Sensitization of the pain pathways is an ongoing process during surgery, despite the patient being general anesthesia. Once central sensitization is established, larger doses of analgesics are required to suppress it. Pre-emptive analgesia may reduce the impact of all these stimuli on the CNS. Woolf and Chong demonstrated that the morphine dose needed to prevent central hyperexcitability, given before brief noxious electrical stimulation in rats, was one tenth the dose required to abolish activity after it had developed. This observation was translated to clinical practice. In a clinical trial of 60 patients undergoing abdominal hysterectomy, those who received 10 mg of morphine intravenously at the time of induction of anesthesia required significantly less morphine for postoperative pain control. Furthermore, pain sensitivity around the wound (secondary hyperalgesia) was also reduced in the morphine pretreated group.

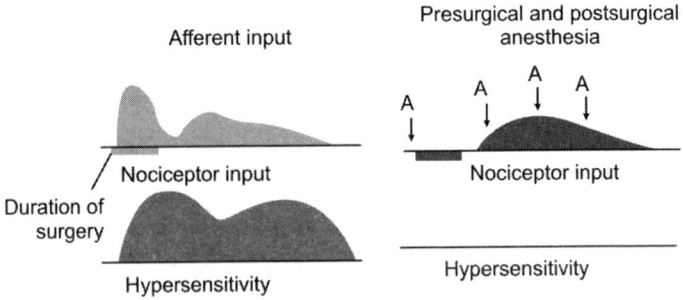

Fig. 22.10: Effect of presurgical and postsurgical analgesia on the development of pain hypersensitivity. A: analgesic administration.

Further Reading

Bach, S; Noreng, M; Tjellden NU. **Phantom limb pain in amputees during the first 12 months following limb amputation, after preoperative lumbar epidural blockade.** *Pain. 1988; 33:297–302.*

Bridges, D; Thompson, SWN; Rice, **ASC. Mechanisms of neuropathic and pain.** *Br J Anaesth 2001; 87: 12–26.*

Dworkin, RH; Backonja, M, et al. **Advances in Neuropathic Pain Diagnosis, Mechanisms, and Treatment Recommendations.** Arch Neurol. *2003;60:1524–1534.*

Gottschalk, A; Smith, DS. **New Concepts in Acute Pain Therapy: Preemptive Analgesia** *Am Fam Physician. 2001;63:1979–85.*

Woolf, CJ; Chong, MS. **Preemptive analgesia—treating postoperative pain by preventing the establishment of central sensitization.** *Anesth Analg. 1993; 77:362–79.*

23

Pituitary Gland

FUNCTIONAL ANATOMY

The pituitary gland is situated in the sella turcica of the sphenoid bone at the base of the skull (Fig. 23.1). Optic chiasma is present just above the pituitary gland. The lateral wall of sella turcica abuts on cavernous sinus, which contains cranial nerves III, IV and VI (Fig. 23.2). These anatomic relations explain why pituitary tumors may produce visual field defects, cranial nerve palsies or radiological evidence of damaged sella turcica.

The pituitary gland consists of two parts, the anterior pituitary gland and posterior pituitary gland. Anterior pituitary constitutes 80% of the gland. Though, pituitary gland is entirely ectodermal in origin but is composed of 2 functionally distinct structures that differ in embryologic development and anatomy: the adenohypophysis (anterior pituitary) and the neurohypophysis (posterior pituitary).

The anterior pituitary develops from Rathke's pouch, which is an upward invagination of oral ectoderm; in contrast, the posterior pituitary develops from the infundibulum, which is a downward extension of

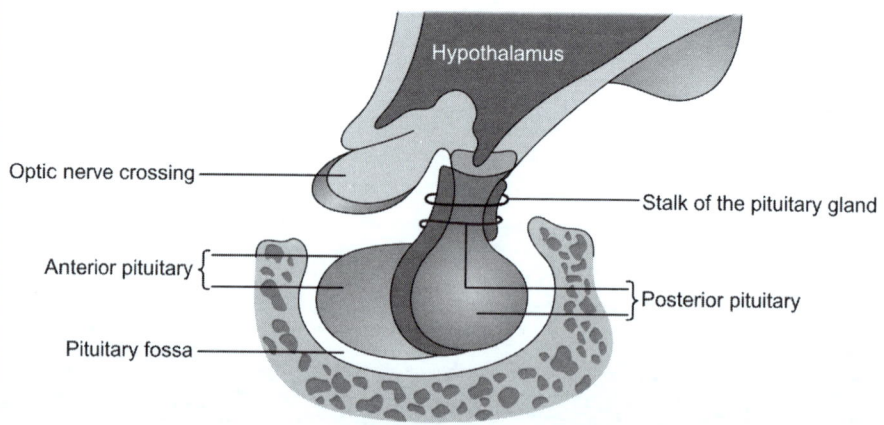

Fig. 23.1: The anatomic location of pituitary gland.

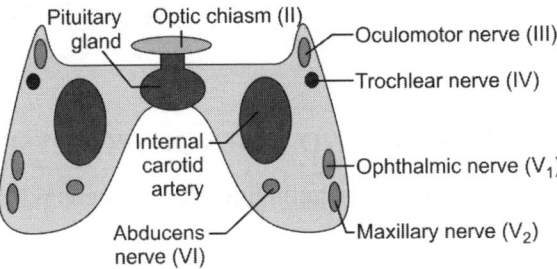

Fig. 23.2: Important structures around the pituitary gland.

neural ectoderm from the floor of the diencephalon. That is why; the two components histologically differ from each other. The anterior pituitary is a glandular structure (Fig. 23.3A) and hence also named adenohypophysis. The posterior pituitary is a neural structure and hence also named as neurohypophysis.

The posterior pituitary gland (neurohypophysis) is actually an extension of hypothalamus. It contains nerve endings of the hypothalamic hypophyseal tract in close proximity to blood capillaries (Fig. 23.3B). On appropriate hypothalamic stimulation, either of the two posterior pituitary

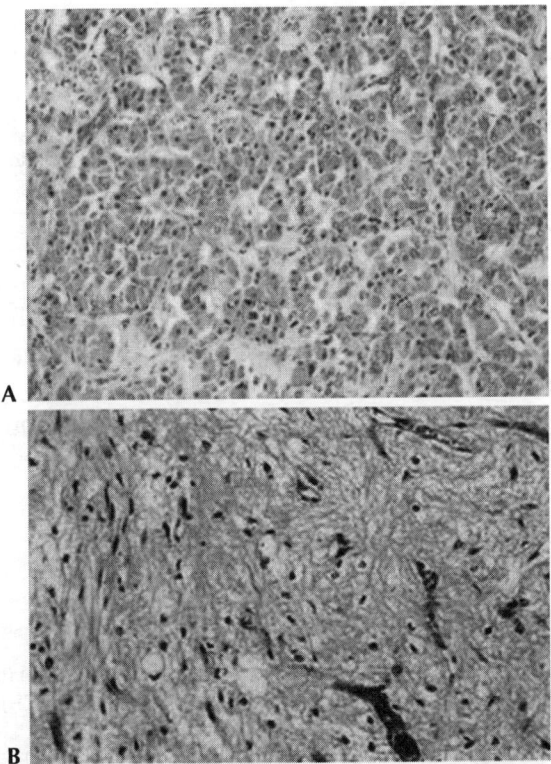

Fig. 23.3(A and B): Histology of pituitary gland.

hormones, antidiuretic hormone (ADH) and oxytocin are released into blood circulation.

ANTERIOR PITUITARY GLAND (ADENOHYPOPHYSIS)

The anterior pituitary gland contains five types of cells which release six types of hormones (Table 23.1).

Hypothalamic Control of Anterior Pituitary Gland

Unlike posterior pituitary gland, anterior pituitary gland has no neural link with the hypothalamus. Still, hypothalamus controls the secretion of anterior pituitary gland. The hypothalamic control is exerted through a number of chemical mediators called releasing hormones and release-inhibiting hormones which reach the anterior pituitary via hypothalamic hypophyseal portal vessels.

The anterior pituitary gland has a peculiar system of blood supply. The bilateral superior hypophyseal arteries break up into a network of capillaries in the median eminence region of hypothalamus. These capillaries converge to form a few long portal vessels which descend along the pituitary stalk. The portal vessels break up into a second network of capillary sinusoids among the cells of anterior pituitary gland (Fig. 23.4). The bilateral inferior hypophyseal arteries supply blood directly to the posterior pituitary gland. Finally, venous blood is drained from the anterior pituitary and posterior pituitary into the cavernous sinus through adenohypophyseal and neurohypophyseal veins, respectively.

Hypophysiotropic Hypothalamic Hormones

All the hypophysiotropic hypothalamic hormones are polypeptides, except PIH which is dopamine. Between GRH and GIH, the former has dominant role. GIH inhibits TSH secretion also. TRH increases secretion of not only TSH but also prolactin.

The lactotrophs are under a continuous inhibitory control of PIH. Section of pituitary stalk in an experimental animal decreases the secretion

Table 23.1: Cell types and secretions of anterior pituitary gland

Cell type	% of total anterior pituitary cells	Hormone(s) secreted
Somatotrophs	50	Growth hormone (Somatotropin)
Thyrotrophs	10	Thyroid stimulating hormone (TSH) (thyrotropin)
Corticotrophs	15	Adrenocorticotropic hormone (ACTH) (corticotropin)
Lactotrophs	10–15	Prolactin
Gonadotrophs	10	Follicle stimulating hormone (FSH), luteinizing hormone (LH)

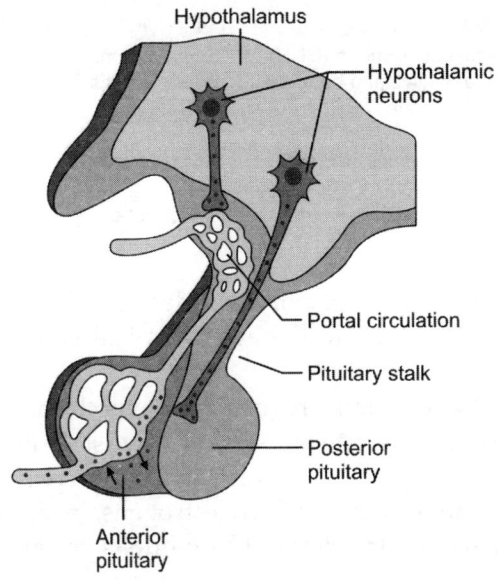

Fig. 23.4: Hypothalamic hypophyseal portal system of blood vessels.

of all anterior pituitary hormones, except prolactin, whose secretion increases.

Growth Hormone (GH)

Human growth hormone is a single polypeptide chain with 191 amino acids. Pulsatile release of GH is a characteristic feature. Circulating levels of GH are very low for most of the day punctuated by 4–8 bursts after meals, exercise and especially during slow wave sleep. The significance of pulsatile release of GH is not clear. About 50–75% of total GH secretion over 24 hours occurs during sleep.

GH is necessary for normal linear growth, but unlike thyroxine, it is not essential during antenatal or perinatal period. Children with congenital deficiency of GH manifest growth retardation only after 1–2 years age. Besides growth promotion, GH has important metabolic functions: protein anabolism, lipolysis and inhibition of peripheral glucose utilization (hyperglycemic effect). GH is one of the counter regulatory hormones which restore normal blood glucose level during long intervals between the meals. Patients with deficiency of GH have a tendency to develop hypoglycemia, whereas those with GH excess develop insulin resistance.

Insulin-like Growth Factors (IGFs)

The linear growth promotion and many metabolic effects of GH are produces indirectly. GH acts on the liver and other soft tissues and

Hypothalamic hormone	Target cell	Action
Growth hormone releasing hormone (GRH)	Somatotrophs	↑ GH secretion
Growth hormone release-inhibiting hormone	Somatotrophs	↓ GH secretion
Thyrotropin releasing hormone (TRH)	Thyrotrophs	↑ TSH secretion
Corticotropin releasing hormone (CRH)	Corticotrophs	↑ ACTH secretion
Gonadotropin releasing hormone (GnRH)	Gonadotrophs	↑ FSH secretion ↑ LH secretion
Prolactin inhibiting hormone (PIH)	Lactotrophs	↓ Prolactin secretion

stimulates the production of polypeptides called insulin-like growth factors. Both IGF-I and IGF-II have chemical structures similar to proinsulin.

Growth hormone secretion is regulated by hypothalamic GRH and GIH. Hypoglycemia, severe exercise, stress, slow wave sleep increase the release of GRH, whereas hyperglycemia and REM sleep increase the secretion of GIH. Gonadal hormones, particularly estrogens, increase the frequency of nocturnal bursts of GH release. These bursts are more prominent at puberty.

Effect of Age on GH Secretion

In the normal population, a gradual and progressive fall in spontaneous growth hormone (GH) secretion occurs with increasing age and is reflected in a parallel fall in circulating insulin-like growth factor (IGF)-I (Fig. 23.5), reduction in lean body mass, increase in body fat and rise in low-density lipoprotein (LDL) cholesterol. Aging is also associated with a progressive failure of body functions and particularly with an increasing lack of physical strength and mobility. This phenomenon is sometimes known as "*somatopause.*" However, at this state of our knowledge, it premature to recommend GH treatment to reverse the age-associated deterioration in body composition and physical performance.

PROLACTIN

Prolactin is secreted by lactotrophs of anterior pituitary gland. Lactotrophs normally constitute 10–25% of the cells in anterior pituitary gland. During pregnancy their proportion rises to about 50% by the end of pregnancy. Gradually increasing blood estrogen levels during pregnancy promote mitosis in the existing lactotrophs as well as conversion of some of the somatotrophs to lactotrophs. As a result, weight and volume of pituitary gland enlarge by about 33%.

During pregnancy, high plasma prolactin levels help in the development of glandular tissue in the breasts; its lactogenic action is inhibited by high plasma estrogens and progesterone levels. After parturition, when the placental source of the sex hormones disappears,

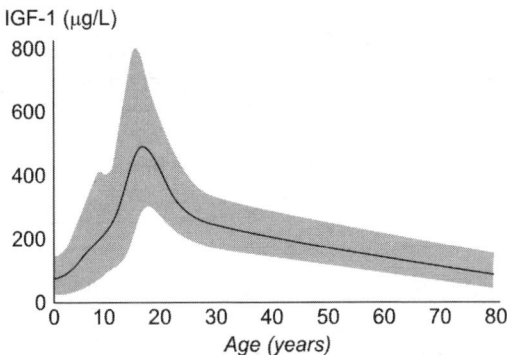

Fig. 23.5: Effect of age on serum IGF-I levels.

lactogenic effect of prolactin begins. Prolactin is essential for the initiation and maintenance of lactation.

Hypertrophy and hyperplasia of lactotrophs during pregnancy results in the enlargement of the anterior pituitary, without a corresponding increase in blood supply. Secondly, the anterior pituitary is supplied by a low pressure portal venous system. Major hemorrhage or hypotension during the peripartum period can result in ischemia of the affected pituitary regions leading to necrosis (Sheehan's syndrome). The posterior pituitary is usually not affected due to its direct arterial supply.

Lactotrophs are present in the anterior pituitary gland in males also. Physiologic levels of prolactin in males enhance luteinizing hormone-receptors in Leydig cells, resulting in testosterone secretion, which leads to spermatogenesis. The neuroendocrine response to sexual activity in humans is characterized by a pronounced orgasm-dependent increase of plasma levels of prolactin, both in males and females. Prolactin provides the body with sexual gratification after sexual acts. The hormone counteracts the effect of dopamine, which is responsible for sexual arousal (Fig. 23.6). This is thought to cause the sexual refractory period. The amount of prolactin can be an indicator for the amount of sexual satisfaction and relaxation. Highly elevated levels of prolactin decrease the levels of sex hormones—estrogen in women and testosterone in men.

Under normal circumstances, the secretion of prolactin is under hypothalamic restraint through PIH. During lactation, the PIH is inhibited by reflexes arising from the suckling baby. High plasma levels of prolactin have feedback inhibition of not only prolactin but GnRH-gonadotropins as well. This fact explains the phenomenon of lactational amenorrhea. More important consequences of this negative feedback effect are seen in patients with hyperprolactinemia—amenorrhea in women and loss of libido and impotence in men. TRH stimulates both thyrotrophs and lactotrophs. Hence hyperprolactinemia may be observed in patients with primary hypothyroidism (↑ TRH and ↑ TSH levels).

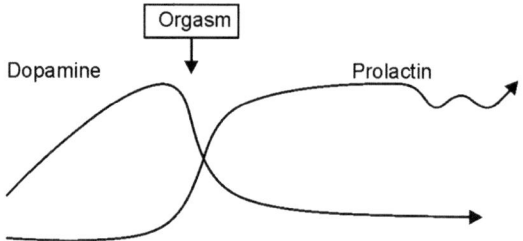

Fig. 23.6: Blood levels of dopamine and prolactin during sexual intercourse.

Adrenocorticotropic Hormone (ACTH)

ACTH is a single polypeptide with 39 amino acids. It is essential for maintenance of normal structure and function of adrenal cortex, particularly its zona fasciculata and zona reticularis. After experimental hypophysectomy, these two zones of adrenal cortex undergo atrophy; aldosterone-secreting zona glomerulus is not affected.

The major factors controlling the release of ACTH include circadian rhythm and stress. The diurnal pattern of ACTH secretion shows a peak at 4–8 am and a nadir around 8 pm. Any type of stress (severe pain, trauma, pyrogens, severe exercise, surgical operation, hypoglycemia or severe emotional stress enhance ACTH (and hence cortisol) secretion. Stress-related secretion of ACTH does not show circadian periodicity.

Plasma free cortisol level has a negative feedback effect on ACTH secretion. Pronged administration of pharmacologic doses of glucocorticoids result in suppression of hypothalamus-pituitary-adrenal cortex axis leading to atrophy of adrenal cortex (Fig. 23.7). Such a patient is unable to increase endogenous production cortisol in response to exposure to any stress. The recovery of adrenal cortical structure and

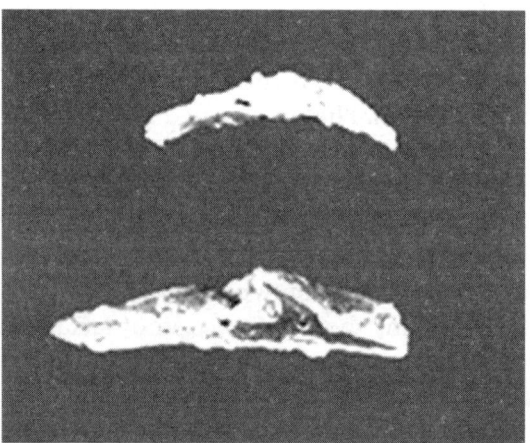

Fig. 23.7: Top: Adrenal gland from a patient who died of a complication following prolonged administration of glucocorticoids. Bottom: Normal adrenal gland.

function takes a few weeks when administration of glucocorticoids is gradually tapered off.

Thyroid Stimulating Hormone (TSH)

TSH is a glycoprotein. It is essential for maintenance of normal structure and function of thyroid gland. TSH stimulates each step of biosynthesis and release of thyroid hormones. Histological evidence of TSH overactivity includes increased height of follicular epithelial cells, decreased concentration of colloid and increased vascularity of thyroid gland.

Unlike other hormones, plasma levels of TSH (as well as, T_3 and T_4) remain constant over days and weeks. Prolonged exposure to cold weather is the only known stimulus for increase in TSH secretion. That explains slightly higher TSH levels in winter than in summer.

The secretion of TSH is under negative feedback control of plasma T_3 and T_4 levels. That explains markedly elevated TSH levels in primary hypothyroidism. In such patients, hypertrophy and hyperplasia of thyrotrophs in adenohypophysis is a characteristic finding. In Graves' disease, Plasma TSH level is almost undetectable.

To interpret thyroid status of an individual, besides T_3 and T_4 levels plasma TSH level is estimated. In primary thyroid failure, plasma TSH level may increase before plasma T_3 and T_4 decline below the normal range.

GONADOTROPINS

Adenohypophysis secretes two gonadotropins: follicle stimulating hormone (FSH) and luteinizing hormone (LH), both in males and females. At the pituitary, GnRH stimulates the synthesis and secretion of both the gonadotropins. These processes are controlled by the size and frequency of GnRH pulses, as well as by feedback from androgens and estrogens. Low-frequency GnRH pulses lead to FSH release, whereas high-frequency GnRH pulses stimulate LH release.

There are differences in GnRH secretion between females and males. In males, GnRH is secreted in pulses at a constant frequency, but, in females, the frequency of the pulses varies during the menstrual cycle, and there is a large surge of GnRH just before ovulation. In males, FSH regulates production of sperms, whereas LH is essential for Leydig cell function (testosterone secretion).

Estimation of plasma gonadotropins levels helps to differentiate primary gonadal failure (high gonadotropin levels) from secondary gonadal failure (low gonadotropins levels). However, gonadotropins measurement is unnecessary in women with normal ovulatory cycles or men with normal sperm count.

Syndromes of Anterior Pituitary Hypersecretion

Pituitary adenomas account for 10–15% of intracranial neoplasms. They can cause syndrome of anterior pituitary hormonal excess, syndrome of anterior pituitary hormone deficiency or structural damage to the surrounding tissues, e.g. visual field defects, ophthalmoplegia, etc.

Hyperprolactinemia

Hypersecretion of prolactin by the lactotrophs is the most common pituitary disorder. A prolactin-secreting adenoma (prolactinoma) is benign and commonest secretory pituitary tumor. Many drugs like antidepressants, antipsychotics, methyl dopa, oral contraceptives, etc. are other causes of hyperprolactinemia.

Hyperprolactinemia in young adults results in hypogonadism (a feedback effect of high plasma prolactin levels on GnRH/gonadotropin secretion), and bilateral galactorrhea. In females, it leads to amenorrhea/oligomenorrhea and infertility. Hyperprolactinemia may account for 10–40% of the cases of amenorrhea. In males, it results in gynecomastia, decreased libido, complete or partial impotence and/or infertility. Galactorrhea is present in about 90% of the females but only about 25% of males with hyperprolactinemia.

In older men or postmenopausal women, prolactinomas produce symptoms and signs of increased pituitary mass, e.g. headache, visual abnormalities, or cranial nerve palsies. If the tumor becomes very large, syndromes of other pituitary hormones deficiency may result.

Acromegaly and Giantism

These disorders are produced by an adenoma of somatotrophs in the anterior pituitary gland. It occurs most often in middle aged adults, when it results in acromegaly, since linear growth cannot occur because of fused epiphyseal plates. Such a tumor occurring before puberty causes giantism. The slowly growing tumor, usually a macroadenoma, causes not only increased GH secretion, but also deficient secretion of other anterior pituitary hormones, especially gonadotropins.

The most characteristic feature of acromegaly is acral enlargement, i.e. enlargement and thickening of extremities (hands and feet). The hands become spade-like, and fingers sausage-shaped. A gradual increase in shoe-size may be the first sign. Soft tissue overgrowth is another prominent feature. Enlargement of facial bones and soft tissues results in characteristic facial features, i.e. thick lips, exaggerated nasolabial folds, broad nose, thick scalp, prominent cheek bones and protrusion of lower jaw with malocclusion (Fig. 23.8).

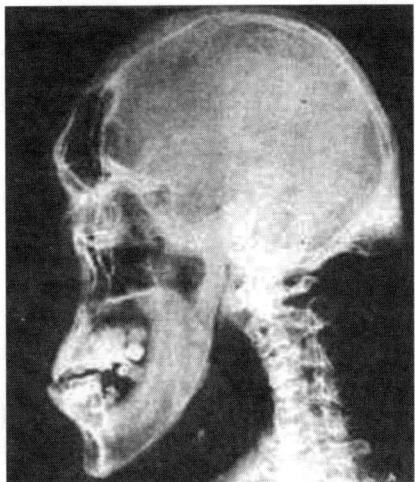

Fig. 23.8: Radiograph of the skull of a patient of acromegaly.

Basal metabolic rate is increased leading to hyperhidrosis and heat-intolerance. Paresthesias due to compression of carpel tunnel are common. Glucose intolerance, diabetes mellitus and hypertension may develop. Visual field defects and cranial nerve palsies may also occur.

Syndromes of ACTH Excess

(Cushing Disease and Nelson's Syndrome)

Cushing syndrome is characterized by centripetal obesity, moon face, weight gain, plethora, hypertension, easy bruisability, and hirsutism. Nowadays, Cushing syndrome is most commonly iatrogenic, i.e. due to prolonged administration of glucocorticoids in pharmacologic doses. Among endogenous causes, about 80% are due to ACTH-dependent bilateral adrenal hyperplasia. This disorder is known as **Cushing disease**. The primary cause is ACTH secreting pituitary microadenoma. Additional features of Cushing disease include hyperpigmentation of scars (ACTH in excess has MSH-like activity), and menstrual abnormalities (excessive secretion of adrenal androgens). *ACTH-independent endogenous Cushing syndrome is caused by adrenal adenoma or adrenal carcinoma.*

In 1960s and 1970s, Cushing disease was treated by bilateral adrenalectomy. Some of such cases, developed symptoms of pituitary mass, i.e. headache, visual field defects, cranial nerve palsies. This disorder was known as Nelson's syndrome. These patients had extremely high ACTH levels. Nelson's syndrome was caused by postoperative absence of feedback effect of cortisol level on ACTH-secreting microadenoma, resulting in accelerated growth of tumor into macroadenoma. Since, nowadays, pituitary microsurgery is the preferred treatment of Cushing disease, Nelson's syndrome is of historical interest only.

Anterior Pituitary Deficiency Syndromes

Hypopituitarism refers to deficiency of one or more hormones of pituitary gland. Isolated GH or gonadotropin deficiency is relatively more common than isolated deficiency of ACTH or TSH. The defect may be in hypothalamus or pituitary gland. When diabetes insipidus is also present, the defect is almost invariably in the hypothalamus.

Damage to anterior pituitary may be due to a pituitary adenoma, pituitary surgery, irradiation, head trauma, or infarction during postpartum stage (Sheehan's syndrome). In a gradually growing pituitary adenoma in an adult, GH secretion first to be lost (lethargy, muscle weakness). Next, gonadotropin secretion is affected (loss of libido and impotence in males, oligomenorrhea/amenorrhea in females). ACTH secretion is next affected, leading to secondary adrenal insufficiency (fatigue, decreased appetite, weight loss, decreased skin and nipple pigmentation). With continued ACTH and gonadotropin deficiency, axillary and pubic hair may be lost. Secretion of TSH is last to be affected, leading to secondary hypothyroidism (cold intolerance and apathy); frank hypothyroidism is usually not seen.

In cases with pituitary adenoma, additional symptoms that arise from the underlying cause may be present. For instance, if the hypopituitarism is due to a growth hormone—producing tumor, symptoms of acromegaly may be present. If the tumor extends to the optic nerve or optic chiasm, there may be visual field defects. Headache is another common symptom.

Posterior Pituitary Gland (Neurohypophysis)

Posterior pituitary gland secretes two hormones, antidiuretic hormone (ADH, vasopressin, arginine vasopressin) and oxytocin. Both hormones are produced in the hypothalamus nuclei: supraoptic nucleus (SON) synthesizes ADH predominantly whereas oxycitocin is mainly synthesized by paraventricular nucleus (PVN). The two hormones are transported in the axons of hypothalamic hypophyseal neural tract to the posterior pituitary gland to be stored at the nerve endings as secretory granules (visible as "Herring bodies" under light microscopy).

The SON and PVN respond to various stimuli, e.g. plasma osmolality, or impulses from the nipple respectively. Neural impulses so generated are transmitted down the axons resulting in release of appropriate hormone from the nerve endings. The two hormones are released independent of each other.

Antidiuretic Hormone

Antidiuretic hormone acts on two types of receptors: V_1 and V_2 receptors (Fig. 23.9). V_1 receptors are present on the smooth muscle of the arterioles

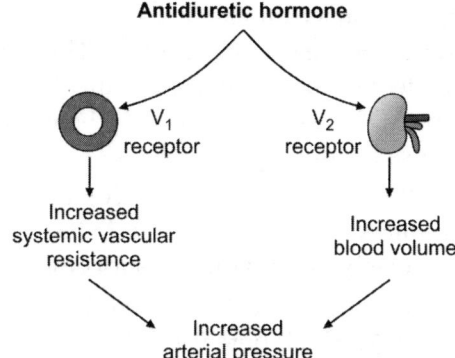

Fig. 23.9: Action of ADH (vasopressin) on V_1 and V_2 receptors.

and mediate vasoconstrictor effect of ADH. These receptors are activated by relatively higher plasma concentrations of ADH than V_2 receptors, e.g. in hemorrhage or other types of hypovolemic shock.

V_2 receptors are located in the basolateral borders of epithelial cells of collecting ducts of the kidney. These receptors are activated even by low plasma concentrations of ADH and mediate antidiuretic response of the hormone. The interstitial cells (I cells) of the collecting ducts contain water channels called aquaporins 2 in the cytoplasm. Binding of ADH with V_2 receptors results in cAMP-mediated translocation of aquaporins to the apical (luminal) border of the 'I' cells (Fig. 23.10). The water channels help in the movement of water from the ductal lumen to ECF. The number of water channels translocated directly varies with the plasma concentration of ADH. Therefore, there is proportionate increase in urinary concentration and a decrease in urinary volume.

The release of ADH is regulated by three mechanisms: via (i) osmoreceptors (ii) low pressure volume receptors and (iii) high pressure baroreceptors.

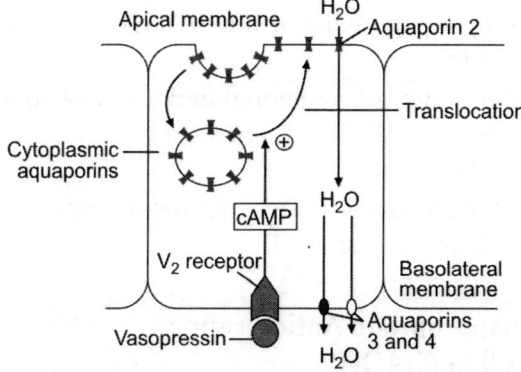

Fig. 23.10: Mechanism of action of ADH via V_2 receptors.

Even 1% increase in plasma osmolality is sufficient to trigger increased release of ADH from the posterior pituitary. The osmoreceptors are equally sensitive to a decrease in plasma osmolality that leads to a prompt decrease in release of ADH. Osmoreceptors are believed to be located in the hypothalamus close to supraoptic nucleus.

Volume receptors (low pressure stretch receptors) are located in the left atrium and pulmonary vessels. A decrease in blood volume increases release of ADH. Conversely, hypervolemia suppresses release of ADH.

High pressure baroreceptors located in carotid sinus and aortic arch also regulate release of ADH. Hypotension due to acute loss of blood is the most potent stimulus for release of ADH. Under such conditions, plasma ADH concentrations as high as 600 pg/ml have been recorded (normal 2–10 pg/ml).

Under conditions of water deprivation or intake of water load, there is a reciprocal change in blood volume and plasma osmolality, which brings about an appropriate change in release of ADH from the posterior pituitary gland. However, there are situations in which there may be conflict between the two stimuli, e.g. there is severe hyperosmolalty as well as increased plasma volume. In such a situation, preservation of osmotic function dominates: plasma osmolality is preserved at the cost of plasma volume regulation. However, after a severe hemorrhage, ADH is released, even if it decreases plasma osmolality.

Finally, AVP is also released in response to stressful stimuli, such as pain or anxiety, and by various drugs.

Diabetes insipidus (DI) is the term used to describe an uncommon condition in which the patient excretes a large volume of dilute urine and has excessive thirst. Restriction of water intake does not decrease urinary water excretion. The condition could be due to a failure of ADH release in response to normal physiological stimuli. Such cases are said to be suffering from central (or cranial or neurogenic) DI. Causes of cranial DI include pituitary or hypothalamic tumor, metastatic brain tumor, head trauma and idiopathic.

Still rarer is DI because of congenital deficiency of ADH-receptors in the kidney (nephrogenic DI). Acquired nephrogenic DI is produced by certain drugs, notably lithium.

Typical patient of DI passes 3 to 6 L or more of urine per day. (Urinary osmolality 100–150 mOsm/kg.)

Syndrome of Inappropriate Antidiuretic Hormone Secretion (SIADH)

This term is used to describe a group of disorders in which there is excessive secretion of ADH associated with hyponatremia, without

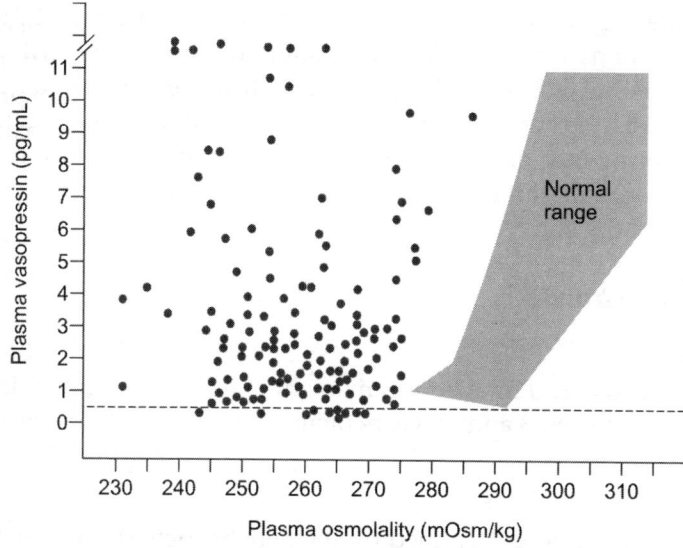

Fig. 23.11: Inappropriate secretion of ADH.

edema. SIADH is the most common cause of euvolemic hyponatremia in hospitalized patients. The causes include:

a. Drug or disease induced release of ADH from neurohypophysis (e.g. head injury or drugs which induce ADH release or potentiate action of ADH.
b. Ectopic production and release of ADH (e.g. small cell carcinoma of lungs, pulmonary tuberculosis or lung abscess).

Inappropriate ADH release results in secretion of concentrated urine despite subnormal plasma osmolality and Na^+ concentration (Fig. 23.11). Urinary Na^+ excretion is maintained near normal despite hyponatremia because of suppression of renin-angiotensin-aldosterone axis and increased secretion of atrial natriuretic peptide (ANP), both induced by hypervolemia. When hypervolemia is severe or acute in onset, body weight increases and symptoms of cerebral edema (e.g. restlessness, irritability, convulsions or coma) supervene.

GROWTH DISORDERS

Physiology of Growth

1. Intrauterine Growth

Intrauterine growth is a remarkable period of growth and development. From conception to birth, the fetal weight increases 440 million times, as compared to 20-fold increase from birth to adulthood. Moreover, a single cell is converted into a complex body with billions of cells working in harmony with each other. Besides the genetic regulatory mechanisms, the intrauterine growth is affected by uterine blood flow and maternal nutrition. Poor maternal nutrition is a common cause of low birth weight. Chronic maternal diseases, eclampsia, alcoholism, viral infections (rubella, toxoplasmosis) adversely affect fetal growth. Many other factors are responsible for low birth weights, e.g. non-white race, low maternal weight gain, small parental size, primiparity, low pre-pregnant weight, female sex of the baby, etc.

2. Postnatal Growth

a. Genetic Factors

There is a good correlation between height of the two parents and height of the child between 3 and 18 years of age.

b. Socioeconomic Factors

The height potential determined by the genetic factors can be achieved only if socioeconomic conditions of the family are optimum. Poor nutrition and poor hygiene are the most common cause of short stature. Better nutrition, particularly greater protein intake in the developed countries has led to a trend towards greater height in successive generations in the last century (Fig. 23.12).

c. Hormones

Growth hormone: Growth hormone promotes protein anabolism throughout life and promotes linear growth during childhood. However, growth hormone does not seem to have any role in regulation of growth during intrauterine and immediate postnatal period. After that, GH has

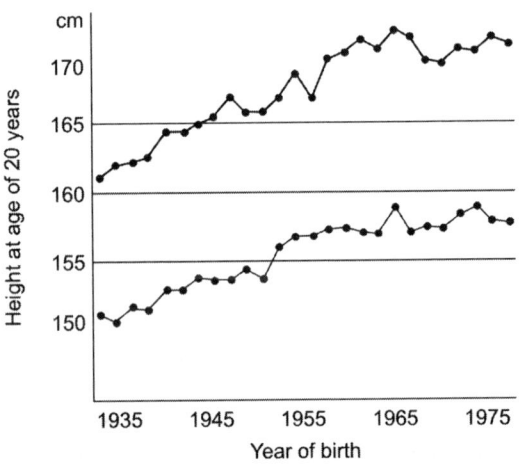

Fig. 23.12: Height of Japanese men (top) and women (bottom), born between 1935 and 1975 on reaching the age of 20 years.

a significant role in modulation of growth till puberty. In the absence of GH, the linear growth in childhood is reduced to 1/2 to 1/3 of normal rate. Congenital deficiency of GH may be due to decreased synthesis of GRH by the hypothalamus or deficient synthesis of GH at pituitary level. Children with congenital deficiency of GH have normal length at birth but growth retardation becomes apparent by 1–2 year age.

Thyroid hormones: In contrast to GH, thyroxine seems to be absolutely necessary for growth in both intrauterine and postnatal growth. In total absence of thyroxine, linear growth ceases almost completely. Besides a direct action on growth, thyroxine deficiency decreases the secretion of GH also.

Development of central nervous system is particularly vulnerable during the period extending from later parts of gestation to several months postnatal. Hypothyroidism during this period retards growth of neuron cell bodies, axons and dendrites as well as delays myelination. The action of thyroxine on neural growth may be direct or more probably through release of nerve growth factor in the central nervous system.

Insulin: Insulin stimulates growth during fetal life as well as postnatal. Insulin-deficient newborns are underweight. Growth failure in juvenile diabetes is also well known. On the other hand, diabetic mothers give birth to hyperinsulinemic over-sized babies. Insulin has a general anabolic effect, i.e., uptake and utilization of substrates necessary for growth.

Glucocorticoids: Even moderate excess of glucocorticoids (2–3 times the normal levels) can result in inhibition of normal growth. This fact may help to differentiate obesity due to Cushing syndrome from nutritional obesity. Growth is retarded in the former and accelerated in the latter disorder, i.e. a child with Cushing syndrome is smaller whereas nutritionally obese is taller than average for that age.

Earlier it was believed that glucocorticoids inhibit growth by suppression of GH secretion. Recent researches have shown normal levels of GH and IGFs in children with Cushing syndrome. Glucocorticoids seem to inhibit growth by a direct action on the tissues. Another important fact is that correction of cortisol excess may not be followed by catch-up growth characteristic of many other causes of growth failure.

Gonadal steroids: Androgens and estrogens are mainly responsible for growth spurt at puberty. Androgens directly stimulate growth and maturation of bones, but presence of normal levels of GH is essential for its action. The growth response to exogenous androgens is markedly reduced in humans with GH deficiency.

Estrogens seem to have biphasic action. They stimulate growth at low concentrations but inhibit it at high concentrations. Administration of pharmacologic doses of estrogens to tall girls leads to attenuation of growth rate.

Short Stature

Short stature is defined as height more than 2 standard deviations below the mean for age and gender, which corresponds to the shortest 2.3% of individuals. This means that almost all of the other children of that age (more than 95% or 19 out of 20) are taller.

All causes of short stature fall into one of three major categories:
- Chronic disease (for example, malnutrition, congenital heart disease, kidney diseases, asthma, sickle cell anemia, thalassemia, inflammatory bowel disease, celiac disease)
- Familial short stature, or
- Constitutional delay of growth and development ("late bloomers").

Worldwide, malnutrition is the most common cause of growth failure and is usually related to poverty. Poor weight gain is often more noticeable than short stature.

Children with familial short stature have short parents. These normal children display normal growth velocity (speed of growth over time), and their bone development is normal (as indicated by the bone age corresponding to the calendar age). Children with familial short stature have normal growth spurts and enter puberty at a normal age. They typically reach an adult height similar to that of their parents.

Children with constitutional growth delay do not have any diseases. These children enter puberty later than their peers. However, because they continue to grow for a longer period of time, they catch up to their peers as they reach their adult height, which is normal and comparable to their parents. Constitutional growth delay is characterized by delayed bone age, normal growth velocity, and a predicted adult height appropriate to the family pattern.

Although rare, endocrine disorders, such as hypothyroidism or growth hormone deficiency also cause growth failure. Short stature is commonly associated with genetic diseases, such as a SHOX gene mutation, Down syndrome, or Turner syndrome. According to one authority on the subject, 98% of all cases of short stature are due to normal variation in growth (constitutional growth delay). GH deficiency and congenital hypothyroidism account for about 0.1% and 0.2% of cases of delayed growth, respectively.

Tall Stature

Many children have height greater than mean + 2DS. It is prudent to exclude familial tall stature, i.e. parents are also tall. Tall children whose parents are not tall need to be investigated for pathological disorders such as GH excess, sexual precocity and virilism. A tall child with delayed puberty should be investigated for Klinefelter syndrome. A child with

Marfan's syndrome is usually above the average height, but not outside the normal range (mean + 2SD).

Further Reading

Juul A, et al. **Serum insulin-like factor-1 in 1030 healthy children, adolescents and adults.** *J Clin Endocrinol Metab 1994; 78:744–752.*

Savine, R; Sonksen, PH. **Is the somatopause an indication for growth hormone replacement?** *J Endocrinol Invest 1999; 22 (5suppl): 142–149.*

Nwosu, BU; Lee, MM. **Evaluation of short and tall stature in children.** *Am Fam Physician. 2008; 78:597–604.*

24

Thyroid Gland

FUNCTIONAL ANATOMY

The thyroid gland is one of the largest endocrine glands. The thyroid gland is found in the neck, below the thyroid cartilage. The isthmus (the bridge between the two lobes of the thyroid) is located inferior to the cricoid cartilage (Fig. 24.1). Histologically, it consists of follicles surrounded by capillary network. The follicles are lined by cuboidal epithelium and the lumen contains a proteinaceous material called colloid (Fig. 24.2). Chemically, colloid is glycoprotein, thyroglobulin, in which thyroid hormones are synthesized and stored. The thyroid gland secretes two hormones, namely, thyroxine (tetraiodothyronine, T_4) and triiodothyronine (T3) (Fig. 24.3).

Biosynthesis and Release of Thyroid Hormones (Fig. 24.4)

The epithelial cell of thyroid follicles is unique in the sense that it is responsible for synthesis, storage and release of thyroid hormones. The

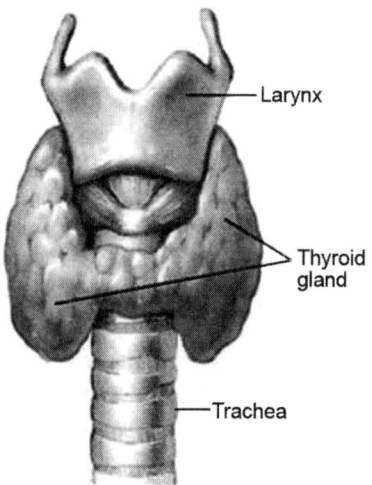

Fig. 24.1: The thyroid gland.

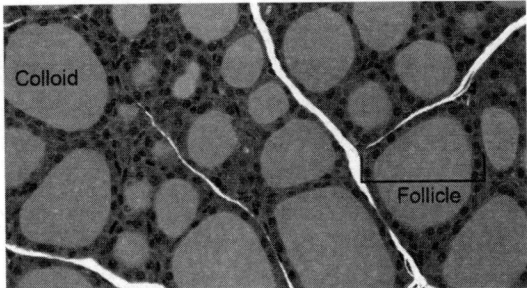

Fig. 24.2: Histology of thyroid gland.

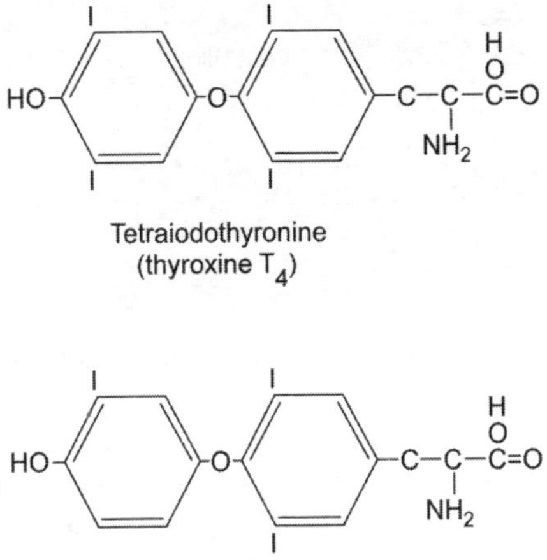

Tetraiodothyronine (thyroxine T_4)

Triiodothyronine (T_3)

Fig. 24.3: Chemical structure of thyroxine (T_4) and T_3.

synthesis and release of thyroid hormones may be considered to consist of five steps. Thyroid stimulating hormone (TSH) secreted by anterior pituitary gland promotes each step:
1. Uptake of iodide (I⁻) from the circulating blood at the basal border of the epithelial cell by an active transport mechanism.
2. Biosynthesis of thyroglobulin by the endoplasmic reticulum—Golgi apparatus and its transfer at the apical border into the follicular lumen.
3. The third step involves oxidation of iodide to iodine near the apical border of epithelial cell and its transfer to some of the tyrosine residues of thyroglobulin molecule to form monoiodotyrosine (MIT) and diiodotyrosine (DIT).
4. The fourth step involves coupling of MIT and DIT molecules to form T_4 (mainly) and T_3. The thyroglobulin molecules have T_4, T_3, MIT and DIT as well as non-iodinated tyrosine residues. Steps 3 and 4 are facilitated by an enzyme thyroperoxidase present at the apical border of the epithelial cells.

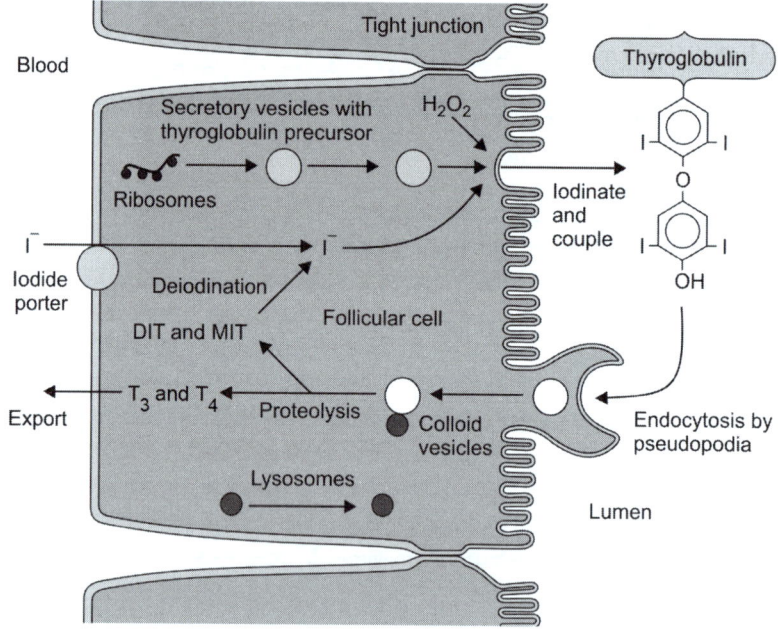

Fig. 24.4: Biosynthesis and release of thyroid hormones.

5. The fifth and final step involves release of T_4 and T_3 into blood circulation at the basal border of the epithelial cell. This steps starts as pinocytosis of a colloid droplet at the apical border, followed by proteolysis of thyroglobulin molecule in the cytoplasm, to yield T_4, T_3, MID, DIT and amino acids. Of these, T_4 and T_3 are released into blood circulation, whereas the remaining components of thyroglobulin are recycled into fresh biosynthesis of thyroid hormones (Fig. 24.4).

Plasma contains T_4 and T_3 in the ratio of 98:2. Thyroid gland is the only endogenous source of thyroxine (T_4) in the body. However, only about 20% of circulating T_3 is secreted by thyroid acini, whereas remaining 80% arises from deiodination of T_4 in the peripheral tissues.

Mode of Action of Antithyroid Agents

Monovalent anions such as chlorates and perchlorates decrease thyroxine synthesis by competitive blockade of iodide uptake by the thyroid gland. More commonly used antithyroid agent, carbimazole blocks the enzyme thyroperoxidase and therefore acts by blocking the steps of iodination of tyrosine residues and coupling reaction.

Iodide itself, when administered in large doses, blocks the iodination and coupling reactions by some unknown mechanism. This action, known as *Chaikoff effect*, is transient lasting only about 10 days. It is therapeutically useful in lowering thyroid activity in cases with thyroid storm or immediately before thyroid surgery.

Excessive intake of certain vegetables (cabbage, turnip, etc.) produces enlargement of thyroid gland ("cabbage goiter"). Such vegetables contain chemicals that inhibit iodide uptake by the thyroid gland.

TRANSPORT OF THYROID HORMONES

Thyroid hormones are transported in blood bound to plasma proteins, chiefly thyroid binding globulin (TBG). The binding of T_3 is less firm than that of T_4. That accounts for rapid onset of action and shorter half-life of T_3 than T_4.

It may be stressed that only the free forms of hormones are available for tissue actions and feedback control. The symptoms and signs of thyroid disorders correlate more closely with concentrations of free T_4 (FT_4) and free T_3 (FT_3) than with total (free + bound) T_4 and T_3. (TT_4, TT_3). Ordinarily, TT_4 is a good indicator of thyroid status of a patient. However, it becomes an unreliable indicator when plasma TBG levels are altered. Plasma TBG levels are elevated in pregnancy and in patients taking estrogens, oral contraceptives and many other drugs. On the other hand, plasma TBG levels are low in patients with nephrosis or those on steroids, androgens and some drugs. In such cases estimation of plasma FT_4 or FT_3 would be more reliable than estimations of TT_4 or TT_3.

Actions of Thyroid Hormones

Thyroid hormones affect almost all tissues of the body.
- *Cardiovascular system:* Thyroid hormones increase heart rate and force of cardiac contraction leading to increased cardiac output, and systolic blood pressure.
- *Calorigenesis:* Thyroid hormones increase oxygen consumption and heat production in almost all body tissues (except brain, and gonads). Excessive calorigenesis tends to increase body temperature which activates heat loss mechanisms, e.g. cutaneous vasodilatation (decreased total peripheral vascular resistance—decreased diastolic BP) and sweating. Thus, heat intolerance, resting tachycardia and wide pulse pressure are characteristic features of hyperthyroidism.
- *Metabolism:* At normal plasma levels, thyroxine acts as an anabolic hormone. At high plasma levels, thyroxine produces protein catabolism (muscle weakness). Thyroxine produces lipolysis (increased plasma FFA level) and lowers plasma cholesterol level
- *Gastrointestinal tract:* Thyroxine increases gastrointestinal motility.
- *Growth and development:* In the perinatal period and early childhood, thyroxine is essential for normal growth and development

of the body, nervous system in particular. Hypothyroidism during this period retards growth of neuron cell bodies, axons and dendrites as well as delays myelination, leading a permanent mental disability. Even in adults, alterations in thyroid function affect mental function.

- **Interaction with sympathetic nervous system:** Thyroxine sensitizes the tissues to the effects of catecholamines. The effect is most prominent in cardiovascular and nervous systems. This interaction explains many symptoms of hyperthyroidism such as tachycardia, palpitation, fine tremor, nervousness, etc. That is why; even though plasma and urinary levels of catecholamines are not elevated, propranolol has been found effective in blocking thyroid storm or just before thyroid surgery.

Regulation of Secretion

Thyroid stimulating hormone (TSH) is the main regulator of morphological and functional state of thyroid gland. TSH stimulates all aspects of biosynthesis and release of thyroid hormones. Excessive TSH-like activity in the blood (Graves' disease) results in hypertrophy of thyroid follicular epithelium and increased vascularity of thyroid gland. This aspect deserves attention during thyroid surgery.

Feedback control: Thyroxine affects so many tissues of the body that it is important to maintain almost constant plasma levels of T4. This is achieved by the classical hypothalamus-anterior pituitary-thyroid axis with negative feedback control (Fig. 24.5).

Biosynthesis of thyroid hormones may be affected by acute fluctuations in the availability of dietary iodide, but fluctuations in plasma T4 and T3

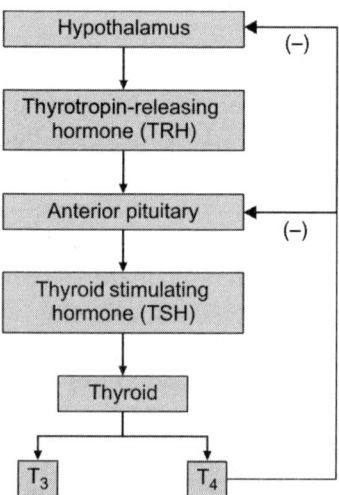

Fig. 24.5: Feedback control in hypothalamus-pituitary-thyroid axis.

are prevented by the unique large intraglandular stores of the hormone. Prolonged exposure to cold environment is the only known stimulus which may mildly increase plasma thyroxine level. This effect explains mild seasonal variations in plasma T_4 and T_3 levels (higher level in winter than in summer). Pharmacologic doses of glucocorticoids (used in some cases of thyroid storm) seem to help by decreasing the peripheral conversion of T_4 to T_3.

HYPERTHYROIDISM

Hyperthyroidism results from excessive secretion of thyroid hormones. Mostly (in 50–60%), it is due to Graves' disease. Other causes of hyperthyroidism include multinodular toxic goiter and autonomous functioning toxic adenoma.

Graves' Disease

Graves' disease is an organ-specific autoimmune disorder characterized by a variety of circulating antibodies, including common autoimmune antibodies. The most important autoantibody is thyroid-stimulating immunoglobulin (TSI). TSI acts as a TSH-receptor agonist. Similar to TSH, TSI binds to the TSH receptor on the thyroid follicular cells to activate thyroid hormone synthesis and release as well as causes hypertrophy and increased vascularity of thyroid gland. This results in the characteristic picture of Graves' thyrotoxicosis, with a diffusely enlarged thyroid, very high radioactive iodine uptake, and excessive thyroid hormone levels. Major secretory product of the thyroid gland remains T_4, but $T_3:T_4$ ratio is increased several fold, reflecting disproportionate production of T_3. In some instances, serum T_3 level alone increase; T_4 level remains normal.

Graves' disease may be associated with other autoimmune disorders, such as pernicious anemia, myasthenia gravis, vitiligo, adrenal insufficiency, and type 1 diabetes mellitus.

Increased plasma levels of thyroid hormones produce symptoms related to various organ systems: Palpitation, tachycardia, nervousness, easy fatigability, hyperkinesia, fine tremor, diarrhea, excessive sweating, and heat intolerance. Catabolic action on muscle proteins produces proximal muscle weakness, manifested by difficulty in climbing stairs. In general, nervous symptoms dominate in younger patients, whereas cardiovascular symptoms and myopathy are dominant features in older subjects in whom angina, atrial fibrillation and congestive heart failure may occur.

The pathogenesis of ophthalmopathy is not clear. It seems to be immunologically-mediated but TSI is not implicated. Within the orbit, there is proliferation of fibroblasts which secrete hydrophilic mucopolysaccharides. The resulting increase in interstitial fluid content combined with chronic inflammatory cell infiltration causes marked swelling of extraocular muscles and an increase in retrobulbar pressure. Consequently, eyeballs are displaced forward (proptosis, exophthalmos). In more severe cases, compression of optic nerve may lead to optic atrophy. Some ophthalmic signs such as stare, lid-lag, and lid-retraction are due to sympathetic overactivity.

Dermopathy (pretibial myxedema), is occasionally seen in patients with Graves' disease. A more appropriate name for this disorder would be thyroid dermopathy. It is characterized by thickness (non-pitting edema) of dermis of anterior aspects of tibia or feet. The dermis is infiltrated with lymphocytes and hydrophilic mucopolysaccharides. Almost all patients of Graves' disease with pretibial myxedema have ophthalmopathy as well.

Thyroid Storm (Hyperthyroid Crisis)

This is a rare, but life-threatening increase in severity of clinical features of hyperthyroidism. Characteristic features of thyroid storm include, fever, agitation, diarrhea, hypertension, confusion, tachycardia or atrial fibrillation and in older patients, cardiac failure. Congestive heart failure is associated with hypotension and shock

Thyrotoxic crisis is usually precipitated by a surgical emergency or any sepsis in an untreated or poorly treated patient of hyperthyroidism. (medical storm). Factor(s) that initiates the medical storm is not clear. It does not appear to be due to an acute increase in the severity of thyroid hyperfunction. It seems to be due to a shift from protein-bound to free form of thyroid hormones, secondary to production of a binding inhibitor by the systemic illness.

Thyroid storm can be a postoperative complication of subtotal thyroidectomy in a patient of hyperthyroidism who was operated without proper preparation with anti-thyroid drugs and iodide therapy (surgical storm). Surgical storm is due to a transient rise in thyroid hormone levels in blood.

Hypothyroidism

Hypothyroidism is mostly due to a disorder in the thyroid gland (primary hypothyroidism). Less than 5% cases are due to panhypopituitarism or isolated TSH deficiency (secondary hypothyroidism) or deficiency of hypothalamic TRH (tertiary hypothyroidism).

Primary hypothyroidism may result from 3 major causes:
- Autoimmune hypothyroidism
- Postablative or post ^{131}I therapy in patients with hyperthyroidism
- Iodine deficiency goiter and hypothyroidism

Autoimmune hypothyroidism is the most common organ-specific autoimmune disorder. Two specific forms of autoimmune hypothyroidism exist: (1) chronic autoimmune thyroiditis, which is also known as Hashimoto's thyroiditis or Hashimoto's disease (Fig. 24.6), and (2) autoimmune atrophic thyroiditis, which is also known as primary myxedema.

The thyroid gland becomes firm, large, and lobulated in Hashimoto's thyroiditis. Enlargement of the thyroid (goiter) is due to lymphocytic infiltration and fibrosis rather than tissue hypertrophy. It is also characterized by invasion of the thyroid tissue by leukocytes, mainly T-lymphocytes. The disorder is primarily caused by the presence of autoantibodies against thyroid peroxidase (TPO) and/or thyroglobulin which cause gradual destruction of follicles in the thyroid gland. Accordingly, the disease can be detected clinically by looking for these antibodies in the blood. Atrophic thyroiditis (primary myxedema) is similar to Hashimoto's thyroiditis, except a goiter is not present.

Post-treatment hypothyroidism: Up to half or more of patients who receive radioactive iodine treatments for an overactive thyroid develop permanent hypothyroidism within a year of therapy. Even subtotal thyroidectomy is followed by hypothyroidism in majority of the patients.

Iodine Deficiency Hypothyroidism

When iodine deficiency is severe, thyroid hormone production falls and the patient may experience a hypothyroid condition. Deficiency of thyroid hormones in the blood results in increased secretion of TSH from the anterior pituitary gland in an effort to increase T_4 production. High plasma TSH levels lead to enlargement of thyroid gland (iodine deficiency goiter, endemic goiter). In such cases, adults have the usual signs and symptoms

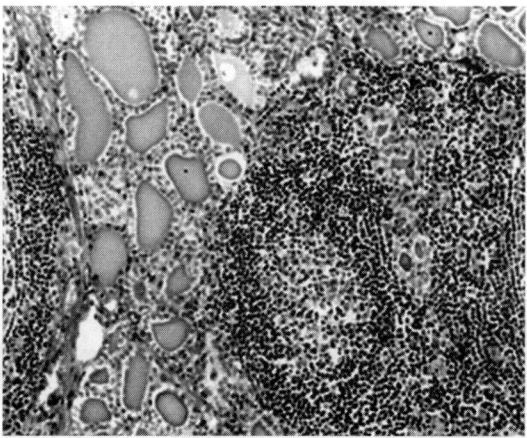

Fig. 24.6: Hashimoto thyroiditis.

of hypothyroidism. However, congenital hypothyroidism (also known as cretinism) in fetuses and young children prevents central nervous system development and maturation, resulting in permanent mental retardation, neurologic defects, and growth abnormalities.

ADULT HYPOTHYROIDISM

Myxedema is the most characteristic feature of adult hypothyroidism. It is caused by increased deposition of connective tissue components (like glycosaminoglycan, hyaluronic acid, and other mucopolysaccharides) in the dermis of the skin as well as many other tissues of the body such as heart, pleural cavity, GIT, etc. The material binds with water to produce mucinous edema (Fig. 24.7).

Skin

Accumulation of myxedematous material in the skin causes thickening of the features and puffy appearance of the face. Myxedema is non-pitting type and most apparent around the eyes, dorsum of hands and feet and supraclavicular fossae. In addition to puffy appearance, the skin is pale and cool as a result of anemia and vasoconstriction (a result of decreased heat production). Carotenemia (due to decreased conversion of carotene to vitamin A) gives yellow tint to the skin. The secretion of sweat glands and sebaceous glands is reduced giving the skin a dry coarse appearance.

Voice

The myxedematous material causes enlargement of the tongue and thickness of pharyngeal and laryngeal mucous membranes resulting in a thick slurred speech and hoarseness of voice.

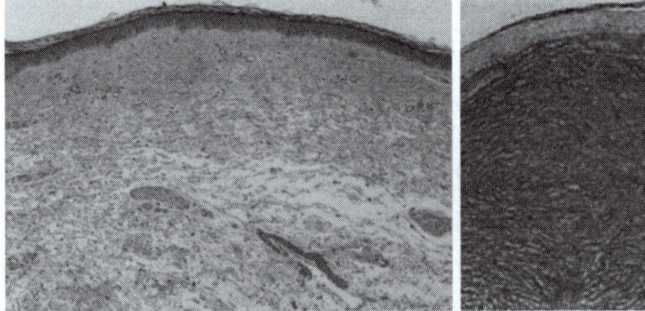

Fig. 24.7: Histological appearance of skin in myxedema. Left: H & E stain. Right: special mucin stain.

Cardiovascular System

In the heart, thyroxine deficiency results in decreased rate and force of contraction of the heart leading to a reduction in cardiac output. Presence of mucinous material in the myocardium causes enlargement of the heart. Enlargement of the heart is also due to pericardial effusion rich in proteins and mucopolysaccharides. Electrocardiogram shows sinus bradycardia, prolonged P-R interval, low amplitude Ps and QRS complexes and flattened or inverted T waves.

Respiratory System

In the respiratory system, pleural effusion is common. In severe cases, myxedematous material involves respiratory muscles results in alveolar hypoventilation and CO_2 retention. The problem is aggravated by depression of respiratory drive to hypoxia and hypercapnia. Respiratory failure is one of the contributory factors in the development of myxedema coma.

Gastrointestinal System

In the gastrointestinal system, decreased appetite and peristaltic activity leads to constipation. In spite of decreased food intake, there is moderate wait gain (not obesity) because of retention of fluid by hydrophilic polysaccharides deposited in the tissues. Total achlorhydria is seen in about 50% cases of myxedema. Consequently, malabsorption of iron and vitamin B_{12} may occur.

Hematological System

Due to a decrease in oxygen consumption and decreased production of erythropoietin, red cell mass is decreased. Anemia is usually mild, normochromic normocytic type. Less common is macrocytic anemia due to vitamin B_{12} deficiency. Hypochromic microcytic anemia may also occur due to deficient iron absorption and menorrhagia.

Nervous System

In a patient with hypothyroidism, slowing of all intellectual functions including speech is noticeable. Lack of initiative, lethargy, and somnolence are prominent. Numbness and tingling in the extremities result from accumulation of mucinous material around peripheral nerves, especially median nerve in the carpel tunnel. Tendon jerks are slow, especially during relaxation (hung up reflex). The phenomenon seems to be due to slow contraction and relaxation of muscle rather than any slowing of conduction velocity. EEG shows slow α-rhythm and generalized loss of amplitude of EEG waves.

METABOLISM

Decreased oxygen consumption, and heat production are reflected in low BMR, decreased appetite, cold intolerance and subnormal basal body temperature. Both synthesis and degradation of lipids are depressed, especially the latter. As a result, there is not only an increase in serum cholesterol but also triglycerides and LDL. HDL concentration is decreased.

Biochemical Profile

Low T_4 and elevated level of plasma TSH are hallmark of primary hypothyroidism. T_3 concentration does not help to differentiate a hypothyroid from a euthyroid patient.

In secondary hypothyroidism due to a pituitary macroadenoma, decreased plasma T_4 level is associated with low-normal or only slightly elevated plasma TSH level. Panhypopituitarism is usually present.

Myxedema Coma (Myxedema Crisis)

Myxedema coma is an extreme complication of hypothyroidism in which patients exhibit progressive mental deterioration. A common misconception is that a patient must be comatose to be diagnosed with myxedema coma. The condition occurs in patients with long-standing, untreated hypothyroidism and is usually precipitated by a secondary insult, such as climate-induced hypothermia, infection, myocardial infarction, or the administration of sedative drugs, especially opioids Myxedema coma is characterized by lethargy, confusion, stupor, delirium, or and rarely coma. Myxedema crisis would be a more appropriate term for this disorder. The basic contributory factors for the development of myxedema crisis include:

- CO_2 retention and hypoxia
- Hypothermia
- Fluid retention and hyponatremia

Further Reading

Limonard EJ, et al. **Thyroid function after subtotal thyroidectomy in patients with Graves' hyperthyroidism.** *Scientific World Journal. 2012 Article ID 548796.*
The Lancet. **"Iodine deficiency—way to go yet"**. *The Lancet 2008; 372: 88.*

25
Adrenal Gland

Each adrenal gland consists of two distinct endocrine organs within single capsule, namely adrenal cortex and adrenal medulla (Fig 25.1). Embryologically, the cortex is of mesenchymal origin whereas medulla is of neuroectodermal origin. Histologically, three zones can be identified in the adrenal cortex:

Zona glomerulosa, the subcapsular outermost zone which produces mineralocorticoids, chiefly, aldosterone.

Zona fasciculata, the middle zone secretes glucocorticoids, chiefly cortisol.

Zona reticularis, the innermost zone secreting adrenal androgens, chiefly dehydroepiandrosterone (DHEA).

The granular argentaffin cells of the adrenal medulla can be easily distinguished from lipid filled cells of adrenal cortex (Fig. 25.1).

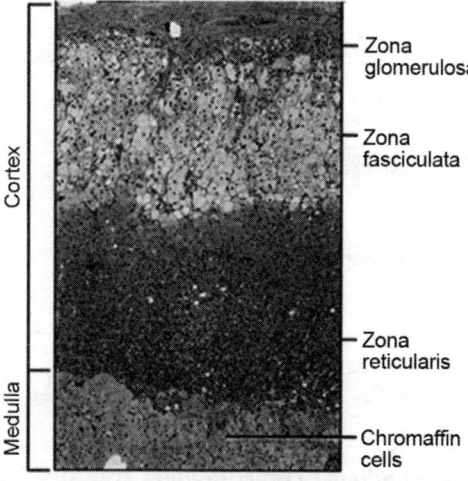

Fig. 25.1: Histology of adrenal gland.

BIOSYNTHESIS OF ADRENAL CORTICOSTEROIDS

All the adrenal corticosteroids are derived from cholesterol. Adrenal cortex can synthesize cholesterol de novo, but it mostly utilizes cholesterol from circulating low density lipoproteins (LDL). Many enzymes are essential for the synthesis of various corticosteroids (Fig. 25.2). An enzyme, cholesterol desmolase pushes cholesterol into adrenal corticosteroid synthesis pathways. Another enzyme, 17α-hydroxylase pushes steroid precursors along several side chain pathways. Activity of enzyme 17–20 lyase directs the precursors towards synthesis of adrenal androgens.

Zona glomerulosa lacks the enzyme 17α-hydroxylase, but it contains another enzyme aldosterone synthase. Therefore, in zona glomerulosa, steroid precursors are pushed straight towards aldosterone, without any production of cortisol or DHEA.

Knowledge of steroid biosynthesis pathways and various enzymes involved in it is important from the point of view of many congenital disorders of adrenal cortex.

Fetal Steroid Biosynthesis

A morphologically and functionally distinct fetal zone exists in human fetal cortex until birth, after which it rapidly involutes. The fetal zone is

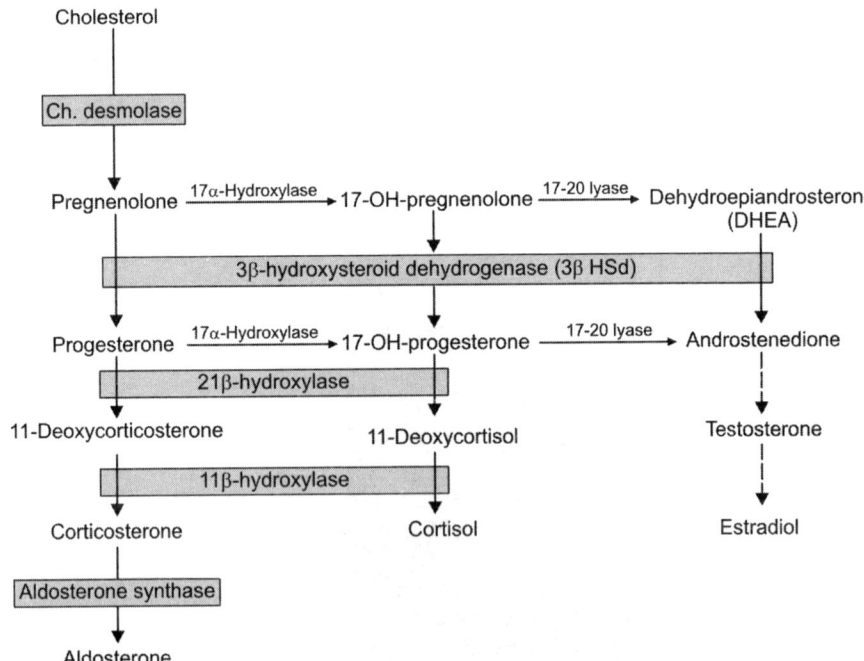

Fig. 25.2: Biosynthesis of adrenal corticosteroids. (Ch. desmolase = cholesterol desmolase).

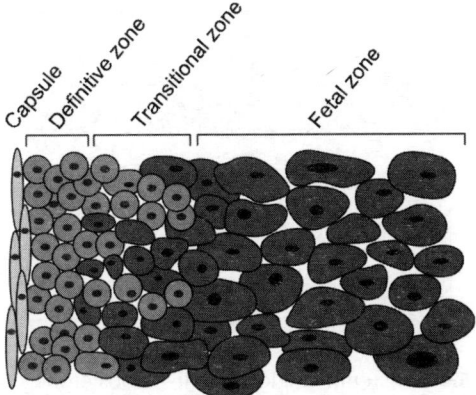

Fig. 25.3: Fetal adrenal cortex (diagrammatic).

much larger than the 'definitive zone' which remains as adrenal cortex postnatal (Fig. 25.3). Fetal zone produces DHEA and DHEAS, but not aldosterone or cortisol, because of the absence of enzyme 3β HSD. Tremendous amounts of DHEA and DHEAS produced by the fetal zone are used as precursors for estrogen synthesis by the placenta. The definitive zone of fetal cortex secretes cortisol and small amount of aldosterone. Even in adult adrenal cortex, DHEAS remains the major adrenalcortical secretory product, but except for a mild androgenic effect in the female, it does not seem to have any physiological role.

REGULATION OF ADRENAL STEROIDOGENESIS

Regulation of Glucocorticoid Secretion

Adrenocorticotropic hormone (ACTH) mainly increases the production and secretion of cortisol and androgens and to a minor extent aldosterone. ACTH has an acute effect which occurs in minutes and a chronic effect which requires many days of elevated ACTH level in plasma. The acute effect is to increase the activity of enzyme cholesterol desmolase in the adrenal cortex. In contrast, chronic effect involves increased synthesis of most of the enzymes of steroidogenic pathways, as well as, general action of producing hyperplasia of adrenal cortical cells. The regulation of ACTH secretion has been discussed elsewhere (*see* Chapter 23).

Regulation of Mineralocorticoid Secretion

Unlike cortisol, aldosterone secretion is controlled by a number of mechanisms, but renin – angiotensin II mechanism (Figs 25.4 and 25.5) and plasma K^+ concentration are the main regulators. These agents increase the release of aldosterone by increasing the activity of enzymes cholesterol desmolase and aldosterone synthase.

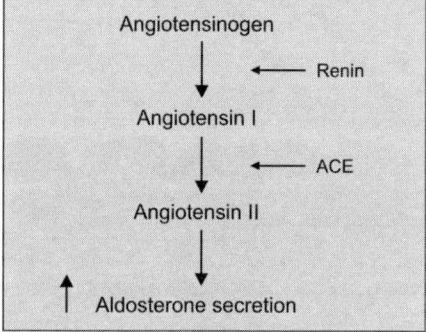

Fig. 25.4: The renin–angiotensin II—aldosterone system.

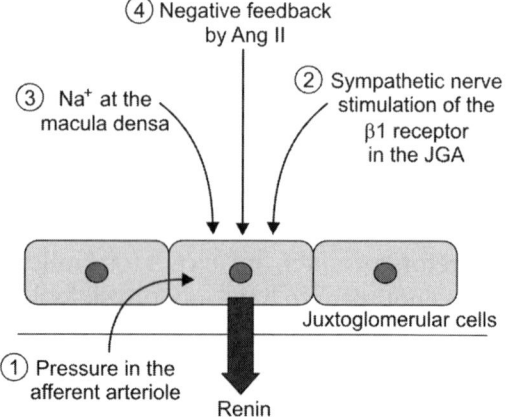

Fig. 25.5: Regulation of renin secretion.

Renin secretion by juxtaglomerular cells (JG cells) of the renal afferent arterioles is increased by (Fig. 25.5):
- A decreased in blood volume (dehydration, hemorrhage)
- A decrease in Na^+ delivery in distal convoluted tubule as sensed by macula densa cells
- Increased sympathetic neural discharge (hemorrhage)

On the other hand, an increase in plasma levels of angiotensin II or atrial natriuretic peptide (ANP) or a decrease in K^+ level inhibit secretion of renin. Plasma K^+ has a direct action on zona glomerulosa cells. Even a mild increase in plasma K^+ level directly increases aldosterone secretion.

Regulation of Adrenal Androgen Secretion

The control of androgen biosynthesis and secretion is not clear, but ACTH seems to be the main regulator. Adrenal androgen secretion is low in childhood but increase after puberty. During severe illness or in old age, adrenal androgen secretion decrease; without any concomitant changes in ACTH secretion. Many researches have tried to prove rejuvenation effects of DHEA in old age, but the results are not convincing.

Transport in Blood

Cortisol is transported in blood bound to plasma proteins, chiefly cortisol binding globulin (CBG) (95%) and in free form (5%). Free cortisol is the physiologically active form of cortisol. It is the free form that gets filtered into glomerular filtrate and appears in the urine. In states of hypersecretion of cortisol, up to 25% of plasma cortisol may exist as free form, because the limited capacity of CBG is saturated. Therefore, increased quantity of free cortisol is excreted in the urine.

High plasma estrogen level increases plasma CBG concentration. Hence, high estrogen states such as pregnancy, oral contraceptive therapy, cause a parallel increase in protein bound cortisol. However, since the plasma concentration of free cortisol is not increased manifestations of glucocorticoid excess do not appear. Most synthetic glucocorticoids have low affinity for CBG. That explains the tendency of some synthetic analogues to cause Cushingoid effects even at low doses.

With a pronounced circadian rhythm, between 15 and 30 mg of cortisol is secreted by the adrenal cortex per day. Liver is the main organ causing its inactivation by reduction followed by conjugation with glucuronic acid. The resultant water soluble compounds are excreted in the urine. Urine also contains a small amount of free cortisol (20–100 µg/day). Only about 50–250 µg of aldosterone is secreted by the adrenal cortex per day. It is chiefly inactivated in the liver. In liver cirrhosis or congestive heart failure with hypoperfusion of liver, hepatic clearance of aldosterone is decreased. About 15–30 mg of adrenal androgens are secreted by the adrenal cortex per day, chiefly as DHEA– sulphate. DHEA is the major precursor of urinary 17-ketosteroids. In men, 2/3rds of urinary 17-ketosteroids are derived from the adrenal androgens, and 1/3rds from the testes. In women, the entire urinary 17-ketosteroids are of adrenal origin.

ACTIONS OF GLUCOCORTICOIDS

Naturally occurring glucocorticoids have a predominant role in intermediary metabolism, though they have a weak action on mineral metabolism also. Cortisol regulates intermediary metabolism of carbohydrates, proteins and fats. It increases blood glucose level by promoting hepatic *gluconeogenesis* and decreasing peripheral utilization of glucose. Cortisol promotes *protein catabolism* in the skeletal muscle.

The keto-acids produced by deamination of amino acids act as substrate for gluconeogenesis. Cortisol increases plasma FFA level by mobilization of stored fat.

Glucocorticoids increase renal free water clearance by a number of mechanisms, i.e. increased GFR, suppression of ADH secretion, and a direct action on renal tubules. This action assumes importance only in cases with adrenal corticoid deficiency states, since the patient has difficulty in excretion of a water load. Glucocorticoids have a weak action of Na^+ and water retention and K^+ excretion in the kidney. However, in Cushingoid states, salt and water retention is one of the important clinical features.

Role during stress: Any type of stress — physical (e.g. surgery, extensive trauma), psychological (e.g. anxiety, depression) or physiological (hypoglycemia, severe exercise)—may produce up to 20-fold increase in the secretion of ACTH and glucocorticoids (Fig. 25.6).

The mechanism(s) by which elevated levels of cortisol protect the body against stress is not clear. In patients with adrenal cortical deficiency on replacement therapy, any stress may lead to hypotension, shock and death, unless the dose of glucocorticoids is increased during the period of stress.

The anti-inflammatory action of glucocorticoids is seen only when administered in pharmacologic doses (or in states of glucocorticoid hypersecretion). Glucocorticoids suppress various aspects of inflammatory response and decrease capillary permeability and exudation as well as fibroblast proliferation. All these actions result from an inhibition of phospholipase A2 leading to a reduction in the release of leukotrienes, thromboxane, prostaglandins and prostacyclin. Glucocorticoids also inhibit the release of interleukin-1. Hence systemic effects of inflammation are suppressed. Whereas, these pharmacologic actions are useful in autoimmune inflammations such as rheumatoid

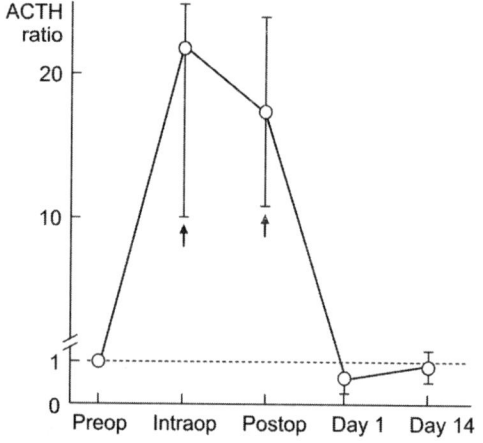

Fig. 25.6: Plasma ACTH levels during surgical operations.

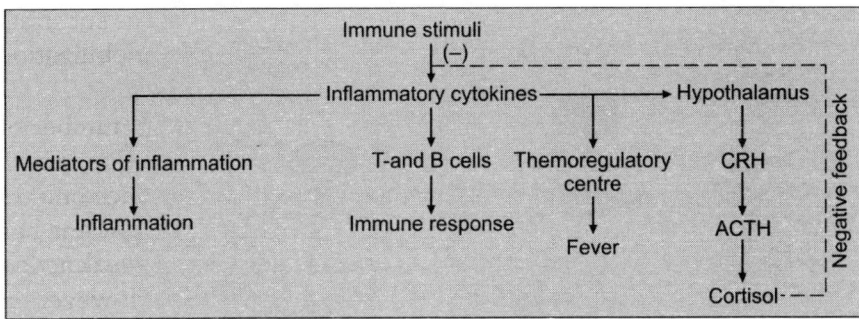

Fig. 25.7: Feedback effect of immune responses.

arthritis or rheumatic heart disease, glucocorticoid administration may mask the symptoms and signs of acute bacterial infections. Acute bacterial infections may also become more fulminating since normal "walling effect" of inflammatory response is absent. Glucocorticoid excess also suppresses the immunological response of T- and B-lymphocytes (Fig. 25.7).

In pharmacologic doses, glucocorticoids have a powerful **anti-allergic action by** inhibiting the actions of histamine by some unknown mechanism. Their importance in the treatment of anaphylactic states cannot be overemphasized.

Glucocorticoids have an important role in growth and differentiation. In embryonic life, glucocorticoids induce surfactant production by type II pneumocytes; and promote differentiation of neural crest epithelium into chromaffin cells of adrenal medulla.

Actions of Mineralocorticoids

Aldosterone acts on Na^+–K^+-ATPase pump at the basolateral border of the cells of distal tubules and collecting ducts of the kidney. The active reabsorption of Na^+ is followed by H_2O retention by osmotic effect. From the luminal border, Na^+ is reabsorbed by a carrier mediated diffusion using Na^+–K^+ antiport and Na^+–H^+ antiport systems. Therefore, increased urinary loss of K^+ and H^+ is an essential component of the action of aldosterone (Fig. 25.8).

Escape Phenomenon

When aldosterone levels are continuously elevated, Na^+ and H_2O retention occurs but not to a stage that edema may occur, because renal tubules "escape" from the action of aldosterone beyond a limit. The exact mechanism of this "escape phenomenon" is not clear. It seems to be related to increased secretion of atrial natriuretic peptide (ANP); or a change in the renal hemodynamics may play a role. *However, it may be remembered that there is no escape for K^+ losing effect of aldosterone.*

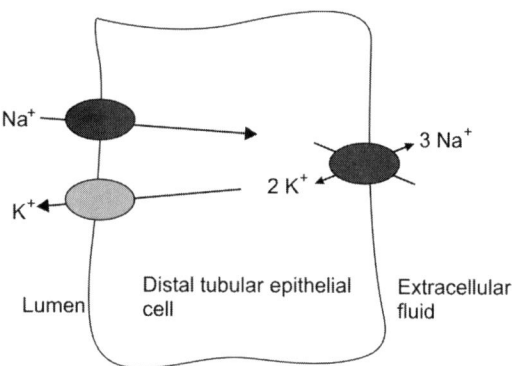

Fig. 25.8: Renal action of aldosterone.

HYPERFUNCTION OF ADRENAL CORTEX

Excessive secretion of adrenal cortical hormones may result in Cushing syndrome (glucocorticoid excess), primary or secondary hyperaldosteronism (aldosterone excess) or virilism (androgen excess). These syndromes do not always occur in 'pure' form; overlapping often occurs.

Cushing Syndrome

The commonest cause of Cushing syndrome nowadays is iatrogenic, i.e. prolonged administration of pharmacologic doses of glucocorticoids. The following discussion refers to the 'spontaneous' Cushing syndrome.

In most cases, there is bilateral adrenal hyperplasia caused by a hypersecretion of ACTH by a microadenoma of anterior pituitary gland or more rarely due to ACTH secretion by a non-endocrine tumor (e.g. carcinoma lung). An individual who has ACTH producing tumor is said to be suffering from **Cushing disease** (as it was originally described by Cushing in1932). All other disorders of glucocorticoid excess are grouped under the heading of **Cushing syndrome.** About 20–25% of cases of Cushing syndrome have adrenal neoplasia (adenoma or carcinoma). This condition is known as **non-ACTH dependent Cushing syndrome.**

Clinical features of Cushing syndrome can be derived from the physiologic or pharmacologic actions of glucocorticoids (Table 25.1).

In a patient of Cushing syndrome all the clinical features may not be present (Table 25.2).

Primary Aldosteronism (Conn's Syndrome)

This disorder is typically due to an aldosterone producing adrenal adenoma or bilateral cortical hyperplasia. Clinical features include hypertension, headache, muscular weakness or muscle cramps. After renal disease, Conn syndrome is said to be second most common cause of secondary hypertension.

Table 25.1: Pathophysiologic basis of clinical features of Cushing syndrome

Clinical sign	Pathophysiologic basis
Centripetal obesity: moon-like face, buffalo –hump, thin limbs	Redistribution of body fat
Increased body weight	Salt and water retention
Easy fatigability, Muscle weakness: proximal myopathy	Muscle protein catabolism
Hypertension	Salt and water retention
Impaired glucose tolerance	Anti-insulin action of glucocorticoids
Abdominal striae	Decreased collagen synthesis: scarring of thin fragile skin
Impotence in men, oligomenorrhea, infertility in women	Suppression of FSH, LH secretion
Easy bruisability	Vessel wall weakness
Back ache, vertebral collapse, fractures	Osteoporosis: decreased osteoblastic activity, decreased intestinal calcium absorption
Hirsutism	Increased androgen production
Psychological disturbance	Cerebral effects of high glucocorticoid levels

Table 25.2: Frequency of clinical features in patients with Cushing syndrome

Feature	Proportion
Obesity or weight gain	95%
Facial plethora	90%
Rounded face	90%
Decreased libido	90%
Thin skin	85%
Decreased linear growth	70–80%
Menstrual irregularity	80%
Hypertension	75%
Hirsutism	75%
Depression or emotional lability	70%
Bruising easily	65%
Clucose intolerance	60%
Weakness	60%
Osteopenia or fracture	50%

The action of excess of aldosterone produces hypernatremia, water retention, hypokalemia, and alkalosis. Hypernatremia and water retention lead to hypertension. Hypokalemia produces muscle weakness and fatigue, whereas muscle cramps are related to alkalosis (alkalotic tetany). Edema does not occur because of 'escape phenomenon', unless congestive heart failure or renal disease is associated. Plasma aldosterone level is increased, whereas plasma renin activity is very low (negative feedback effect).

Secondary Hyperaldosteronism

Elevated plasma aldosterone level and hypokalemia are also features of a number of disease states associated with peripheral edema, e.g.

324 Pathophysiology

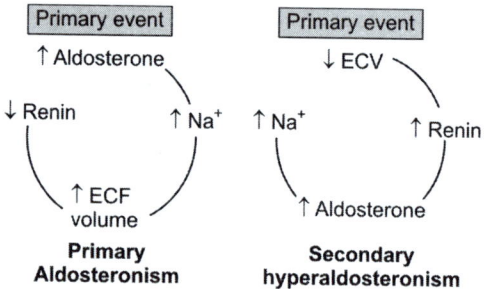

Fig. 25.9: Pathophysiologic difference in increase in plasma aldosterone level in primary aldosteronism and secondary hyperaldosteronism.

congestive heart failure, liver cirrhosis and nephrotic syndrome. The primary event in secondary hyperaldosteronism is a decrease in effective circulating volume (Fig. 25.9).

Syndromes of Adrenal Androgen Excess (Congenital Adrenal Hyperplasia)

Congenital adrenal hyperplasia (CAH) refers to any of several autosomal recessive diseases resulting from mutations of genes for enzymes mediating the biochemical steps of adrenal corticosteroid biosynthesis. It results in abnormal plasma concentrations of cortisol, aldosterone and androgens.

In patients with complete deficiency of 21β-hydroxylase, synthesis of cortisol and aldosterone is inhibited resulting in increased plasma levels of ACTH by feedback action. Increased plasma levels of ACTH produce adrenal hyperplasia as well as increased the activity of cholesterol desmolase. Consequently, more of cholesterol is pushed into the open pathway of adrenal androgen biosynthesis (Fig. 25.10).

Among these enzyme defects, partial deficiency of 21β-hydroxylase is most common, i.e. seen in 90–95% cases of CAH. The decreased synthesis of cortisol and aldosterone is compensated by increased ACTH secretion leading to adrenal hyperplasia. Since pathway of adrenal androgen biosynthesis is fully open, androgen synthesis is increased. High plasma androgen levels produce virilism (compensated form). Virilization is usually apparent at birth in a female baby or within 2–3 years of life in a male baby.

Congenital deficiency of 11β-hydroxylase (5% cases of CAH) results in deficiency of cortisol and aldosterone but excessive secretion of 11-deoxycortisol and 11-deoxycorticosterone (Fig. 25.2). Since the latter is an active mineralocorticoid, the patient suffers from salt and water retention, hypertension, cortisol deficiency and androgen excess (hypertensive form of CAH).

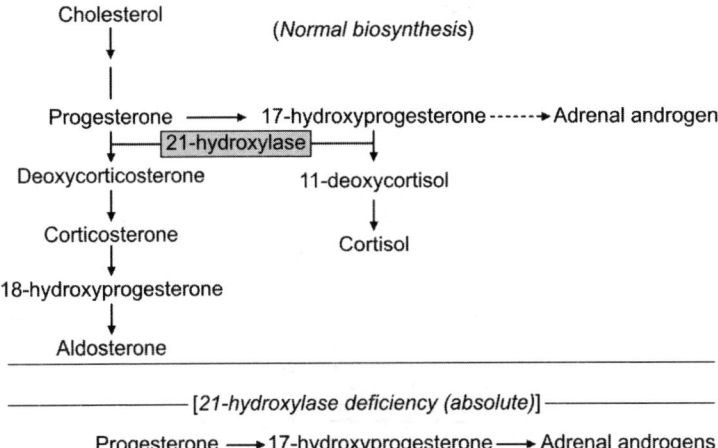

Fig. 25.10: Effect of deficiency of 21-hydroxylase on adrenal corticoid hormone secretion (lower panel) as compared to normal biosynthesis of adrenal cortical hormones (upper panel).

ADRENOCORTICAL INSUFFICIENCY

In **primary adrenal insufficiency**, adrenal glands fail to produce all the adrenocortical hormones. Plasma ACTH level is elevated. Causes include an autoimmune disorder, tuberculosis or bilateral adrenalectomy.

Symptoms result from deficiency of both glucocorticoids and mineralocorticoids: hypoglycemia, dehydration, weight loss, and disorientation. Symptoms may also include weakness, tiredness, dizziness, low blood pressure that falls further when standing (orthostatic hypotension), cardiovascular collapse, muscle aches, nausea, vomiting, and diarrhea. Since the symptoms are vague, it is the pigmentation of skin and mucous membranes (an effect of high ACTH levels) which usually alert the physician to the possibility of the disorder.

Secondary adrenocortical insufficiency results from deficient ACTH production, because of a hypothalamic-pituitary disease or more commonly following sudden withdrawal of chronically administration pharmacologic doses of glucocorticoids. In cases of secondary adrenal insufficiency, aldosterone secretion is usually normal. Moreover, hyperpigmentation does not occur.

ADRENAL MEDULLA

Adrenal medulla and sympathetic nervous system constitute an anatomic and physiologic unit, referred to as sympathoadrenal system. Norepinephrine (NE) is the only catecholamine released at adrenergic postganglionic sympathetic nerve endings. Adrenal medulla releases both

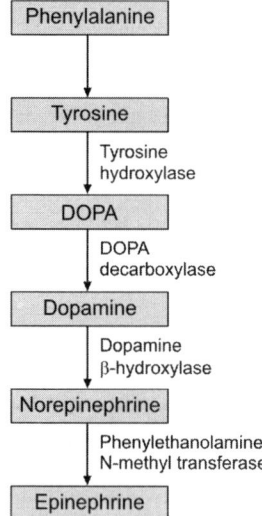

epinephrine (E) and NE in the ratio of about 80:20. Adrenal medulla also releases another catecholamine, namely dopamine, whose physiological function is not yet known.

The reactions involved in the biosynthesis of catecholamines are given above. The enzyme phenyl ethanolamine N-methyl transferase (PNMT) is present only in adrenal medulla and epinephrine-secreting neurons in CNS. Postganglionic sympathetic neurons do not contain PNMT and therefore cannot synthesize/release NE.

Effects of Adrenergic Receptor Stimulation

A1 receptor stimulation produces *vasoconstriction* in coronary, skeletal, cutaneous, renal and gastrointestinal blood vessels. It also produces pupillary dilatation and relaxation of intestinal smooth muscle.

A2 receptor stimulation produces vasoconstriction, platelet aggregation and inhibition of insulin release.

B1 receptor stimulation produces *increased rate and force of contraction of the heart*, intestinal relaxation and lipolysis (in adipose tissue).

B2 receptor stimulation produces bronchodilatation, vasodilatation in skeletal and pulmonary vessels, intestinal relaxation, calorigenesis, glycogenolysis, and hyperglycemia. β-blockers are widely used in clinical medicine.

Sympathoadrenal Response in Some Pathophysiologic States

Volume depletion, because of hemorrhage or dehydration, brings about a strong sympathetic neural response. If hypotension is pronounced, adrenal medulla is also recruited; adrenal catecholamines reinforce the effects of increased sympathetic neural discharge.

Congestive heart failure is characterized by selective increase in sympathetic neural charge. Whereas chronotropic and inotropic effects on the heart improve cardiac output, selective arteriolar constriction in the skin, subcutaneous tissue and abdominal viscera helps to divert blood to vital organs such as brain and heart.

Hypoglycemia produces selective and marked increase in epinephrine secretion from adrenal medulla rather than a generalized increase in sympathoadrenal discharge. Epinephrine increases hepatic output of glucose as well as increases plasma levels of alternative fuels such as FFA and ketone bodies. Most of the clinical manifestations of hypoglycemia (tachycardia, palpitation, nervousness, tremor, cold sweat) are related to the effects of increased plasma epinephrine level on CVS and CNS. In patients with longstanding diabetes, the adrenal medullary response to hypoglycemia is blunted leading to *hypoglycemia unawareness*. Such patients are at risk of developing severe hypoglycemia leading to cerebral damage.

Acute stress of any type results in strong activation of sympathoadrenal system. Beneficial effects of increased sympathoadrenal discharge during severe exercise, hypoglycemia, cold exposure or hemorrhage are obvious. If this response is not able to maintain homeostasis, other stress hormones, mainly cortisol are released by activation of hypothalamus-pituitary adrenal cortex axis (Fig. 25.11). If the stress becomes chronic (e.g. burns, multiple fractures) adrenal medullary discharge subsides but adrenal cortical response continues till stress subsides.

In spite of dramatic increase in adrenal medullary discharge seen on exposure to acute stress, adrenal medulla, unlike adrenal cortex, is not essential for survival. Following bilateral adrenalectomy, replacement

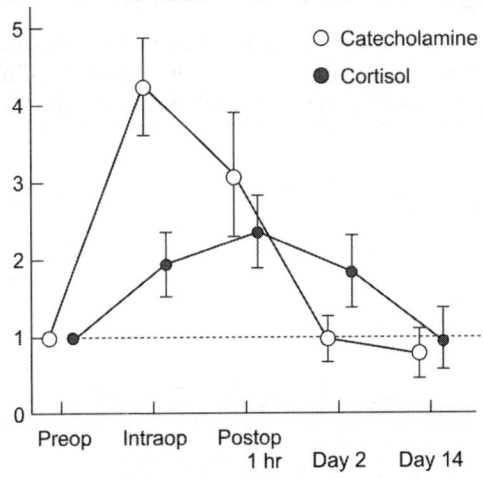

Fig. 25.11: Time-course of changes in plasma cortisol and catecholamine levels during and after surgery.

therapy with glucomineralocorticoids is sufficient for maintenance of normal health.

Pheochromocytoma

Pheochromocytoma is a rare tumor of adrenal medullary chromaffin cells. It accounts for less than 0.1% of all cases of hypertension. Still rarer is a tumor arising from extra-adrenal chromaffin cells, e.g. in sympathetic chain or prevertebral sympathetic ganglia. Adrenal pheochromocytoma produces both E and NE but NE predominates. Extra-adrenal pheochromocytoma produces NE only. Unlike adrenal pheochromocytoma, the secretion from extra-adrenal tumor is not related to sympathetic neural discharge.

Hypertension is the commonest manifestation of pheochromocytoma. In over 60% of the cases, hypertension is sustained, often severe, and resistant to treatment. Even though hypertension is sustained, blood pressure is labile. Many patients have distinct crisis or paroxysms. In the rest 40% it is episodic, with paroxysms of severe hypertension, headache, palpitation, apprehension and profuse sweating. The paroxysms may be precipitated once or twice daily by any activity that displaces abdominal viscera. Other clinical features include fever, mild to moderate weight loss (due to tissue hypermetabolism). Orthostatic hypotension is often present. It seems to be related reduced blood volume or blunting of baroreceptor reflexes due to sustained increase in blood pressure. Both of these factors predispose the patient to develop hypotension and shock during any trauma or surgery. Impaired glucose tolerance may occur due to suppression of insulin secretion.

> **Further Reading**
>
> Findling, JW; Raff, H. **Clinical review: Cushing's syndrome: Important issues in diagnosis and management.** *Endocrinol Metab 2006; 91:3746–3753.*
>
> Boscaro, M, et al. **Cushing's syndrome.** Lancet 2001; 357:783–791.

26

Endocrine Pancreas

The endocrine pancreas is constituted by about one million islets distributed throughout the exocrine pancreatic acini, each of which measures about 0.2 mm in diameter (Fig. 26.1).

PHYSIOLOGICAL CONSIDERATIONS

The islets of Langerhans' contain four types of cells:
A cells (α cells) that secrete glucagon (15–20%)
B cells (β cells) that secrete insulin (65–80 %)
D cells (δ cells) that secrete somatostatin (3–10%)
PP cells that secrete pancreatic polypeptide (3–5%).

INSULIN

Insulin consists of two polypeptide chains joined together by two disulfide bridges. It is synthesized in the B (β) cells of the islets of Langerhans. The human pancreas secretes about 40–50 units of insulin per day in a normal adult. Insulin secretion is increased by:
- Increased plasma glucose level

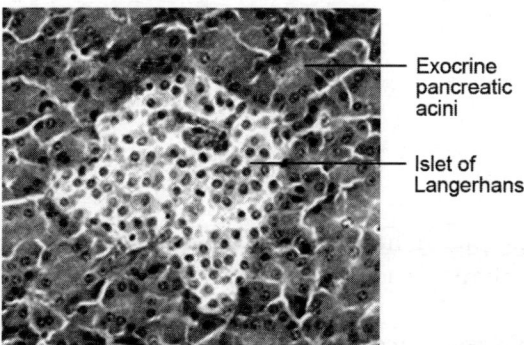

Fig. 26.1: Exocrine and endocrine pancreas (islet of Langerhans).

- Increased plasma amino acid level
- Vagal stimulation
- Enteric hormones such as GIP, CCK, gastrin

In postprandial state, all the four factors named above are activated. Inhibitors of insulin secretion include hypoglycemia and sympathetic stimulation.

Actions of Insulin

In Liver

Promotes

- Glycogenesis
- Glycolysis
- Synthesis of triglycerides, cholesterol and VDLD
- Protein synthesis

Inhibits

- Glycogenolysis
- Ketogenesis
- Gluconeogenesis

In Skeletal Muscle

Promotes

- Protein synthesis
- Glycolysis

Inhibits

Glycogenolysis

In Adipose Tissue

Promotes

Lipogenesis

Inhibits

Lipolysis

Glucagon

Glucagon is a single chain polypeptide synthesized by A (α) cells of the islets of Langerhans. It is a single polypeptide chain. Its secretion is promoted by:
- Decreased plasma glucose level
- Increased plasma amino acid level

Actions

In the liver, it promotes glycogenolysis, gluconeogenesis and ketogenesis.
In adipose tissue, it promotes lipolysis.

BLOOD GLUCOSE HOMEOSTASIS

In fasting state, normal range of plasma glucose is 70–110 mg/dl (4.4–6.1 mmol/L. Postprandial, it rises but normally remains <140 mg/dl (7.8 mmol/L). Plasma glucose levels in mg/dl and equivalent values in mmol/L are depicted in Fig. 26.2. Maintenance of plasma glucose level within the normal range is critical for survival, because plasma glucose is the predominant fuel utilized by central nervous system. Even a brief period of hypoglycemia produces profound dysfunction of the brain, which if prolonged can be fatal. That may be the reason why the body is provided with only one hypoglycemic hormone (insulin) as compared to four hyperglycemic hormones (also known as counter-regulatory hormones), namely, glucagon, epinephrine, cortisol and growth hormone. Therefore, physiologically, hypoglycemia is rare, but mild hyperglycemia occurs after every meal.

Postprandial State

After a meal, the absorption of end products of digestion causes an increase in blood glucose level that results in increased secretion of insulin

Blood glucose	
mmol/L	mg/dL
2	35
3	55
4	75
5	90
5.5	100
6	110
7	120
8	150
9	160
10	180
11	200
12	215
13	235
14	250
15	270
16	288

Fig. 26.2: Comparison of blood sugar values in mmol/L and mg/dL.

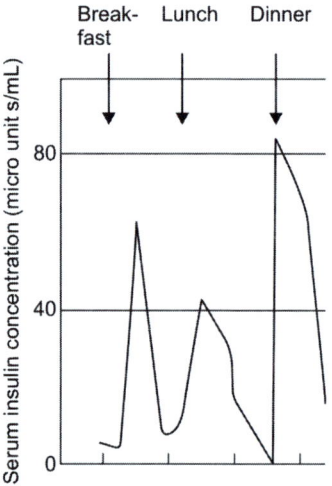

Fig. 26.3: Insulin secretion occurs after each meal.

(Fig. 26.3), as well as, inhibition of glucagon release. Consequently, blood glucose is metabolized to yield energy as well as stored as glycogen in the liver and skeletal muscle. When the glycogen stores are saturated, all the extra glucose is converted to fatty acids in the liver, and transported to adipose tissue to be stored as triglycerides. As a result of all these changes, the elevated blood glucose level is brought to normal within 2 hours after a meal.

Postabsorptive State

About six hours after food intake, glucose delivery to the circulation ceases. Since, glucose utilization continues, plasma glucose level tends to fall. However, plasma glucose remains within the normal range due to release of one or more counter-regulatory hormones. At first, glucagon secretion increases. If fasting is prolonged, or glucagon secretion is inadequate to maintain normal plasma glucose level, secretion of adrenal catecholamines, chiefly epinephrine increases. Increased secretion of adrenal catecholamines is indicated by clinical features such as palpitation, tachycardia, cold sweating, anxiety, etc. If fasting is prolonged, cortisol and growth hormone secretion is also recruited.

Increased secretion of counter-regulatory hormones results in improvement in blood glucose level by a number of mechanisms, such as glycogenolysis (glucagon, epinephrine), gluconeogenesis (glucagon, cortisol) and lipolysis, leading to increased plasma FFA and ketogenesis as well as inhibition of glucose utilization in the peripheral tissues. FFA and ketone bodies become the chief fuel for the body except the brain, where glucose remains the chief substrate for energy production.

PATHOPHYSIOLOGY OF DIABETES MELLITUS

Insulin deficiency, relative or absolute, produces abnormalities in metabolism of carbohydrates, fats and proteins–hyperglycemia, ketosis and increased protein catabolism (Fig. 26.4). Untreated diabetes mellitus (DM) is liable to result in acute complications such as ketotic coma or hyperosmolar coma or chronic complications such as neuropathy, and microvascular and macrovascular complication which may affect almost every organ in the body.

1. Hyperglycemia and its Consequences

Hyperglycemia is one of the cardinal features of DM. It results from decreased tissue glucose utilization coupled with increased rate of gluconeogenesis. When the blood glucose is chronically elevated, the following complications are likely to occur:

i. *Glycosuria, Polyuria, and Polydipsia*

When the blood glucose level exceeds its renal threshold value, it appears in the urine (*glycosuria or glucosuria*). Renal excretion of osmotically active glucose molecules leads to excretion of a large amount of water in the urine *(osmotic diuresis or polyuria)*. The resultant tissue dehydration activates the thirst mechanisms, producing *polydipsia*. Appreciable amounts of Na$^+$ and K$^+$ are lost in the urine as a side effect of osmotic diuresis.

Glucose transport in nervous tissue in general is independent of insulin. However, in ventromedial nucleus (VMN) of hypothalamus, known as

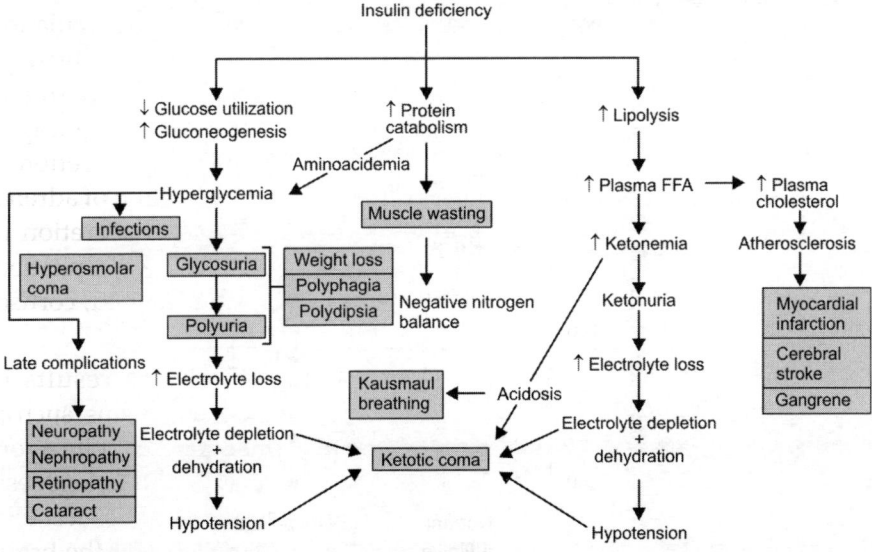

Fig. 26.4: Pathophysiology of diabetes mellitus and its complications.

the satiety center for food intake, glucose transport is insulin-dependent. Consequently, in DM, despite hyperglycemia, VMN remains deficient of glucose and hence not activated. This accounts for *hyperphagia* in a patient with DM. Despite hyperphagia, there is *loss of body weight* in DM. Loss of weight is partly accounted for by the loss of glucose (energy) in the urine and partly because of mobilization of fats and proteins (muscle wasting) for energy production.

From the information given in the textbooks of physiology, it is commonly assumed that renal threshold of glucose (RTG) is fixed at 180 mg/dl. Actually, this is a mean value and there are considerable variations in RTG in normal individuals (just as every individual does not have GFR of 125 ml/dl). The information is important in diabetics where in one study, the mean value was found to be 130 mg/dl. Therefore, in old diabetics, degree of glycosuria does not accurately reflect the plasma glucose level. *Hence, urinary glucose excretion cannot be used to regulate antidiabetic therapy.*

ii. Impaired Phagocytic Function

Hyperglycemia impairs all aspects of leukocyte phagocytic function (adherence, diapedesis, phagocytosis and intracellular killing, Fig. 26.5). Although the exact level above which leukocyte function is impaired is not defined, in vitro evidence suggests a blood concentration of 200 mg/dl as a possible threshold. Humoral immunity and lymphocyte function are also affected. That explains the increased incidence and severity of infections in diabetics. Susceptibility to infections increases with longer

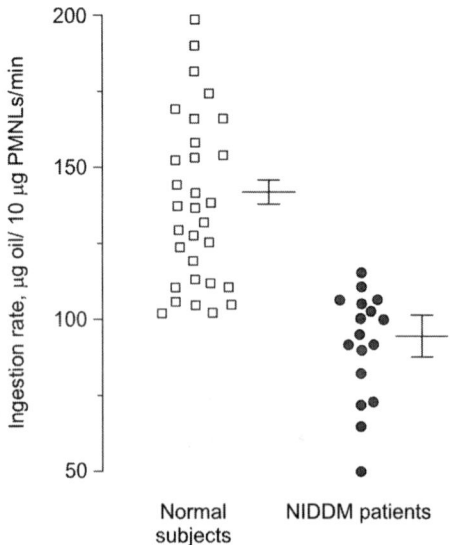

Fig. 26.5: Phagocytic activity in diabetes mellitus.

Endocrine Pancreas

duration and greater severity of diabetes. The presence of glucose in the urine predisposes a diabetic patient especially to urinary tract infections.

iii. Hyperosmolar Effects

As plasma glucose level increases above the renal threshold, progressively increasing degree of glycosuria prevents plasma glucose level from exceeding 300–500 mg/dl. Any intercurrent illness may increase glucose production secondary to release of stress hormones. If the fluid ingestion is simultaneously impaired, decreased extracellular fluid volume reduces glomerular filtration rate. As a result, urinary excretion of glucose is impaired. Because of increased production and decreased urinary excretion, plasma glucose may exceed 600 mg/dl (plasma osmolality > 320 mOsm/kg, normal: 285–295 mOsm/kg).) The hyperosmolality causes tissue dehydration, especially in CNS. The condition called non-ketotic hyperosmolar coma may be fatal. Non-ketotic coma is usually precipitated by an infection, myocardial infarction, stroke or another acute illness complicating a poorly controlled diabetes mellitus.

Plasma osmolality can be calculated as follows:

$$\text{Plasma osmolality (mOsm/kg)} = 2(\text{serum Na}) + \frac{\text{Glucose (mg/dl)}}{18} + \frac{\text{BUN (mg/dl)}}{2.8}$$

iv. Glycosylation (Glycation) of Hemoglobin

In normoglycemic individuals, glucose molecules get non-enzymatically to a small proportion (< 7%) of hemoglobin A. Glucose is attached to terminal valine of each β chain (Fig. 26.6). The attachment occurs continually over the entire lifespan of the erythrocyte and is dependent on blood glucose concentration and the duration of exposure of the erythrocyte to blood glucose.

The product is called glycosylated (glycated) hemoglobin (HbA_1). Three variants of HbA_1 are known, namely, HbA_{1a}, HbA_{1b} and HbA_{1c}.

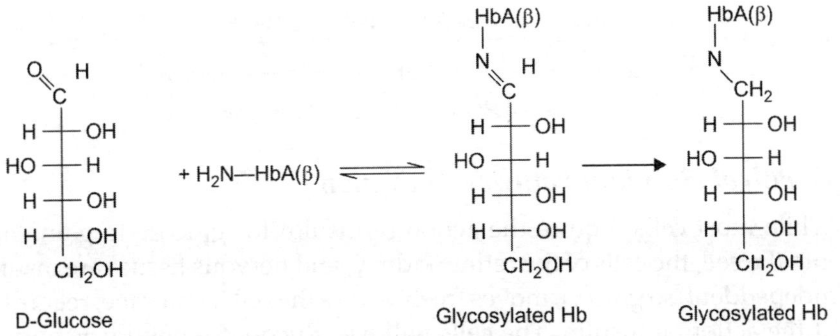

Fig. 26.6: Glycosylation of hemoglobin.

Table 26.1: Derived relationship of HbA$_{1c}$ to estimated average glucose (eAG)

HbA$_{1c}$ (%)	eAG (mg/dl)
5	97
6	126
7	154
8	183
9	212
10	240
11	269
12	298

Glycosylation does not practically affect any physiological function of hemoglobin, but its estimation has an important role in the diagnosis and treatment of diabetes mellitus. The concentration of HbA$_{1c}$ reflects average plasma glucose level of the individual during the previous 6–8 weeks. Therefore, periodic measurement of HbA$_{1c}$ has become an important tool to assess the glycemic control of a diabetic patient.

Until now, the use of HbA$_{1c}$ was not recommended for diagnosis of diabetes. In a recent announcement, the International Expert Committee, which includes representatives from the ADA, International Diabetes Federation, and European Association for the Study of Diabetes (EASD), has recommended HbA$_{1c}$ for diagnosis of diabetes with cut point at 6.5% (Table 26.1).

v. Advanced Glycation end Products (AGE)

Chronic hyperglycemia also results in non-enzymatic glycosylation of tissue proteins such as lens proteins, fibrin, collagen and lipoproteins. The glycated tissue proteins form cross-linked proteins termed advanced glycation end-products. AGE production occurs especially in insulin-independent tissues, e.g. endothelium. AGEs affect nearly every type of cell and molecule in the body, and are thought to be one factor in aging and some age-related chronic diseases. They are also believed to play a causative role in the vascular complications of diabetes mellitus.

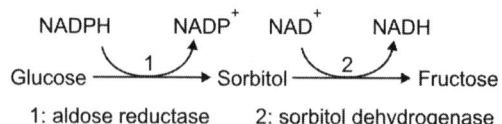

1: aldose reductase   2: sorbitol dehydrogenase

vi. Polyol (Sorbitol) Pathway Activation

While most cells require the action of insulin for glucose to gain entry into the cell, the cells of the retina, kidney, and nervous tissues are insulin-independent, so glucose moves freely across the cell membrane, regardless of the action of insulin. The cells will use glucose for energy as normal, and any glucose not used for energy will enter the polyol pathway. When blood glucose is normal (about 100 mg/dl or 5.5 mmol/l), this interchange causes no problems, as aldose reductase has a low affinity for glucose at normal concentrations.

When plasma glucose levels are chronically elevated, the enzyme aldol reductase is activated in the tissues in which glucose transport is not insulin-dependent, such as the lens, retina, renal glomeruli and peripheral nerves. Since sorbitol reductase is not present, sorbitol accumulates in these tissues.

Excessive activation of the polyol pathway increases intracellular and extracellular sorbitol concentrations, increased concentrations of reactive oxygen species, and decreased concentrations of nitric oxide and glutathione. High concentrations of sorbitol also produce osmotic stress. Each of these imbalances can damage the concerned tissue.

The AGE and activation of polyol pathway are believed to contribute equally to the pathogenesis of chronic complications of diabetes mellitus such as lens cataract, retinopathy, neuropathy and nephropathy, as well as macrovascular complication such as MI, stroke and gangrene. In a patient with diabetes mellitus, nearer the plasma glucose is kept to normal, fewer and less severe are the chronic complications.

2. Ketosis and its Consequences

Deficiency of insulin produces a great reduction in lipogenesis and accelerates the process of lipolysis. As a result, plasma level of FFA is more than doubled. Due to some unknown reason, diabetic patients have constantly elevated plasma glucagon level, even when hyperglycemia is very severe, This contributes to the mobilization of FFA. Free fatty acids provide energy to the glucose-starved insulin-sensitive tissues like skeletal muscle. However, excessive mobilization of FFA results in excessive formation of ketone bodies (acetoacetic acid, β-hydroxybutyric acid and acetone). In patients of DM, ketone formation exceeds the rate of their utilization leading to ketosis, which in turn leads to many metabolic defects:

i. Diabetic Ketoacidosis (DKA)

It is a potentially life threatening complication in patients with diabetes mellitus. It happens predominantly in those with type 1 diabetes, but it can occur in those with type 2 diabetes under certain circumstances, such as intercurrent illness or poor compliance with insulin therapy. Vomiting, dehydration, deep gasping breathing, confusion and occasionally coma are typical symptoms of DKA. Deep gasping breathing (dyspnea or Kussmaul breathing) results from the effect of metabolic acidosis on respiratory centers. The patient's breath smells of acetone. Urine becomes highly acidic.

When the capacity of the kidneys to replace plasma cations accompanying the organic anions by H^+ and NH_4^+ is exhausted, excessive amounts of Na^+ and K^+ are lost in the urine. The electrolyte and water loss leads to dehydration, hypovolemia and hypotension. Finally, acidosis and dehydration may depress the consciousness to the level of coma (ketotic coma, Fig. 26.4).

Following are typical reports of biochemical investigations in the blood of a patient of ketotic coma as compared to that of hyperosmolar coma:

Blood investigation	Ketotic coma	Hyperosmolar coma
Glucose, mg/dl	500	800
Sodium, mEq/l	132	142
Potassium, mEq/l	4.5	5
Chloride, mEq/l	90	98
Bicarbonate, mEq/l	8	20
Urea, mg/dl	35	100
Osmolality, mOsm/kg	295	332
pH	7.01	7.30

ii. *Chronic Dyslipidemia and its Consequences*

Many lipoprotein abnormalities are seen in the untreated, hyperglycemic diabetic patient. The non-insulin-dependent diabetic (NIDDM) patient with mild fasting hyperglycemia commonly has mild hypertriglyceridemia due to overproduction of TG-rich lipoproteins in the liver, associated with decreased high-density lipoprotein (HDL) cholesterol levels. The more hyperglycemic untreated NIDDM and insulin-dependent diabetic (IDDM) patient have mild to moderate hypertriglyceridemia due to decreased adipose tissue and muscle lipoprotein lipase (LPL) activity. These patients also have decreased HDL cholesterol levels associated with defective LPL catabolism of TG-rich lipoproteins. Treatment of diabetes with oral sulfonylureas or insulin corrects most of the hypertriglyceridemia and some of the decrease in HDL cholesterol. The abnormality in adipose tissue LPL activity corrects slowly over several months of therapy. The treated IDDM patient often has normal lipoprotein levels. The treated NIDDM patient may continue to have mild hypertriglyceridemia, increased intermediate-density lipoprotein levels, small dense low-density lipoproteins (LDL) with increased apoprotein B, and decreased HDL cholesterol levels.

Dyslipidemia is chiefly responsible for the macrovascular complications of DM, such as coronary artery disease, cerebral stroke and gangrene (*see* Chapter 10).

3. Increased Protein Catabolism and its Consequences

There is a relative paucity of information regarding the effects of diabetes on protein metabolism compared with our knowledge of the effects on carbohydrate or fat metabolism.

Emaciation in diabetic patients has been noticed by physicians for hundreds of years. In the ancient Sanskrit literature, diabetes mellitus was described as "honey-urine disease," associated with gross emaciation and wasting. Sir William Osler, almost 100 years ago, described the disease in terms of "progressive emaciation," involving massive urinary losses of both glucose and urea. Insulin deficiency produces profound whole-body protein catabolism. Such findings are consistently seen in DM type 1. However, in studies in protein metabolism in DM type 2, the results have not been conclusive. The effects of increased protein catabolism are depicted below.

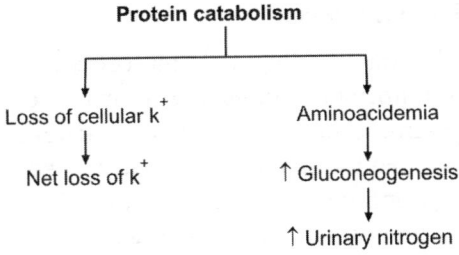

HYPOGLYCEMIA

As discussed above, hyperglycemia is a cardinal feature of untreated DM. However, due to difficulty in regulating the dose schedule of anti-diabetic drugs (insulin or even oral agents), episodes of hypoglycemia occur frequently in such patients. About 4% of deaths in IDDM are said to occur because of hypoglycemia rather than complications of DM. In a patient with DM, hypoglycemia may occur following an overnight fast, missing a meal or heavy exercise.

Fall of blood sugar below 80 mg/dl shuts off insulin secretion. At about 70 mg/dl blood glucose level, glucagon secretion begins to increase. At still lower level, CNS mediated sympathoadrenal discharge is activated which is results in a non-specific sense of arousal, anxiety, palpitation, tachycardia, shakiness, hunger and cold sweating. At still lower levels of blood sugar, cerebral manifestations of hypoglycemia occur. These include impaired mentation, lethargy, confusion, tremor, vertigo, paresthesias, incoordination of movements, slurred speech, diplopia, and other visual defects. At still lower level of blood sugar (<30 mg/dl), convulsions, coma and death occurs (Fig. 26.7). The onset of autonomic symptoms is important because it makes the patient aware of their condition and enables them to take appropriate corrective action before cognitive impairment occurs.

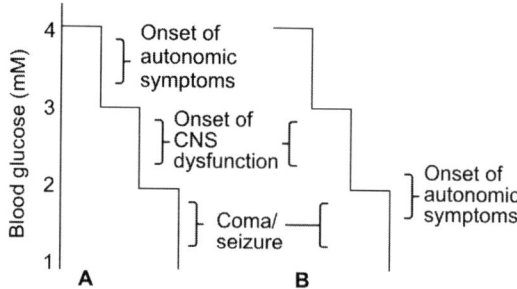

Fig. 26.7: Response to hypoglycemia. (A) Normal response and (B) hypoglycemia unawareness.

Hypoglycemia Unawareness

Some patients with long-standing diabetes lose their ability to secrete the major counter-regulatory hormones, glucagon and epinephrine, and fail to have hypoglycemia-related autonomic warning symptoms. Many investigators confirmed that patients with advanced diabetic autonomic neuropathy have attenuated counter-regulatory hormonal responses to hypoglycemia. Another cause of failure of the counter-regulatory hormone response to hypoglycemia has also been recently described. It seems, in some diabetics with frequent hypoglycemic episodes, there is a decreased central recognition of hypoglycemia and the brain does not activate counter-regulation.

This complication in old diabetic known as *hypoglycemia unawareness* is potentially dangerous, because there is no warning of the existence of hypoglycemia and the patient does not take any remedial measures. The blood sugar levels may fall to a level that cerebral manifestations/coma/death occurs.

Further Reading

Walford, M. Page, MM and Allison, SP. **The influence of renal threshold on the interpretation of urine tests of glucose in diabetic patients.** *Diabetic car.* 1980; 3:672–674.

Delamaire, M, et al. **Impaired leucocyte functions in diabetic patients.** *Diabet Med.* Jan 1997;14:29–34.

Clement, S, et al. **Management of diabetes and hyperglycemia in hospitals.** *Diabetes Care.* 2004;27:553–91.

American Diabetes Association: **Summary of Revisions for the 2009 Clinical Practice Recommendations.** *Diabetes Care* 2009; 32(S1):S3–S5

International Expert Committee Report on the **Role of the A1C Assay in the Diagnosis of Diabetes.** *Diabetes Care* 2009 32:1327–1334.

Solano, MP; Goldberg, RB. **Lipid management in type 2 diabetes mellitus.** *Clinical Diabetes* 2006; 24:127–132.

27
Metabolic Bone Disease

FUNCTIONAL ANATOMY

Structurally, bone may be spongy or compact type. Compact bone forms dense walls of the shaft of long bones, whereas spongy bone fills up the cavity (Fig. 27.1).

Compact Bone

Osteon or **Haversian system** is the fundamental functional unit of compact bone. Osteons are roughly cylindrical structures that are typically several millimeters long and around 0.2 mm in diameter. Osteons are composed of parallel columns made up of concentric bony layers or lamellae arranged around central canals called Haversian canals. Haversian canals run along the longitudinal axis of long bones and are connected to each other, with endosteum and periosteum via Volkmann canals which pierce the columns at right angles to the Haversian canals (Fig. 27.1).

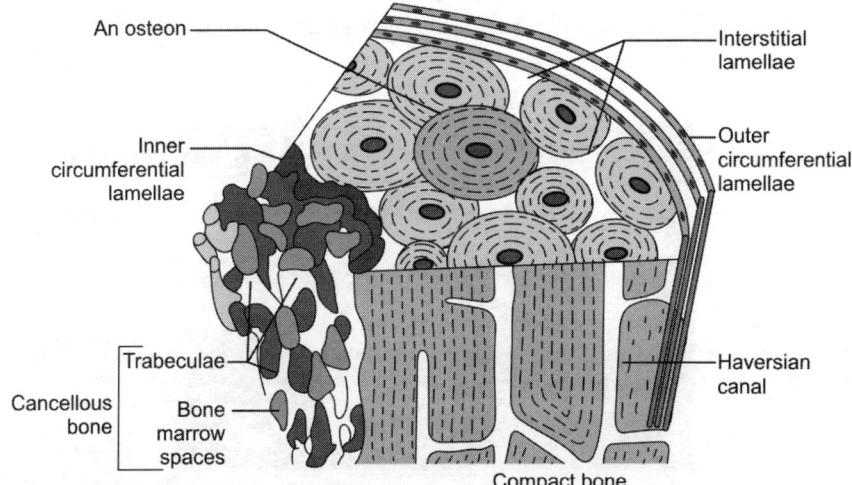

Fig. 27.1: Architecture of compact and cancellous (spongy) bone.

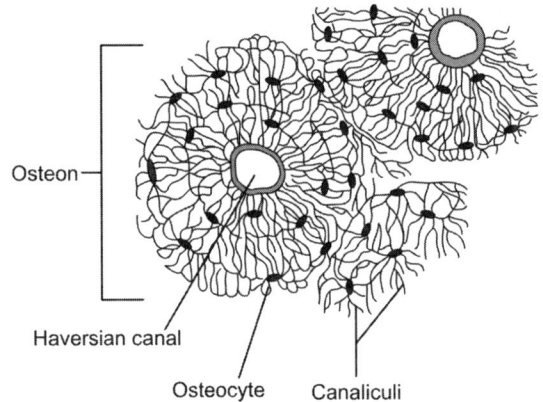

Fig. 27.2: Histological structure of an osteon.

Each Osteon or Haversian system begins as a blood channel at the periphery of which osteoblasts lay down lamellae of bone. During deposition of lamellae, the osteoblasts are trapped as osteocytes in spaces called lacunae. Between adjacent lacunae are minute interconnected canaliculi which contain fine cytoplasmic extensions of osteocytes (Fig. 27.2). The periosteum and endosteum of long bones contain osteoprogenitor (stem) cells which can differentiate into osteoblasts or osteoclasts.

Cancellous (spongy) bone is composed of a network of bony trabeculae, separated by interconnected spaces called bone marrow. The trabeculae are thin and consist of irregular lamellae of bone with lacunae containing osteocytes (Fig. 27.2). The Haversian systems are not seen in spongy bone. The osteocytes exchange metabolites with blood sinusoids in the bone marrow through the canaliculi present around the lacunae. The trabeculae are covered with a thin layer of connective tissue called endosteum which contains osteoblast; osteoclast and osteoprogenitor (stem) cells (Fig. 27.3).

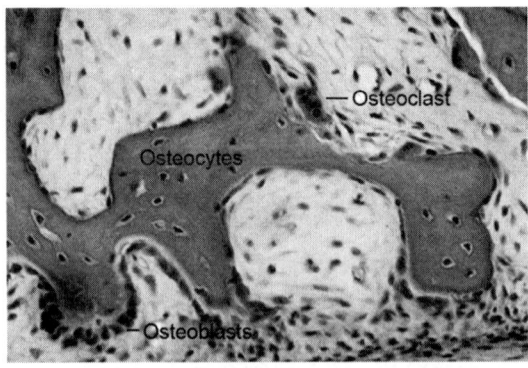

Fig. 27.3: Spongy bone.

Remodeling of Bone

Bone is an active tissue in which bone deposition and bone resorption continues throughout life. By this process a bone can adjust to the degree of bone stress. The thickness and even the shape of a bone can change according to the mechanical forces acting on it (Fig. 27.4).

Bone Formation

Bone is continuously deposited by osteoblasts. These cells are present in periosteum and endosteum. Osteoblasts secrete the protein collagen and the ground substance. Collagen polymerizes into collagen fibers. The resultant organic tissue is known as the **osteoid**. As the osteoid is being formed, some of the osteoblasts trapped into it and are now called osteocytes. Soon after osteoid is formed, hydroxy-apatite crystals are deposited on the surface of collagen fibers. The exact mechanism causing precipitation of calcium-phosphate from the ECF is not clear. Osteoblastic activity is associated with increased concentrations of the enzyme alkaline phosphatase. It is believed that the enzyme hydrolyses phosphate esters and increases the concentration of phosphate. As a result, calcium phosphate solubility product ($Ca^{++} \times PO_4^-$) increases to such a critical value that the salt precipitates out. Some unknown property of collagen may also be helping in binding of calcium salt.

Bone Resorption

Osteoclasts, the multinucleated cells that contain numerous mitochondria and lysosomes, are responsible for the resorption of bone. Attachment of the osteoclast to the osteon begins the process. The osteoclasts secrete collagenase and other enzymes important in the resorption process. High levels of calcium, magnesium, phosphate and products of collagen will be released into the extracellular fluid as the osteoclasts tunnel into the

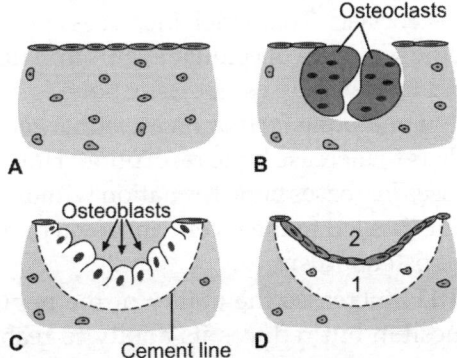

Fig. 27.4: Stages of bone remodeling: Quiescent phase (A); resorption phase (B); formation phase (C) and Quiescent phase after remodeling (D). The new bone may restore original surface or attain a new shape (1, 2).

mineralized bone. Osteoclasts require weeks to resorb bone, whereas osteoblasts need months to produce new bone. Therefore, any process that increases the rate of bone remodeling results in net bone loss over time.

Because osteoblasts and osteoclasts inhabit the surface of bones, trabecular bone is more active, so is more subject to bone turnover and remodeling. Not only is bone density decreased, but the microarchitecture of bone is also disrupted. Common osteoporotic fracture sites, the wrist, the hip and the spine, have a relatively high trabecular bone to cortical bone ratio. These areas rely on trabecular bone for strength, so the intense remodeling causes these areas to degenerate most when the remodeling is imbalanced.

As people get older, the rate of resorption tends to exceed the rate of replacement, leading to conditions like osteoporosis. Furthermore, in periods of rapid remodeling (e.g., after menopause), bone is at an increased risk for fracture because the newly produced bone is less densely mineralized, the resorption sites are temporarily unfilled, and the isomerization and maturation of collagen are impaired. In addition, certain medical conditions such as hormone imbalances can cause bone resorption to increase.

ROLE OF PARATHYROID HORMONE IN BONE METABOLISM

Parathyroid hormone (PTH) regulates calcium and phosphate flux across cellular membranes in bone and kidney, resulting in increased serum calcium and decreased serum phosphate. In bone, PTH increases the activity and number of osteoclasts, the cells responsible for bone resorption. However, this stimulation of osteoclasts is not a direct effect. Rather, PTH acts on the osteoblast (the bone-forming cell) to induce a membrane-bound protein called **RANK ligand (RANKL)**. This factor acts on osteoclasts and osteoclast precursors to increase both the numbers and the activity of osteoclasts. This action increases bone turnover or bone remodeling, a specific sequence of cellular events initiated by osteoclastic bone resorption and followed by osteoblastic bone formation. Although both bone resorption and bone formation are enhanced by PTH, the net effect of excess PTH is to increase bone resorption. However, PTH in low and intermittent doses increases bone formation without first stimulating bone resorption. This has led to the recent approval of recombinant PTH for the treatment of osteoporosis.

In the kidney, PTH increases the ability of the nephron to reabsorb calcium and magnesium but reduces its ability to reabsorb phosphate, amino acids, bicarbonate, sodium, chloride, and sulfate. Another important action of PTH on the kidney is its stimulation of 1,25–dihydroxyvitamin D (1,25$[OH]_2$D) production.

Role of Vitamin D in Bone Metabolism

Calcitriol (1,25 (OH)$_2$ cholecalciferol, or 1,25(OH)$_2$D) is the most potent agent with respect to stimulation of intestinal calcium and phosphate transport and bone resorption. Calcitriol appears to act on the intestine both by induction of new protein synthesis (e.g., calcium-binding protein) and by modulation of calcium flux across the brush border and basolateral membranes by a means that does not require new protein synthesis. The molecular action of calcitriol on bone has received less clear. However, like PTH, calcitriol can induce RANK ligand in osteoblasts and proteins such as osteocalcin, which may regulate the mineralization process. The metabolites 25(OH)D and 24,25(OH)$_2$D are far less potent stimulators of intestinal calcium and phosphate transport or bone resorption. Specific receptors for 1,25(OH)$_2$D exist in target tissues.

Role of Osteocytes in Bone Metabolism

The role of osteoblasts and osteoclasts in the remodeling of bone discussed above has been since long. However, the role of **osteocytes**, the most abundant cells in bone, has received attention recently. Many reports point to a mechanosensory function whereby osteocytes regulate bone remodeling in response to shear or strain forces, but their possible role in calcium and phosphate homeostasis is less clear. Several paracrine and endocrine factors, notably parathyroid hormone (PTH), prostaglandins, glucocorticoids and estrogen, have emerged as potential regulators of osteocyte function(s) and/or survival. These observations indicate that osteocytes play a critical role in regulating and maintaining normal skeletal and mineral homeostasis.

METABOLIC BONE DISEASE

This term is used to include disorders in which the entire skeleton is involved. Osteoporosis is the most prevalent metabolic bone disease. Others include rickets and osteomalacia, Paget's disease and osteitis fibrosa.

Osteoporosis

Osteoporosis is a state of reduced mass per unit volume with normal ratio of minerals to matrix. Osteoporosis may be confused with osteomalacia. The normal human skeleton is composed of a mineral component, calcium hydroxyapatite (60%), and organic material, mainly collagen (40%). In osteoporosis, the bones are porous and brittle (Fig. 27.5), whereas in osteomalacia, the bones are soft. This difference in bone consistency is related to the mineral-to-organic material ratio. In osteoporosis, the mineral-to-collagen ratio is within the normal range,

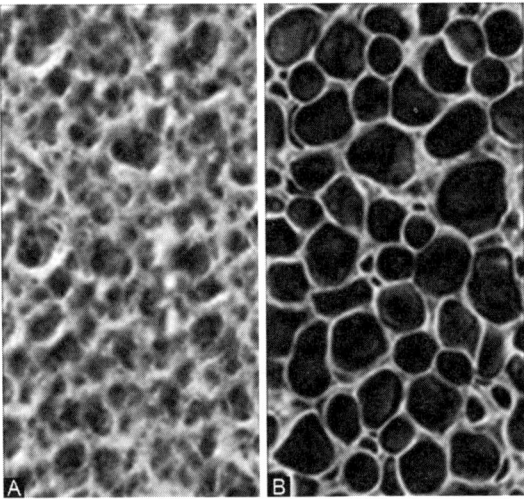

Fig. 27.5: Architecture of bone: Normal (A) and in osteoporosis (B).

whereas in osteomalacia, the proportion of mineral composition is reduced relative to organic content. Osteoporosis itself has no symptoms; its main consequence is the increased risk of bone fractures. Osteoporotic fractures occur in situations where healthy people would not normally break a bone; they are therefore regarded as fragility fractures. Typical fragility fractures occur in the vertebral column, rib, hip and wrist. The most characteristic feature of osteomalacia is pain when weight or pressure is applied to a bone. Severe osteomalacia may result in deformities or fractures of bones.

Osteoporosis seen in cases with immobilization or hormonal disorders such as Cushing syndrome or thyrotoxicosis is known as secondary osteoporosis. Senile osteoporosis in men and postmenopausal osteoporosis is far more common. In over 25% of women over the age of 60 years, osteoporosis is severe enough to be detected radiologically.

Senile/Postmenopausal Osteoporosis

The exact cause of senile/postmenopausal osteoporosis is not known. However, certain risk factors have been identified:

1. Peak Bone Mass

Peak bone mass has been identified as one of the most important factor in the pathogenesis of osteoporosis. Maximum bone mass is attained in both men and women at around the age of 30 years. A failure to attain optimal bone strength by this point is one factor that contributes to osteoporosis later in life. After the age of 30 years, the remodeling process involves slightly greater bone resorption than bone deposition. Thus, the age-related bone loss gradually sets in. By the age of 60 years in men, and approximately a decade earlier in women, the loss of bone mass becomes significant. Osteoporosis sets in earlier in those with low peak bone mass. The racial difference in peak bone mass is reflected in the incidence of severe osteoporosis. In the American population, peak bone mass is significantly greater in blacks than whites. The incidence of fracture femoral neck (severe osteoporosis) is significantly greater in whites than blacks. Indians in general have low peak bone mass. Twin and family studies have shown that genetic factors play an important role in regulating bone mineral density and bone turnover.

2. Gonadal Hormonal Deficiency

Aging and loss of gonadal function are the 2 most important factors contributing to the development of osteoporosis. Estrogen or testosterone deficiency, regardless of age of occurrence, results in accelerated bone loss. The exact mechanisms of this bone loss potentially are numerous, but, ultimately, an increased recruitment and responsiveness of osteoclast precursors and an increase in bone resorption, which outpaces bone formation, occurs. Studies have shown that bone loss in women accelerates rapidly in the first years after menopause (Fig. 27.6).

Blood gonadal hormone levels decline with age both in male and females. However, the postmenopausal precipitous fall in blood estrogen level observed in females (Fig. 26.7) does not occur in blood testosterone levels in male; blood testosterone levels in males decline more gradually (Fig. 27.8). These facts may be correlated in the relation between bone mass and age in men and women (Fig. 27.6).

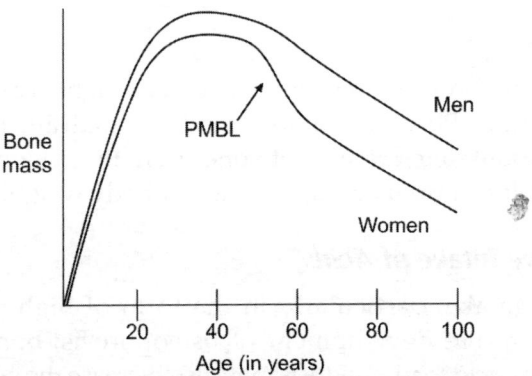

Fig. 27.6: Age and sex related loss of bone mass. (PMBL: postmenopausal bone loss).

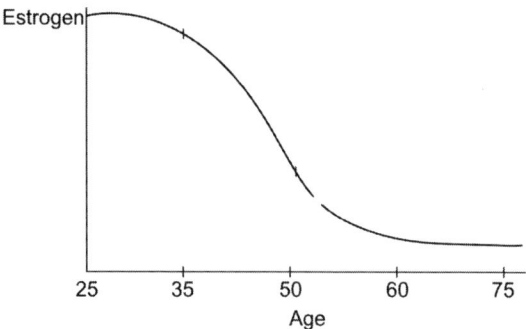

Fig. 27.7: Blood estrogens levels in females in relation to age.

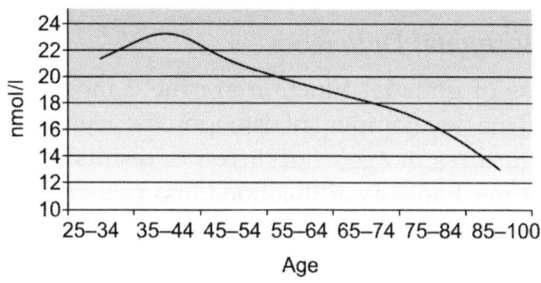

Fig. 27.8: Blood testosterone levels in males in relation to age.

3. Dietary Calcium and Vitamin D

Dietary calcium intake during the first three decades of life is an important factor since it determines the value of peak bone mass. However, in postmenopausal women, the benefit of increased dietary calcium in decreasing the rate of bone mass loss is controversial. Recent meta-analysis evidences support the use of calcium, or calcium in combination with vitamin D supplementation, in the preventive treatment of osteoporosis in people aged 50 years or older.

4. Exercise

At any age, immobilization with decreased weight bearing leads to rapid bone resorption. Physical activity, muscle strength and body weight seem to be important determinants of bone strength. Osteoporotic subjects in general are less muscular and have lower body weight.

5. Excessive Intake of Acids

High acid intake, particularly in the form of high protein diet may contribute to the development of osteoporosis; bone is involved in buffering the acid load. Acidosis may also increase the osteoclastic activity by a direct action.

OSTEOMALACIA AND RICKETS

The basic defect common to both osteomalacia and rickets is deficient mineralization of the bone with normal or slightly greater than normal organic (osteoid) component (Fig. 27.9). The soft bones are liable to deformities in shape as well as fractures. This is in contrast to osteoporosis in which both inorganic and organic components are deficient to a similar extent and fractures are hallmark of severe osteoporosis.

The primary defect in osteomalacia and rickets is a deciency of activated vitamin D (calcitriol), which promotes calcium absorption from the gastrointestinal tract and facilitates mineralization of bone.

Osteomalacia/rickets may result from:
- Insufficient solar exposure (insufficient cutaneous synthesis of vitamin D)
- Insufficient intake of vitamin D
- Malabsorption syndrome
- Chronic biliary obstructive jaundice
- Celiac disease
- Chronic pancreatitis
- Chronic renal disease
- Chronic liver disease
- Antiepileptic drugs

Solar exposure results in synthesis of previtamin D_3 by the action of ultraviolet B radiation on 7-dehydrocholesterol present in the epidermis and dermis. Vitamin D_3 circulates in the blood bound to vitamin D binding

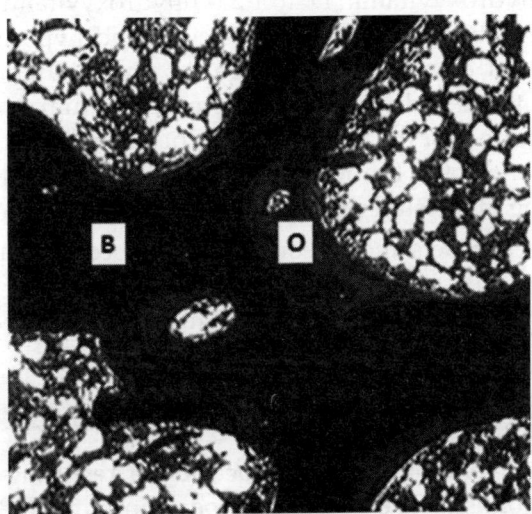

Fig. 27.9: Spongy bone from a patient with osteomalacia showing excess of osteoid (O) and bone (B).

protein. Vitamin D_3 is converted to 25-hydroxycholecalciferol [(25(OH) D_3] in the liver. 25(OH) D_3 is the major circulating form that is used for assessing the vitamin D status of an individual. 25 (OH) D_3 is further hydroxylated in the kidneys resulting in the production of 1,25 dihydroxycholecalciferol [(1,25 (OH)$_2$$D_3$], the biologically active form of vitamin D. Being fat-soluble, vitamin D_3 is also present in dairy products and cod liver oil. Vitamin D_2 is obtained by ultraviolet radiation of ergosterol present in yeast. Vitamin D_2 has been extensively used to fortify milk with vitamin D. In the body, vitamin D_2 is metabolized just like vitamin D_3.

In view of vitamin D metabolism discussed above, it is easy to understand why osteomalacia is common in individuals with inadequate solar exposure (purdah-observing women) or those with malabsorption of dietary fats or chronic liver or renal disease.

In early decades of 20th century, osteomalacia and rickets were rampant all over the world including industrialized countries. The disease was brought under control in the Western world by compulsory fortification of milk with vitamin D_2. Recently interest in vitamin D deficiency state has been revived because of the observations that osteomalacia, in mild form, is very common in old age, or in people of Asian origin (dark skinned) living in countries with limited sunshine.

Osteomalacia is often a component of renal osteodystrophy, the collection of bone disorders that occur in varying degrees of severity in almost all patients with chronic renal failure (CRF). The development of osteomalacia and rickets ("renal rickets") in CRF is due to the loss of renal parenchyma accompanied by a decreased renal enzymatic capacity to convert 25-hydroxyvitamin D_3 to 1,25-dihydroxyvitamin D_3, resulting in impaired intestinal absorption of calcium and hypocalcemia; and a decreased renal excretion of inorganic phosphates, resulting in hyperphosphatemia and a reciprocal decrease in serum calcium to a level below that required for the mineralization of osteoid. This stimulates the increased secretion of PTH and secondary hyperplasia of the parathyroid gland, resulting in the superimposed bone changes of osteitis fibrosa.

Drug-induced rickets and osteomalacia may occur in association with the use of the anticonvulsive drug phenytoin and is attributed to phenytoin's interference with vitamin D metabolism in the liver.

PATHOPHYSIOLOGY OF VITAMIN D DEFICIENCY STATES

Vitamin D deficiency leads to hypocalcemia resulting in secondary hyperparathyroidism. The consequent parathormone-induced increase in osteoclastic activity tends to improve plasma Ca^{++} but it aggravates skeletal demineralization.

Bone pains and proximal limb muscle weakness are early symptoms of osteomalacia. Presence of unmineralized osteoid underneath the heavily innervated periosteal membrane is perceived by the patient as throbbing aching bone pain, especially if pressure is applied. Proximal muscle weakness manifests as waddling gait and a difficulty in climbing stairs. The exact mechanism of osteomalacic myopathy is not clear. The histology shows non-specific muscle fiber atrophy without degenerative changes. The clinical and electromyographic examinations together show clear evidence of a myopathy. Severe osteomalacia tends to produce narrowing of pelvic outlet (due to inward pressure from the hips) leading to difficult labor and fetal morbidity, but such complications are rarely seen nowadays. Fracture of femur neck, pubic ramus, spine or ribs may occur, especially when osteomalacia is associated with osteoporosis, e.g. in aged individuals.

In rickets, the region of epiphyseal cartilage of a growing bone shows characteristic irregular and disordered columns of chondrocyte proliferation. Mechanical stress at the unmineralized osteoid leads to characteristic bulging at epiphyseal cartilage. This pathology is responsible for many of the characteristic clinical signs of rickets, e.g. rachitic rosary and Harrison's groove. Insufficiently mineralized bones are soft resulting in deformities in the legs (knock-knee; bow-legs) as well as posterior flattening of the skull.

Paget's Disease

Paget's disease affects 3–4% of population in the Western world, particularly men above the age of 40 years. The disorder is rare in India, Japan, China and the Middle East.

The exact etiology of Paget's disease is not known. At present, it is believed to be caused by a viral infection since intranuclear inclusions in the osteoclasts are the hallmark of the disease. Such inclusions are not observed in other metabolic bone diseases. The evidence that environmental factors may play a role in Paget's disease is based on the fact that the number of people who are affected by the condition has fallen sharply over the last 50 years. If Paget's disease was only caused by genetic mutations, the number of new cases that are recorded by the authorities each year would either stay relatively stable or would increase.

One suggested environmental factor is the measles virus. The virus may lie dormant for many years before being 're-activated' and attack the osteoclast cells, causing them to malfunction. Therefore, the fall in the number of cases of Paget's disease could be because of a corresponding fall in the number of measles infections owing to the measles vaccination programs. However, no virus has been cultured from pagetic tissue, and extracted ribonucleic acid (RNA) has not confirmed a viral presence.

The fundamental defect in Paget's disease is derangement of the process of remodeling. There is accelerated rate of bone resorption as well as new bone formation. At early stages of the disease osteoclastic activity is dominant, when calcium balance may be negative. Later on osteoclastic activity decreases and it is replaced by increased osteoblastic phase. Unlike other metabolic bone diseases, entire skeleton is not involved in the pathological process. Typically only one or at the most few bones are affected. Increased bone turnover correlates with the increased plasma alkaline phosphatase activity.

The structure of the newly formed bone is abnormal (Fig. 27.10). In the mature lesion, there is a mixture of lamellar and woven bones, which transforms the matrix into a chaotic "mosaic" pattern of irregularly juxtaposed pieces of lamellar bone, interspersed with woven bone. The result is structurally weakened bone.

Pelvic bones are most commonly affected followed by femur, skull and spine. Small bones are usually not affected. A common feature of Paget's disease is skeletal deformity. This clearly evolves over a period of many years (probably decades) in most patients. The deformity is most visible in the skull and lower extremities. Bone pain is usually absent even in patients with extensive disease.

Osteitis Fibrosa Cystica

Osteitis fibrosa cystica is characterized by subperiosteal resorption of the distal phalanges, tapering of the lateral ends of clavicles, salt-and-pepper appearance of the skull, and brown tumors of the long bones. Fibrosis within the trabeculae is evident. Early changes in bone include demineralization, with progression in late stages to marked bone resorption and peritrabecular fibrosis (Fig. 27.11). The so-called "brown tumors" are large areas of bony resorption with hemorrhage in advanced hyperparathyroidism. This metabolic bone disease used to seen in advanced cases of primary hyperparathyroidism. Now that the estimation of plasma calcium level has become routine and plasma parathormone levels can be

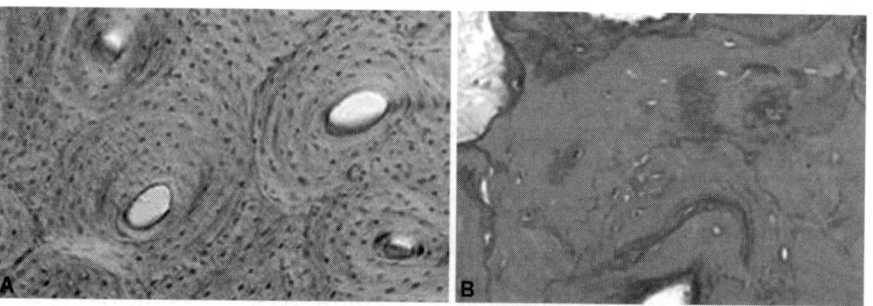

Fig. 27.10: Compact bone: Normal (A) and in Paget's disease (B)

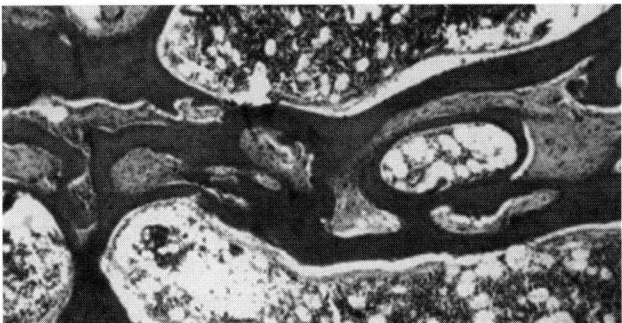

Fig. 27.11: Osteitis fibrosa cystica.

Table 27.1:	Blood chemistry in metabolic bone disease. (N = normal; E = elevated; D = decreased)			
	Plasma calcium	Plasma phosphate	Plasma alkaline phosphatase	Plasma parathormone activity
Osteoporosis	N	N	N	N
Osteomalacia	D	D	E	E
Paget's disease	N	N	E/N	N
Osteitis fibrosa cystica	E	D	E	E

assessed, primary hyperparathyroidism is usually diagnosed before the bony lesions progress to the stage of osteitis fibrosa cystica.

Most of the symptoms of primary hyperparathyroidism are due to hypercalcemia and are nonspecific, e.g. muscle weakness, fatigue, volume depletion, nausea and vomiting. Neuropsychiatric manifestations are particularly common and may include depression or confusion. In addition, the chronically increased excretion of calcium in the urine can predispose to the formation of renal stones.

In cases of primary hyperparathyroidism, the characteristic biochemical features are elevated plasma levels of calcium, alkaline phosphatase and parathormone, decreased plasma inorganic phosphate and hypercalciuria. In Table 27.1, changes in blood chemistry in various types of metabolic bone disease are compared.

Further Reading

Cranney, A, et al. **Parathyroid hormone for the treatment of osteoporosis: a systematic review.** CMAJ 2006;175:52–59

Gallacher, SJ; Dixon, T. **Impact of treatments for postmenopausal Osteoporosis on bone quality: A Systematic Review** Calcified Tissue International. 2010;87: 469–484.

Hollick, MF. **Vitamin D deficiency.** N Engl J Med 2007; 357:266–281.

Irani, PF. **Electromyography in nutritional osteomalacic myopathy.** *J NeurolNeurosurg Psychiatry 1976; 39:686–693.*

Sahota, O. **Reducing the risk of fracture with calcium and vitamin D.** *BMJ. 2010; 340: b5492.*

Tang, et al. **Use of calcium or calcium in combination with vitamin D supplementation to prevent fractures and bone loss in people aged 50 years or older.** *Lancet 2007;370:657–666.*

28
Acute Renal Failure

PHYSIOLOGICAL CONSIDERATIONS

Urine Formation

Structure of a nephron is shown in Fig. 28.1. Urine is formed by the following 3 processes: (1) Glomerular filtration followed by (2) tubular reabsorption and (3) tubular secretion. In brief, large amount of protein-free plasma fluid is filtered into the Bowman's capsules of the nephron. As the fluid passes through the proximal convoluted tubule, useful constituents of the glomerular filtrate are reabsorbed and waste products are not reabsorbed. Further reabsorption of useful materials occurs in distal convoluted tubule. This process constitutes tubular reabsorption. In addition, in the distal tubule, some waste products are transferred from the blood to the tubular lumen. This process is called tubular secretion. Waste products present in the lumen of a nephron after tubular reabsorption and secretion, dissolved in small amount of water, constitute urine. It leaves the collecting ducts in to enter the ureters.

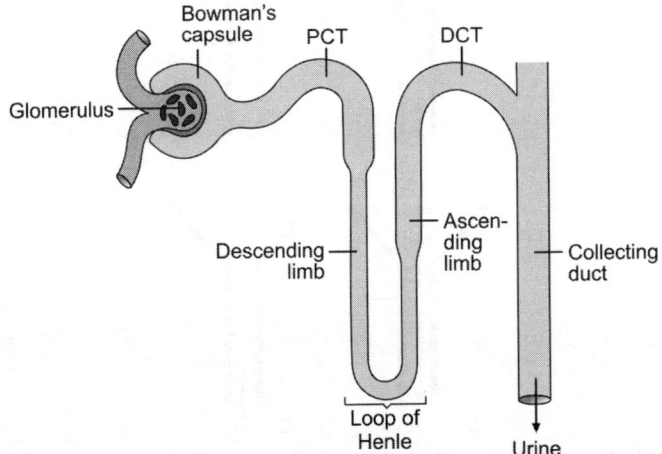

Fig. 28.1: Structure of a nephron.

GLOMERULAR FILTRATION

The two kidneys receive an average blood flow of 1250 ml/min. This enormous blood flow is related to their role in excretory function rather than their metabolic requirements. Of 650 ml of plasma flowing through the two kidneys, 125 ml is filtered out of glomerular capillaries into the Bowman's capsules each minute. This is the normal glomerular filtration rate (GFR). The composition of glomerular filtrate is similar to that of the interstitial fluid filtered out of the systemic capillaries. It contains all the electrolytes and solute constituents, in same concentrations as present in the plasma except that it is practically devoid of proteins and blood cells.

Tubular Mechanisms

As mentioned earlier, the glomerular filtrate (125 ml/min) contains all the constituents of plasma except proteins. This fluid passes through the remaining parts of the nephron (i.e. PCT, loop of Henle, and DCT) and the collecting ducts, where it is subjected to various *reabsorptive and secretory processes*.

The **tubular handling** of a substance may involve:
a. No change: no reabsorption nor secretion (Fig. 28.2A)
b. Complete tubular reabsorption (Fig. 28.2B)
c. Partial tubular reabsorption (Fig. 28.2C)
d. Tubular secretion (Fig. 28.2D)

a. *No change:* Neither reabsorption nor secretion. Totally waste product such as creatinine is handled this way.

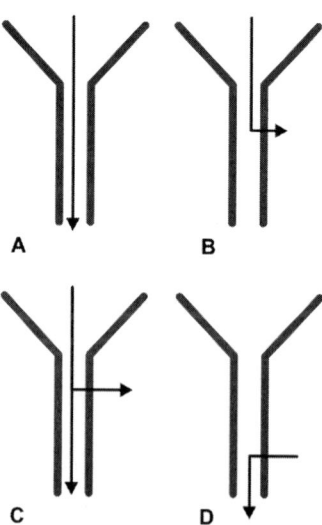

Fig. 28.2: Tubular handling of substances in glomerular filtrate. (A) Complete excretion; (B) complete reabsorption; (C) partial reabsorption; (D) secretion

b. *Complete reabsorption:* Substances of nutritive value such as glucose, amino acids, electrolytes (Na$^+$, K$^+$, Cl$^-$, HCO$_3^-$) and vitamins are completely or almost completely reabsorbed, mostly in the PCT.

Water is reabsorbed in all the segments of the nephron except the ascending limb of the loop of Henle. However, 7/8th of the glomerular filtrate water is reabsorbed in the PCT alone.

c. *Partial reabsorption:* Waste products such as urea, uric acid, sulphate, phosphates, etc. are only partially reabsorbed.

d. *Tubular secretion:* The process of tubular secretion is just opposite to that of tubular reabsorption. In tubular reabsorption, substances are recovered from the tubular fluid whereas in tubular secretion, substances are added to the tubular fluid. Only two natural constituents of plasma are secreted by the distal tubular cells namely, K$^+$ and H$^+$ ions.

ACUTE RENAL INJURY/ ACUTE RENAL FAILURE

Acute kidney injury (AKI), previously called acute renal failure (ARF), is a rapid loss of kidney function. The term AKI is intended to emphasize the reversible nature of most renal insults. AKI is diagnosed on the basis of clinical history, such as decreased urine production, and characteristic laboratory findings, such as elevated blood urea nitrogen and creatinine. Depending on its severity, AKI may lead to a number of complications, including metabolic acidosis, high potassium levels, changes in body fluid balance, and effects to other organ systems.

From the point of view of pathophysiology, ARI may be classified as follows:
1. *Prerenal azotemia (prerenal ARI):* It is an adaptive response to severe volume depletion and hypotension, with structurally intact nephrons
2. *Renal azotemia (intrinsic ARI):* It occurs in response to cytotoxic, ischemic, or inflammatory insults to the kidney, with structural and functional damage to the nephrons.
3. *Postrenal azotemia (postrenal ARI):* It includes disorders associated with obstruction of the urinary tract.

With proper and timely treatment, most forms of ARI are reversible, since kidney is a unique organ which can recover completely even after almost complete loss of renal function.

Prerenal ARI

Causes

- *Hypovolemia:* Hemorrhage, burns, dehydration, diuretics.
- *Low cardiac output:* Myocardial infarction, pericardial tamponade, pulmonary embolism, CHF.

- *Shock:* sepsis, anaphylaxis.
- *Iatrogenic renal hypoperfusion:* Cyclooxygenase inhibitors, ACE inhibitors, catecholamines.

Prerenal AKI represents the most common form (50 to 80%) of acute kidney injury and often leads to *intrinsic AKI (renal AKI)*, if it is not promptly corrected. All the conditions mentioned above cause renal hypoperfusion due to a decrease in the true or effective circulatory volume. A decrease in circulating blood volume activates high pressure arterial baroreceptors leading to a reflex increase in sympathetic discharge, severe renal vasoconstriction and a tendency to reduced GFR. The compensatory renal responses include autoregulatory renal mechanisms, activation of renin-angiotensin-aldosterone mechanism, greater secretion of ADH and increased synthesis of renal prostaglandins. These responses may maintain normal GFR despite decreased renal blood flow. When the renal hypoperfusion is severe, the renal compensatory mechanisms fail, resulting in a severe reduction in GFR and azotemia results (Fig. 28.3).

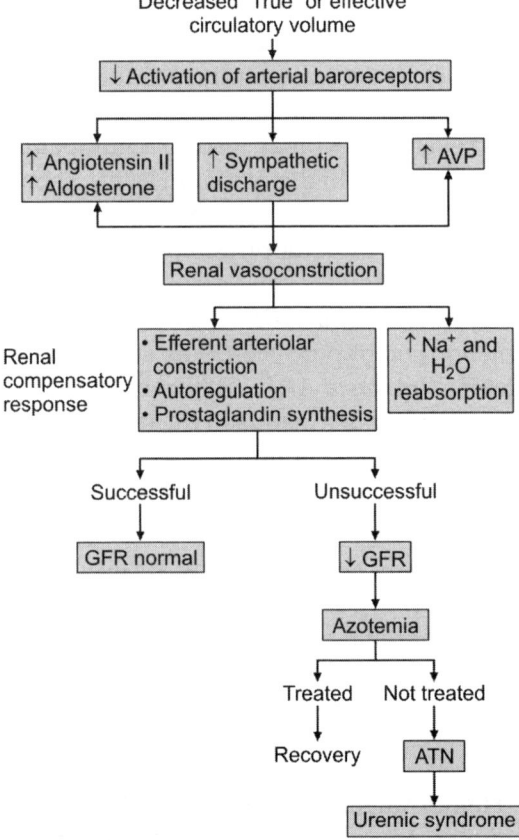

Fig. 28.3: Pathophysiology of prerenal azotemia

Any further delay in treatment of hypovolemia results in such an intense renal vasoconstriction that the renal tubular epithelium undergoes ischemic necrosis (acute tubular necrosis, ATN).

RELATION BETWEEN GFR AND PLASMA LEVELS OF CREATININE AND UREA

Azotemia is an elevation of blood urea nitrogen (BUN) (reference range, 8–20 mg/dl) and serum creatinine (normal value, 0.7–1.4 mg/dl) levels. Figure 28.4 shows the relationship of the glomerular filtration rate (GFR) to steady-state serum creatinine and blood urea nitrogen (BUN) levels. As shown in this figure, in early renal disease, substantial decline in GFR may lead to only a slight elevation in serum creatinine. Elevation in serum creatinine is apparent only when the GFR falls to about 70 ml/min.

Some formulas have been used to calculate *creatinine clearance (GFR)* values from serum creatinine values. As seen from Fig. 28.5, the relation between creatinine clearance and serum creatinine is non-linear. Therefore, such formulas have doubtful validity, especially in early stages of renal failure.

Renal ATI [Renal (Intrinsic) Azotemia]

One specific clinical disorder called the *acute tubular necrosis (ATN)* accounts for most of the cases of intrinsic azotemia. It is produced by injury to renal parenchyma. Acute tubular necrosis may occur due to extrinsic nephrotoxins, e.g. nephrotoxic drugs or endogenous nephrotoxins such as myoglobin in crush syndrome or hemoglobin in

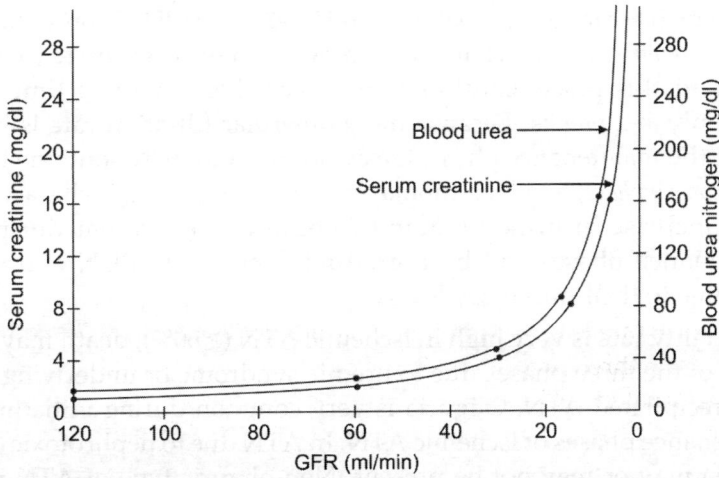

Fig. 28.4: Relation between GFR and serum creatinine or blood urea levels

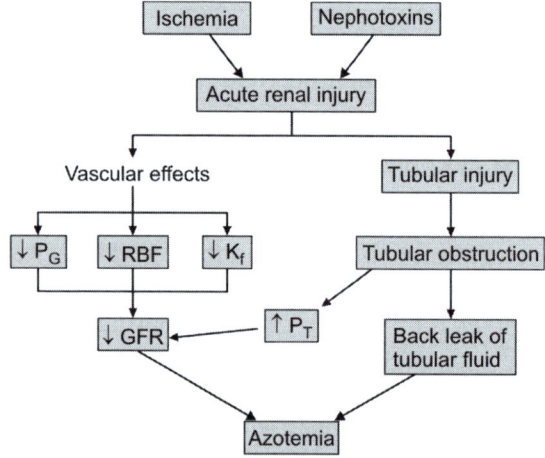

Fig. 28.5: Pathophysiology of azotemia in acute tubular necrosis. P_G: hydrostatic pressure in glomerular capillaries. K_f: Glomerular filtration coefficient P_T: hydrostatic pressure in Bowman's capsule. RBF: renal blood flow

cases with mismatched blood transfusion. However, inflammatory conditions of renal parenchyma such as glomerulonephritis and interstitial nephritis may also produce intrinsic azotemia. The following discussion chiefly concerns acute tubular necrosis:

Acute Tubular Necrosis (ATN) (Fig. 28.5)

ATN usually occurs after an acute ischemic or toxic event in the kidney and it has a well-defined sequence of events. The *initiation phase* is characterized by an acute decrease in GFR to very low levels, with a sudden increase in serum creatinine and blood urea (BUN) concentrations. The *maintenance phase* is characterized by a sustained severe reduction in GFR, and this phase continues for a variable length of time, most commonly 1–2 weeks. Because the glomerular filtration rate is so low during the maintenance phase, the creatinine and BUN continue to rise. The *recovery phase*, in which tubular function is restored, is characterized by an increase in urine volume (if oliguria was present during the maintenance phase) and by a gradual decrease in BUN and serum creatinine to their pre-injury levels.

Mortality rate is very high in ischemic ATN ($\geq 60\%$); death may occur in any of the three phases due to uremic syndrome or underlying cause that precipitated ATN. Oliguria is very common during initiating and maintenance phases of ischemic ATN. In ATN due to nephrotoxic drugs, oliguria may or may not be present. Non-oliguric type of ATN runs a milder and shorter course with lower mortality rate.

Initiation Phase

Ischemic ATN is often occurs as a continuum of prerenal azotemia, i.e. renal parenchymal injury occurs because of severe renal hypoperfusion or it can be the period of nephrotoxic assault. Ischemic ATN results when hypoperfusion overwhelms the kidney's autoregulatory defenses. Renal hypoperfusion initiates cell injury that often, but not always, leads to cell death. Injury of tubular cells is most prominent in the outer medullary region of the kidney (in the straight portion of the proximal tubules and in the thick ascending limb of the loop of Henle). This region is relatively hypoxic even under normal circumstances (with a partial pressure of oxygen being 10–20 mm Hg as compared with 50–60 mm Hg in the cortex). The initiating phase is characterized by severe reduction in GFR and increase in plasma creatinine levels (azotemia). In addition, ischemia leads to decreased production of vasodilators (i.e. nitric oxide, prostacyclin) by the tubular epithelial cells, leading to further vasoconstriction and hypoperfusion.

On a cellular level, ischemia causes depletion of adenosine triphosphate (ATP), an increase in cytosolic calcium, free radical formation, metabolism of membrane phospholipids, and abnormalities in cell volume regulation. The decrease or depletion of ATP leads to many problems with cellular function, not the least of which is active membrane transport. With ineffective membrane transport, cell volume and electrolyte regulation are disrupted, leading to cell swelling and intracellular accumulation of sodium and calcium. Typically, phospholipid metabolism is altered, and membrane lipids undergo peroxidation. In addition, free radical formation is increased, producing toxic effects. Damage inflicted by free radicals apparently is most severe during reperfusion.

Maintenance Phase

The maintenance phase of ATN (oliguric phase) is characterized by a stabilization of GFR at a very low level, and it typically lasts 1–2 weeks. Complications mostly develop during this phase. Severe renal vasoconstriction (RBF 25–50% of normal) has been documented in experimental and clinical ARF and has been considered in the past as a dominant causative factor (Fig. 28.6C). Reduction in total renal blood flow alone does not appear to account for the profound reduction in GFR, because improvement of renal blood flow by volume expansion or administration of vasodilators does not correct the GFR. Therefore, some other mechanisms also seem to be involved in the reduction of GFR (Fig. 28.6B and D):

i. *Tubular obstruction:* In cases with ATN, casts are frequently seen in tubular lumen. They arise from the precipitation of sloughed microvilli and other cellular debris derived from necrotic proximal tubular cells

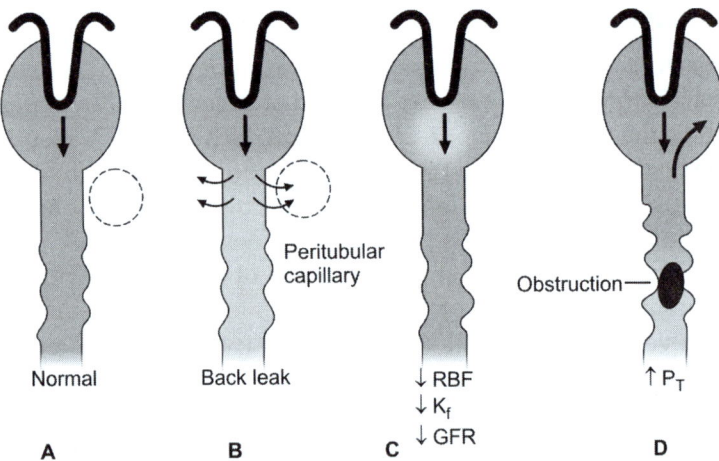

Fig. 28.6: Various pathophysiological mechanisms in ATN leading to reduced effective GFR

or precipitation of filtered proteins such as hemoglobin or myoglobin. The consequent tubular obstruction increases the tubular hydrostatic pressure upstream from the obstruction. The hydrostatic pressure in the Bowman's capsule may exceed the glomerular capillary hydrostatic pressure leading to cessation of glomerular filtration (Fig. 28.6D).

ii. *Tubular back leak:* The exfoliation of tubule cells leave behind denuded areas of the basement membrane, and loss of tight junctions in the attached proximal tubule cells. These changes produce back leak of tubular fluid into the renal interstitium and then into the blood. The glomerular filtrate passes back to the blood circulation without undergoing any reabsorptive or secretory process in renal tubules (Fig. 28.6B). Thus even if the glomerular filtration is not greatly reduced, the clearance of most of the solutes is reduced markedly.

Recovery Phase

If the patient survives the first two phases of ATN, the recovery phase begins with the restoration of disrupted tubular continuity, dissolution/ or mobilization of intratubular casts and recovery of renal perfusion to near normal. Typically the urinary output gradually increases from day to day. If the fluid and salt restriction has not been rigidly maintained during the oliguric phase, **a diuretic phase** follows. Five to ten liters of urine may be formed each day. The mechanism of the diuresis is not completely understood, but it may in part be due to the delayed recovery of tubular cell function in the setting of increased glomerular filtration. In addition, continued use of diuretics (often administered during initiation and maintenance phases) may also add to the problem. Tubular functional capacity is still limited, particularly sodium reabsorption and response to ADH.

Biochemical Abnormalities in ARI

During the oliguric phase of ARI, urinary volume is < 400 ml/24 hr; complete anuria is rare. Urinary osmolality is fixed at 300 mOsm/kg. Urinary Na^+ concentration is relatively high (50 mEq/L). Fractional excretion of Na^+ ($FENa^+$) is more than 3%. Continued ingestion of salt and water in the face of reduced renal excretory capacity leads to salt and water retention, edema, and hypertension. Volume expansion may precipitate life threatening congestive heart failure. Hyperkalemia occurs frequently. Besides the basic abnormality of reduced renal excretion, hyperkalemia is exacerbated if there is extensive tissue injury, hemolysis or increased tissue catabolism because of release of K^+ from the intracellular fluids. Loss of renal excretion of H^+ leads to metabolic acidosis. Severe tissue injuries, systemic illness or starvation, if present, add to the problems.

Hyperphosphatemia and hypocalcemia are usually present during the oliguric phase. Hypocalcemia may lead to tetany or cardiac dysfunction. The exact mechanism of hypocalcemia is not clear. It may be a reciprocal effect of hyperphosphatemia or due to deficient renal production of 1, $25(OH)_2D_3$.

In the **diuretic phase**, tubular dysfunction may persist and is manifested by Na^+ wasting, polyuria (possibly massive) unresponsive to vasopressin, or hyperchloremic metabolic acidosis. Hence excessive diuresis may produce volume depletion unless fluid replacement keeps pace with urinary fluid losses. Approximately 25% of deaths in ATN occur during the diuretic phase.

From therapeutic point of view, it is important to differentiate prerenal azotemia from azotemia due to ATN. The following laboratory indices are helpful in the differential diagnosis (Table 28.1):

Table 28.1: Laboratory indices to differentiate prerenal and renal types of acute renal failure

Laboratory test	Prerenal ARI	Renal ARI
FENa, percent*	<1	>1
BUN to creatinine ratio	>20:1	10 to 20:1
Urine specific gravity	>1.020	1.010 to 1.020
Urine osmolality, mOsm/ kg	>500	300 to 500
Urine sodium concentration, mEq per L (mmol per L)	<10 (10)	>20 (20)
Urine sediment	Hyaline casts	Granular casts

*FENa = fractional excretion of sodium; BUN = blood urea nitrogen.

Note: Fractional excretion of sodium (FENa) can be calculated as follows:

$$FENa\% = \frac{\text{Quantity of } Na^+ \text{ excreted} \times 100}{\text{Quantity of } Na^+ \text{ filtered}}$$

$$= \frac{UNa \times V \times 100}{PNa \times \text{Creatinine clearance}}$$

$$= \frac{UNa \times V \times 100}{PNa \times \frac{Ucr \times V}{Pcr}}$$

$$= \frac{Una \times Pcr \times 100}{PNa \times Ucr}$$

where,
 UNa = Urinary Na⁺ concentration
 Ucr = Urinary creatinine concentration
 Pna = Plasma Na⁺ concentration
 Pcr = Plasma creatinine concentration

Postrenal ARI

Approximately 5–10% cases of acute azotemia are due to obstruction to the urinary tract. Since normal kidney function can be achieved by a single kidney, postrenal ARI can occur if there is:
- Obstruction of bladder neck (prostate pathology) or urethra.
- Bilateral ureteric obstruction, or
- Unilateral ureteric obstruction in a patient with only one functioning kidney.

Prostatic disease is the most common cause of postrenal ARI. Continued formation of urine against the backdrop of obstruction to outflow causes an increase in intraluminal pressure upstream the site of obstruction. Thus, there is a gradual distension ureters, renal pelvis and calyces (hydronephrosis). Ultimately, when the intraluminal pressure in the Bowman's capsule becomes equal to hydrostatic pressure in the glomerular capillaries, filtration ceases. Cessation in glomerular filtration leads to azotemia, acidosis, fluid overload, and hyperkalemia. *Postrenal azotemia is the most common cause of complete anuria, because the basic cause is mechanical.* In prerenal and renal types of ARI, complete renal shutdown seldom occurs.

With relief of obstruction within 48 hours of onset, there is evidence that relatively complete recovery of GFR can be achieved within a week, while little or no further recovery occurs after 12 weeks. Prolonged obstruction can lead to tubular atrophy and irreversible renal fibrosis.

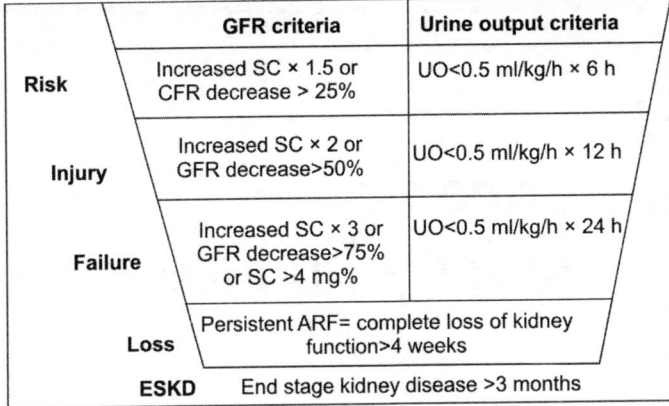

Fig. 28.7: RIFLE criteria of acute renal injury (ARI, or ARF)

RIFLE Criteria in ARI

Management of cases of ARI has presented many problems because of the absence of exact definitions of various stages of acute renal failure. A group of research workers (Acute Dialysis Quality Initiative Group) have come out with what is known as RIFLE Criteria. RIFLE is an acronym comprising Risk, Injury, Failure, Loss and End-stage kidney disease. According to this system of classification, there are three grades of increasing severity of acute kidney injury- risk (class **R**), injury (class **I**) and failure (class **F**)—and two outcome classes (Loss and End-stage kidney disease) (Fig. 28.7). In this classification, *serum creatinine and GFR values are described in reference to the base-line values recorded before the onset of renal insult. If the base-line values are not available, urinary output values can be conveniently used.*

Further Reading

Agraharkar, M; Safirstein, RL. **Pathophysiology of acute renal failure**. In: Greenberg A, Coffman T, (eds). Primer on Kidney Diseases. 3rd ed. San Diego, Calif: Academic Press; 2001:243–86.

Lameire, N; Van Biesen, W; Vanholder, R. **Acute renal failure**. Lancet 2005. 365 : 417–30.

Venkataraman, R.; Kellum, JA. **Definition of acute renal failure: The RIFLE criteria.** J Intensive care Med 2007;22:1.

29
Chronic Kidney Failure

Chronic renal failure (CRF), or more appropriately chronic kidney disease (CKD), refers to a decline in the glomerular filtration rate caused by a variety of diseases, such as diabetes, glomerulonephritis, and polycystic kidney disease. Patients with CKD have a high prevalence of hypertension. Whether hypertension is a cause or a result of CKD remains debatable. Chronic renal failure is a continuous process that begins when some nephrons begin to be lost and ends when the remnant nephrons can sustain life no longer.

Classification: Staging of chronic kidney disease is a way of quantifying the severity of CKD. Chronic kidney disease has been classified into 5 stages (Table 29.1).

RENAL HANDLING OF DIFFERENT SOLUTES IN CHRONIC KIDNEY DISEASE

The body has adequate renal reserve. Consequently, homeostasis of practically all the solutes is maintained till GFR falls below 50% of normal (Stage 3 of CKD). With further deterioration of renal function, it may be expected that plasma concentrations of all the solutes would show a progressive increase. Actually, this holds true only in case of a few waste products such as urea and creatinine whose excretion is mainly controlled

Table 29.1: Stages of chronic kidney disease

Stage	Description	Glomerular filtration rate (ml/min)
At increased risk	**Risk factors** for kidney disease (e.g., diabetes, high blood pressure, family history, older age, ethnic group)	More than 90
1	Kidney damage (protein in the urine) and **normal** GFR	More than 90
2	Kidney damage and **mild** decrease in GFR	60 to 89
3	**Moderate** decrease in GFR	30 to 59
4	**Severe** decrease in GFR	15 to 29
5	**Kidney failure** (dialysis or kidney transplant needed)	Less than 15

by glomerular filtration, with very little role of tubular reabsorption or secretion (Fig. 29.1A).

In case of substances such as phosphates, urate, H^+ and K^+, their normal plasma concentrations are maintained till GFR falls below 25% of normal (stage 4 CKD, Fig. 29.1B). With GFR falling from 50 to 25%, progressive decrease in filtered load of these substances can be compensated by greater excretion or lesser reabsorption in the tubules. However, capacity of this adaptation is limited. When the GFR falls below 25% of normal, their plasma concentrations begin to increase particularly when GFR falls below 10% of normal (Stage 5 CKD).

In case of Na^+, plasma concentration is maintained within the normal range throughout the course of chronic renal disease (Fig. 29.1C). This is possible because of the fact that fractional excretion of sodium increases in direct proportion to the decline in GFR. However, this statement is true as long as the patient maintains "normal" intake of sodium and water. The diseased kidney has very limited capacity to conserve sodium or water. Sodium or water cannot be conserved when intake is limited, or their excretion cannot be increased when there is extra intake load of sodium or water (Fig. 29.2).

PATHOPHYSIOLOGY OF UREMIA

The multiple organ failure in a uremic patient is due to the accumulation of some toxin(s) in the blood. This fact has been confirmed by the observation that serum of a uremic patient exerts toxic effects on a variety of biological reactions. However, the exact nature of the toxin(s) has not yet been identified. The final end product of carbohydrate and fat

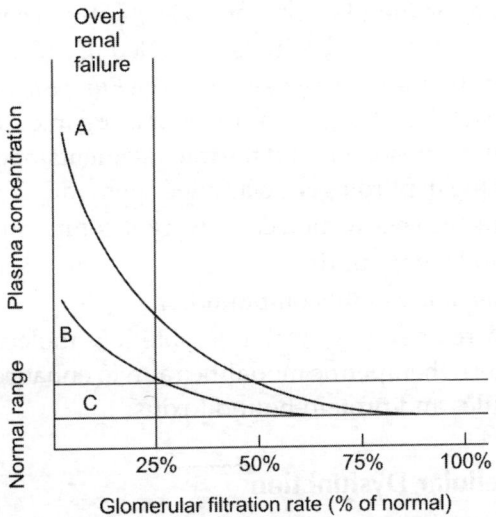

Fig. 29.1: Renal handling of various types of solutes.

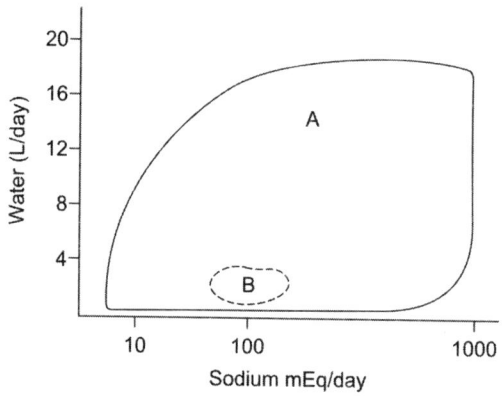

Fig. 29.2: Renal excretory capacity of sodium and water in a normal individual (A), and a patient of end-stage renal failure.

metabolisms is CO_2 (and water), which can be easily excreted by the lungs. The products of protein metabolism consist of a number of nitrogenous waste products which can be excreted only by the kidneys. Their accumulation in the blood consequent to renal failure is believed to be the cause of uremic toxicity. Uremic symptoms correlate only roughly and in an inconsistent manner with the concentrations of blood urea levels. Only a few symptoms such as anorexia, malaise, vomiting, and headache have been attributed to elevated blood urea level. A large number of other nitrogenous products of amino acid metabolism, singly, or in combination, seem to account for other abnormalities seen in uremia. Only a few solutes have an established role as uremic toxins. Hemodialysis therapy does keep patients alive, but does not completely relieve uremic symptoms. The fact that transplantation reverses this residual syndrome constitutes strong evidence for the ill effects of toxic solutes accumulation despite dialysis. These accumulated solutes are called uremic toxins

Many uremic toxins were reviewed by the *European Uremic Toxin Work Group* in the year 2000. Besides a number of inorganic substances, such as water, potassium, phosphate, and the trace elements, about 92 toxins were identified and the nephrologists classified them into three major groups:
- Small water soluble low molecular weight compounds.
- Protein-bound compounds.
- Middle molecular weight compounds.

Dialysis can remove only water soluble low molecular compounds. So, many modern therapeutic modalities aim to enhance removal of both middle molecules and protein-bound toxins.

1. General Cellular Dysfunction

The most basic abnormality in uremia, at cellular level, is partial inhibition of Na^+–K^+ pump, leading to a reduction in transmembrane potential, an increase in intracellular Na^+ and a decrease in intracellular K^+ concentrations. The most prominent result is an osmotically-induced overhydration of the cells. That is why; salt and water retention is one of the important features of uremic syndrome. This abnormality can be corrected temporarily by dialysis or permanently by renal transplantation. Overhydration of cerebral neurons is believed to be one of the factors contributing to the development of uremic encephalopathy. Additional factors decreasing *intracellular K^+* concentration include metabolic acidosis, poor dietary intake of K^+, excessive losses due to vomiting, diarrhea or diuretics.

2. Hypothermia

The sodium-potassium pump is the major consumer of ATP and hence the major cause of thermogenesis. Therefore, uremic patients have reduced energy metabolism, reduced BMR, subnormal body temperature and increased tendency to develop hypothermia.

3. Anemia and Immune Dysfunction

Anemia is a regular feature of uremia. Normochromic normocytic anemia principally develops from decreased renal synthesis of erythropoietin, the hormone responsible for bone marrow stimulation for red blood cell production. Anemia associated with renal failure can be observed when the glomerular filtration rate (GFR) is less than 50 ml/min or when the serum creatinine is greater than 2 mg/dl. Diabetic patients may experience anemia with a GFR of less than 60 ml/min. In the course of the disease, it becomes more severe as the GFR progressively decreases with the availability of less viable renal mass. No reticulocyte response occurs. Other, relatively minor contributory factors include increased hemolysis because of decreased RBC life span, and tendency of gastrointestinal bleeding from the uremia-induced platelet dysfunction, and nutritional deficiencies.

Anemia is associated with fatigue, reduced exercise capacity, impaired cognitive and immune function, and reduced quality of life. Anemia is also associated with the development of cardiovascular disease, the new onset of heart failure, or the development of more severe heart failure already present. Anemia is associated with increased cardiovascular mortality.

Atrophy of lymphoid tissue leading to lymphopenia is common. Neutrophil count is usually normal. Uremic patients have impaired acute inflammatory response because of functional defects in neutrophils, monocytes and lymphocytes. Therefore, uremic patients are more prone to infections but febrile response is less than normal. Platelet dysfunction results in easy bruisability and prolonged bleeding time. Clotting defects may also occur.

4. Renal Osteodystrophy

In a uremic patient, a number of abnormalities of the calcium, phosphate and vitamin D metabolisms, such as hypocalcemia, hyperphosphatemia, increased PTH levels, and metabolic acidosis ultimately lead to renal bone disease (renal osteodystrophy). Renal osteodystrophy is characterized by areas of osteomalacia and osteoporosis, and even osteosclerosis in various bones. These changes are seen more often in children or adults with slowly progressive chronic renal failure.

The clinically active form of vitamin D, $1,25(OH)_2 D_3$ is responsible for GI absorption of calcium and phosphorus. During renal failure, $1,25(OH)_2 D_3$ levels are reduced which leads to decreased calcium absorption from the GI tract and results in low serum calcium levels. Hypocalcemia stimulates the parathyroid gland to secrete more of PTH, a process termed *secondary hyperparathyroidism*. In addition, metabolic acidosis results in bone decalcification and osteoporosis by a direct action.

In addition to the calcium abnormalities, hyperphosphatemia occurs as excretion of phosphate decreases with progressive renal failure. Hyperphosphatemia stimulates parathyroid gland hypertrophy and stimulates increased production and secretion of PTH. Elevated PTH levels have been associated with uremic neuropathy and other metabolic disturbances, which include altered pancreatic response, poor erythropoiesis, and cardiac and liver function abnormalities. The direct deposit of calcium and phosphate in the skin, blood vessels, and other tissue, termed metastatic calcification, can occur when the calcium-phosphate product is greater than 70.

Renal osteodystrophy may present with nonspecific signs and symptoms, including weakness, bone pain, and skeletal deformity. Presentation varies markedly with age. Adults may present with findings of osteomalacia, while children typically show growth retardation. As a result, complications differ depending on the patient's age. The most common complication of renal osteodystrophy is fracture, which may be insufficiency fractures through osteomalacic bone or pathologic fractures through brown tumors.

5. Acidosis

Acidosis is another major metabolic abnormality associated with uremia. Metabolic acid-base regulation is controlled primarily by tubular cells of the kidney, while respiratory compensation is accomplished in the lungs. Failure to secrete hydrogen ions and impaired excretion of ammonium may initially contribute to metabolic acidosis. As kidney disease continues to progress, accumulation of phosphate and other organic acids, such as sulfuric acid, hippuric acid, and lactic acid, creates an increased anion-gap metabolic acidosis. In uremia, metabolic acidemia may contribute to other clinical abnormalities, such as hyperventilation, anorexia, stupor, congestive heart failure, and muscle weakness. Uremic patients are likely to go into severe acidosis on exposure to exogenous acids, e.g. high protein diet or endogenous acids such as lactic acid.

6. Hyperkalemia

As renal function declines, the nephron is unable to excrete a normal potassium load, which can lead to hyperkalemia if dietary intake remains constant. In addition, other metabolic abnormalities, such as acidemia, may contribute to decreased potassium excretion and lead to hyperkalemia. The *extracellular K^+* concentration begins to rise progressively with the degree of azotemia. Hyperkalemia is common when drugs, such as potassium-sparing diuretics, ACE inhibitors, angiotensin-receptor blockers, beta-blockers, or nonsteroidal anti-inflammatory drugs are used in the setting of renal failure. Serum K^+ level of greater than 6.5 mEq/L is a clinical emergency.

7. Cardiovascular Dysfunction

Left ventricular hypertrophy is a common disorder found in approximately 75% of patients of chronic renal failure who have not yet undergone dialysis. Left ventricular hypertrophy is associated with increased ventricular thickness, arterial stiffening, coronary atherosclerosis, and/or coronary artery calcification. Patients are at increased risk for cardiac arrhythmias due to underlying hyperkalemia and metabolic acidosis. Renal dysfunction may contribute to associated fluid retention, which may lead to uncontrolled hypertension and congestive heart failure.

Pericarditis is commonly seen in the later stages of uremia. Uremic pericarditis has a prevalence of 6–10% in patients with acute or chronic renal failure, and it continues to be associated with significant morbidity and occasional mortality. Uremic pericarditis is thought to result from inflammation of the visceral and parietal layers of the pericardium by metabolic toxins that accumulate in the body owing to kidney failure. It may occur even in patients on regular dialysis.

8. Fluid and Electrolyte Imbalance

In most cases of CRF, both total body sodium and water are increased and therefore the expansion of ECF volume may not be apparent. However, the patient is intolerant to both excessive salt intake and salt depletion (Fig. 29.3). Excessive salt intake aggravates hypertension, congestive heart failure, ascites or edema.

Uremic patients also have impaired mechanisms for salt and water conservation. There are more prone to volume depletion in states of sodium losses (vomiting, diarrhea, fever) which may lead to orthostatic hypotension or circulatory shock. Volume depletion may produce further deterioration of renal function.

9. Uremic Neuropathy

Uremic neuropathy is a distal sensorimotor polyneuropathy caused by uremic toxins. The severity of neuropathy is correlated strongly with the severity of the renal insufficiency. Uremic neuropathy is considered a dying-back neuropathy or central-peripheral axonopathy associated with secondary demyelination.

Paresthesias are the most common and usually the earliest symptom. Increased pain sensation is a prominent symptom. Weakness of lower extremities and atrophy follow the sensory symptoms. As disease progresses, symptoms move proximally and involve the upper extremities. Muscle cramps and restless legs syndrome were reported by 67% of uremic patients. These symptoms also can be seen in uremic patients without neuropathy. Patients report that crawling, prickling, and itching sensations in their lower extremities are relieved partially by movement of the affected limb. Autonomic dysfunction can often be demonstrated by autonomic nerve function tests. Patients may complain of dizziness. It usually is associated with postural hypotension.

10. Uremic Encephalopathy

Uremic encephalopathy (UE) is one of many manifestations of renal failure. Its exact cause is unknown. Accumulating metabolites of proteins and amino acids affect the entire neuraxis. No single abnormality can be precisely correlated with the clinical features of UE. Besides accumulation of products of protein catabolism, uremia results in elevation of several hormones such parathyroid hormone (PTH), insulin, growth hormone, glucagon, thyrotropin, prolactin, luteinizing hormone, and gastrin. In healthy dogs, high levels of PTH produce CNS changes like those seen in uremia. PTH is thought to promote the entry of calcium into neurons, which leads to the changes observed. Early symptoms include an inability to concentrate, drowsiness and insomnia. Mild behavioral changes, loss of memory and errors of judgment soon follow. Flapping tremor, chorea, stupor, seizers and coma are seen in terminal stages.

11. Malnutrition

Malnutrition usually occurs as renal failure progresses and is manifested by anorexia, weight loss, loss of muscle mass, low cholesterol levels, low

BUN levels in the setting of an elevated creatinine level, low serum transferrin levels, and hypoalbuminemia. However, whether uremia stimulates protein catabolism directly remains controversial. Co-morbid diseases, such as diabetes, congestive heart failure, or other diseases, that require reduced food intake or restrictions of certain foods may contribute to anorexia.

Numerous epidemiologic studies have shown that a decreased serum albumin concentration is a very strong and independent predictor of mortality among dialysis patients.

12. Endocrine Abnormalities

As mentioned above, uremia results in elevation of levels of several hormones such parathyroid hormone (PTH), insulin, growth hormone, glucagon, thyrotropin, prolactin, luteinizing hormone, and gastrin. Other endocrine abnormalities that may occur in the setting of uremia include changes in carbohydrate metabolism, decreased thyroid hormone secretion, and abnormal sexual hormone regulation.

Reduced insulin clearance and increased insulin secretion can lead to increased episodes of hypoglycemia and normalization of hyperglycemia in diabetic patients. Glycemic control may appear to be improved; however, this may be an ominous sign of renal function decline. Appropriate decrease in doses of antihyperglycemic medications may be prescribed as renal function declines to avoid hypoglycemic reactions.

The kidney extracts substantial amounts of low and medium molecular weight polypeptide hormones from the renal circulation by a process which probably involves both glomerular filtration plus luminal reabsorption and direct peritubular uptake, although the relative contribution of the two mechanisms under physiologic conditions is not known. The bulk of the extracted hormone is catabolized in the renal parenchyma since urinary excretion is negligible. Renal catabolism contributes an important fraction of the total metabolic clearance of polypeptide hormones, which accounts in part for their increased circulating levels in renal failure.

Levels of thyroid hormones, such as thyroxine, may become depressed, while reverse triiodothyronine levels may increase because of impaired conversion of triiodothyronine to thyroxin.

Reproductive hormone dysfunction is common and can cause impotence in men and infertility in women. Renal failure is associated with decreased spermatogenesis, reduced testosterone levels, increased estrogen levels, and elevated luteinizing hormone levels in men, all of which contribute to impotence and decreased libido. In women, uremia reduces the cyclic luteinizing hormone surge, which results in anovulation and amenorrhea. Infertility is common and pregnancy is rare in women with advanced uremia and renal failure, but this may be reversed with renal transplantation.

13. Skin

The classic skin finding in persons with uremia is *uremic frost*, which is a fine residue, thought to consist of excreted urea left on the skin after evaporation of water. The skin may have a velvety appearance and feel, particularly in patients who are pigmented. Patients who are uremic also may have an unhealthy color of the skin due to the combined effect of anemia and accumulation of urochrome, the pigment that gives urine its color. Patients may become hyperpigmented as uremia worsens. Uremic pruritus remains one of the most frustrating, common, and potentially disabling symptoms in patients with end-stage renal disease. The exact cause is not yet clear.

> ### Further Reading
>
> Brouns, R; De Deyn, PP. **Neurological complications in renal failure: a review.** *Clin Neurol Neurosurg. 2004;107:1–16.*
>
> Jacobson, HR. **Chronic renal failure: pathophysiology.** *Lancet. 1991; 338:419–23*
>
> Meyer, TW; Hostetter, TH."**Uremia**". *N Engl J Med 2007; 357:1316–1320.*
>
> Vanholder, R et al. **A Bench to Bedside View of Uremic Toxins.** *J Am Soc Nephrol 2008;19:863–870.*

30
Acid-Base Disorders

THE CONCEPT OF pH

An **acid** is a chemical species that can donate a proton (H^+), and a **base** is a species that can accept (gain) a proton. Pure water undergoes extremely small degree of dissociation to yield H^+ and OH^-

$$H_2O \leftrightarrow H^+ + OH^-$$

The concentration of H^+ in water is 10^{-7} mEq/L. Water is regarded as neutral. Acids are solutions with H^+ concentration greater than 10^{-7} (e.g., 10^{-6} or 10^{-5} mEq/L). Alkalis or bases are solutions with H^+ concentration less than 10^{-7} (e.g. 10^{-8} or 10^{-9} mEq/L). Expression of H^+ concentration in the body fluids as described above is cumbersome; hence a symbol pH came to be used:

$$pH = \log \frac{1}{[H^+]}$$

Thus pH of pure water is written as 7. The arterial blood has an average pH of 7.4 (normal range 7.35–7.45). A decrease of arterial pH value below 7.35 is known as acidosis, whereas the term alkalosis is used to describe arterial pH values higher than 7.45. Arterial pH value below 6.8 or above 8 is not compatible with life. In fact, arterial pH is maintained within a narrow range, transiently with the help of acid-base buffers in the body fluids, and finally by the kidneys and the lungs.

Acid-base Buffers

An acid-base buffer is defined as a solution containing two or more chemical compounds that prevent marked changes in H^+ concentration, when moderate amount of an acid or a base is added to the solution. Acid-base buffers are usually a combination of a weak acid and its salt with a strong base, e.g. H_2CO_3 and $NaHCO_3$. If a small amount of acid is added to the carbonic acid-bicarbonate buffer, the following reaction takes place

$$HCl + NaHCO_3 \Rightarrow H_2CO_3 + NaCl$$

Thus strong acid HCl, an acid which undergoes complete dissociation and yields a large number of H⁺ has been converted to a weak acid (H_2CO_3), which dissociates poorly to yield few H⁺ ions. Therefore, in spite of addition of HCl, the H⁺ concentration of the solution is only mildly increased.

If a small amount of a strong base is added to the carbonic acid-bicarbonate mixture, the following reaction takes place:

$$NaOH + H_2CO_3 \Rightarrow NaHCO_3 + H_2O$$

Thus, a strong base has been converted into a weak base and the decrease in H⁺ concentration of the solution is minimized.

1. Carbonic Acid-bicarbonate Buffer System

The importance of carbonic acid-bicarbonate buffer lies in the facts that (i) it is present as the chief buffer in the extracellular fluid, and (ii) both of its components are subjected to regulatory control in the body: carbonic acid (CO_2) by the lungs and bicarbonate by the kidneys. Under normal circumstances, our body maintains ratio of one part carbonic acid (1.2 mmol/L) to 20 parts bicarbonate (24 mEq/L). With this ratio, the pH of blood would be 7.4, as shown by Henderson-Hasselbalch equation:

$$pH = pK^1 + \log \frac{\text{base}}{\text{acid}}$$

2. Proteins and Hemoglobin

- Most powerful buffer
- 75% of all intracellular buffering
- Hemoglobin an important extracellular buffer due to large concentration of hemoglobin in blood

The plasma proteins in general and hemoglobin in particular constitute an important buffer system. Proteins are composed of amino acid chains. The terminal amino acids possess carboxyl (–COOH) and amino (–NH_2) groups. At pH 7.4, the weak acidic carboxyl group ionizes as follows and donates H⁺ to the medium:

$$\text{Protein} \leftrightarrow \text{Proteinate}^- + H^+$$

The proteinate anions form salt with Na⁺ in the extracellular fluid; with K⁺ in the intracellular fluid. On addition of a strong acid, the reaction mentioned above shifts to the left. On addition of a base, the reaction shifts to the right. Thus, in either case, the change in H⁺ concentration of the fluid is minimal.

Hemoglobin has an additional property which makes it a very efficient buffer. Oxygenated hemoglobin ionizes to a greater extent than deoxygenated hemoglobin. Thus, in the venous blood, when the addition of CO_2 increases the concentration of H⁺ in the blood, the ionization of hemoglobin is reduced. Hence, appearance of H^+ on account of CO_2 is compensated by disappearance of H^+ on account of deoxygenation of hemoglobin. That is why, although the concentration of hemoglobin in the blood is twice that of plasma proteins, the former has six-time stronger buffering action than the latter.

3. Phosphate Buffer

This buffer system is composed of NaH_2PO_4 and Na_2HPO_4. On addition of an acid or a base, the following reactions take place:

$$Na_2HPO_4 + HCl \Rightarrow NaH_2PO_4 + NaCl$$
$$NaH_2PO_4 + NaOH \Rightarrow Na_2HPO_4 + H_2O$$

In the ECF, phosphate concentration is too low for its effectiveness as an acid-base buffer. However, in the renal tubules its concentration increases remarkably because the proportion of its reabsorption is far lower than reabsorption of water. *Therefore, phosphates constitute an important buffer in the kidney and help in excretion of H^+ by the kidneys.*

4. Ammonia Buffer

In the renal tubules, epithelial cells of distal tubules and collecting ducts secrete ammonia (NH_3) that acts as an important buffer. It accepts H^+ to become NH_4 which is excreted in the urine.

The bicarbonate system is primarily extracellular and the fastest to respond to pH imbalance, but it has less total buffering capacity than intracellular system. Intracellular buffering has a very large capacity; about 75% of the body chemical buffering capacity.

REGULATION OF HYDROGEN ION BALANCE

- Buffer systems response—very rapid (in seconds), incomplete
- Respiratory responses—rapid (in minutes), incomplete
- Renal responses—slow (in hours to days), complete

Under normal circumstances, tremendous amounts of hydrogen ions (H^+) are being continuously added to the body fluids. Carbon dioxide accounts for the addition of over 12,000 mEq H^+ per day. Nonvolatile (fixed) acids account for another 60 mEq/day. Almost all the CO_2 is excreted by the lungs, whereas the kidney is responsible for the excretion of non-volatile acid products of protein metabolism. Lactic acid produced during severe exercise or keto acids produced in severe diabetes are also excreted by the kidney.

Fruits are the main dietary source of the alkali. They contain sodium and potassium salts of weak organic acids, whose metabolism produces $NaHCO_3$ or $KHCO_3$ (and CO_2). Normally, the alkali content of the diet is very small and all the normal individuals excrete acidic urine except for transient postprandial alkaline tide.

Role of Respiration

In response to changes in blood pH, respiratory responses occur within minutes by stimulation/depression of respiratory centers in the CNS.

In spite of addition of 12,000 mEq H^+ per day to the blood, the pH of arterial blood remains remarkably constant at 7.4. Similarly pCO_2 of the arterial blood is kept constant at 40 mm Hg. This is made possible by two factors:

i. In the venous blood, CO_2 is converted to H_2CO_3 and further to H^+ and HCO_3^-. Hydrogen ions are immediately buffered by the blood buffers, chiefly hemoglobin and plasma proteins.

ii. As the venous blood passes through the lungs, CO_2 is regenerated by reversal of the reactions mentioned above (i) and excreted very efficiently. The pulmonary ventilation is so delicately adjusted that it exactly matches the CO_2 produced is the body. Even during severe exercise, when CO_2 production increases 20 folds, CO_2 excretion is so efficient that arterial pCO_2 does not increase at all. Such a delicate control is made possible by the fact that ventilation is controlled by both CO_2 as well as H^+ concentration through central and peripheral chemoreceptors.

a. Effect of CO_2

CO_2 is a highly diffusible gas. It can easily cross the blood–brain and blood-CSF barriers, and stimulate the medullary central chemoreceptors. In contrast, H^+ cannot cross these barriers easily. Therefore central chemoreceptors are most sensitive to changes in arterial pCO_2 and less so to changes in H^+ concentration.

b. Effect of pH

An increase in H^+ concentration of arterial blood also stimulates pulmonary ventilation, chiefly through the peripheral (sino-aortic) chemoreceptors. Therefore, the respiratory system helps in regulation of acid-base balance of the body even when the increase in H^+ concentration is not due to CO_2 but due to non-volatile acids like sulphuric acid, phosphoric acid or lactic acid.

Role of Kidneys

The kidneys regulate pH by either acidification or alkalinization of the urine. The renal response occurs over hours/days, and is capable of nearly complete restoration of acid/base balance.

As mentioned above, about 60 mEq of H^+ is added to the blood every day as non-volatile acids. They cannot be excreted by the lungs. They are excreted by the kidneys in an indirect manner. In the kidneys, most of the excretory products are initially filtered into the glomerular filtrate. All that is necessary for their excretion is that renal tubules reabsorb them partially or not all. In contrast, the concentration of H^+ in the blood is so small, that they cannot be excreted in this manner. Actually, most of the H^+ produced in the body do not remain as such. They are immediately buffered by HCO_3^- and other buffers. The kidney generates new hydrogen ions equivalent to the amount metabolically produced and actively secretes them into the urinary tubules, where they are buffered by phosphate and ammonium ions.

The generation of H^+ in the renal tubules is accompanied by production of HCO_3^- which diffuses into the blood circulation and replenishes the amount of HCO_3^- lost during initial buffering of the acids. In case excess of base ($NaHCO_3$) is ingested, it is excreted by the kidney by filtration followed by partial or complete non-reabsorption.

In primary pulmonary diseases such as emphysema, pulmonary excretion of CO_2 is diminished and therefore arterial pCO_2 and H^+ concentration tend to rise (respiratory acidosis). In such circumstances, renal excretion of H^+ is the only means of maintaining body pH near normal (renal compensation). Similarly in chronic renal failure, renal excretion of H^+ is diminished leading to metabolic acidosis. In such a condition, excessive loss of CO_2 by hyperventilation is the only means of maintaining body pH near normal (respiratory compensation).

Anion Gap Concept

In the plasma, total cations (Na^+, K^+, Ca^{++}, Mg^{++}, etc.) are always counter-balanced by total anions (Cl^-, HCO_3^-, PO_4^-, SO_4^-, etc.). Of these ions, only Na^+, K^+, Cl^-, and HCO_3^- are routinely measured. Therefore the concentration of *measured anions* is always less than the concentration of *measured cations*. The difference is known as the anion gap:

$$\text{Anion gap} = \{[Na^+] + [K^+]\} - \{[Cl^-] + [HCO_3^-]\}$$

Example:

Anion gap = {140 mEq/L + 4 mEq/L} – {100 mEq/L + 28 mEq/L} = 16 mEq/L

The anion gap concept is useful in the differential diagnosis of metabolic acidosis. In one group of disorders producing metabolic acidosis, the anion gap becomes larger than normal. Such disorders are said to produce *high anion gap metabolic acidosis*. In the other group of disorders, the anion gap remains normal. Such disorders are said to produce *normal anion gap metabolic acidosis* (*see* details below). *Estimation of anion gap is also a useful tool to assess mixed acid-base disorders.*

In clinical practice, since K⁺ concentration does not vary grossly, the anion gap is usually calculated as follows:

Anion gap = [Na⁺] − {[Cl⁻] + [HCO$_3^-$]}

Calculated in this way, the normal anion gap is 12 ± 4 mEq/L.

ACID-BASE DISORDERS IN CLINICAL PRACTICE

A. Primary Acid-base Disorders

1. Metabolic Acidosis (MA)

The primary abnormality in metabolic acidosis is a decline in plasma HCO$_3^-$ concentration. This metabolic abnormality may arise because of:

a. Increased H⁺ load on the body in the form of lactic acidosis, ketoacidosis or ammonium chloride administration.
b. Deficient renal H⁺ excretion.
c. Loss of HCO$^-_3$ from GI tract or kidneys.

Metabolic acidosis may be classified into two major groups: (i) high anion gap MA and (ii) normal anion gap (hyperchloremic) MA.

High Anion Gap MA

There are four prominent causes of high anion gap MA:

1. Lactacidosis

- Circulatory shock
- Severe hypoxia

2. Ketoacidosis

- Diabetic ketoacidosis
- Alcoholic ketoacidosis
- Starvation

3. Renal Failure

Acute or chronic

4. Exogenous Acids

Salicylic acid, methyl alcohol

In uncompensated stage of such MA, the acid-base picture is:

$$\downarrow pH = pK^1 + \log \frac{\downarrow base}{acid}$$

Acidosis stimulates central and peripheral chemoreceptors causing hyperventilation (respiratory compensation). The renal compensation consists of excretion of highly acidic urine (H⁺ excretion). Renal compensation is not possible if MA is due to renal failure.

The respiratory compensation decreases the arterial pCO_2, whereas renal compensation generates HCO_3^- (a side effect of H⁺ secretion), which partially restores the depleted HCO_3^-. The acid-base status of a case of compensated MA is as follows:

$$pH = pK^1 + \log \frac{\downarrow \text{base}}{\downarrow \text{acid}}$$

The two most important causes of high anion gap MA in clinical practice are diabetic ketoacidosis and renal failure. The two disorders can be differentiated by the study of serum K⁺ level, which is elevated in renal failure and subnormal in diabetic ketoacidosis. A typical pattern of acid-base status and electrolyte status of patients of these two types of disorders is given below.

	Diabetic	Uremic
Na⁺ (mEq/L)	125	135
K⁺ (mEq/L)	3.5	5.4
HCO_3^- (mEq/L)	5	12
Cl⁻ (mEq/L)	90	101
pH	7.01	7.32
PCO_2 (mmHg)	20	24

Normal Anion Gap (Hyperchloremic) MA

- Diarrhea
- Renal tubular acidosis

High anion gap MA is characterized by a decrease in plasma HCO_3^- level, but no significant change in plasma Cl⁻ level. In hyperchloremic type of MA, a decrease in plasma HCO_3^- is accompanied by a significant increase in plasma Cl⁻ and hence the name hyperchloremic. This type of MA is typically seen in patients suffering from diarrhea or renal tubular acidosis (RTA). In diarrhea HCO_3^- is lost from the gut in exchange for Cl⁻. In RTA, the failure of bicarbonate reabsorption from the renal tubules results in greater reabsorption of Cl⁻. In either case, plasma Cl⁻ level is significantly elevated. A typical pattern of acid-base status and electrolyte pattern in a case of RTA is given below.

Na⁺(mEq/L)	140
K⁺(mEq/L)	2.5
HCO_3^-(mEq/L)	15
Cl⁻(mEq/L)	115
pH	7.30
PCO_2 (mmHg)	30

The anion gap in the three cases with MA given above is calculated below:

Anion gap = $[Na^+] - [(Cl^-) + (HCO_3^-)]$
Diabetic: 125 − [90 + 5] = 30 mEq/L (high anion gap)
Uremic: 135 − [101 + 12] = 22 mEq/L (high anion gap)
RTA: 140 − [115 + 15] = 10 mEq/L (normal anion gap)

2. Metabolic Alkalosis

- Excessive sodium bicarbonate ingestion
- Persistent vomiting

Metabolic alkalosis occurs as a result of net gain of bicarbonate (e.g. ingestion of $NaHCO_3$ for peptic ulcer) or more often due to loss of non-volatile acids (e.g. HCl in prolonged vomiting). The primary acid-base picture in uncompensated stage is as follows:

$$\uparrow pH = pK^1 + \log \frac{\uparrow base}{acid}$$

For metabolic alkalosis, there is respiratory as well as renal compensation. Alkalosis inhibits the peripheral chemoreceptors, resulting in hypoventilation and elevation of $PaCO_2$. In the kidney, metabolic alkalosis results in decreased secretion of H^+ by the renal tubules. Hence filtered bicarbonate is not completely absorbed. The urinary losses of bicarbonate decrease the extent of elevation of plasma bicarbonate. Hence the change in pH of blood is minimized. The acid-base status of a case of compensated metabolic alkalosis is as follows:

$$pH = pK^1 + \log \frac{\uparrow base}{\uparrow acid}$$

Metabolic alkalosis due to persistent vomiting is accompanied by not only loss of acid but also fluid from the stomach. The resulting hypovolemia becomes a strong stimulus for sodium reabsorption in the kidneys through Na^+–K^+ as well as Na^+–H^+ antiport systems. Therefore, when metabolic alkalosis is accompanied by hypovolemia, the renal response tends to aggravate alkalosis rather than correct it. It leads to hypokalemia as well. A fairly typical pattern of acid-base status and electrolytes in a patient with persistent vomiting is given below.

Na^+ (mEq/L)	140
K^+ (mEq/L)	3.2
HCO_3^- (mEq/L)	42
Cl^- (mEq/L)	84
pH	7.52
pCO_2 (mmHg)	52

3. Respiratory Acidosis

The primary abnormality in respiratory acidosis is elevation of $PaCO_2$ due to alveolar hypoventilation. Alveolar hypoventilation also reduces PaO_2. Therefore hypoxemia is always accompanies hypercapnea.

Acute respiratory acidosis is defined as hypercapnea developed in the time prior to renal compensation, i.e. less than 24 hours. In acute respiratory acidosis, the acid-base status is as follows:

$$\downarrow pH = pK^1 + \log \frac{\text{base}}{\uparrow \text{acid}}$$

Acute respiratory acidosis may be caused by:
- Acute airway obstruction (severe asthma)
- Central respiratory drive depression
  - Drugs—narcotics, benzodiazepines, barbiturates
  - Neurologic disorders—encephalitis, brainstem disease, trauma, poliomyelitis.

Chronic respiratory acidosis is most commonly present in
- Chronic obstructive pulmonary disease
  - Emphysema
  - Chronic bronchitis
- Chest wall deformities
  - Kyphoscoliosis
  - Fibrothorax
  - Thoracoplasty
- Neuromuscular disorders
  - Amyotrophic lateral sclerosis
  - Muscular dystrophies—Duchenne and Becker dystrophies
  - Diaphragm paralysis
  - Guillain-Barré syndrome
  - Myasthenia gravis

The renal compensation involves H^+ excretion, as well as increased generation of HCO_3^-. The resultant increase in plasma bicarbonate concentration partially restores the blood pH towards normal:

$$pH = pK^1 + \log \frac{\uparrow \text{base}}{\uparrow \text{acid}}$$

Renal compensation results in elevation of plasma HCO_3^- by 3.5 mEq/L for every 10 mmHg increase in pCO_2. A fairly typical pattern of acid-base and electrolyte status of a patient with chronic respiratory acidosis is given below.

Na^+ (mEq/L)	137
K^+ (mEq/L)	4.5
HCO_3^- (mEq/L)	40
Cl^- (mEq/L)	90
pH	7.31
pCO_2 (mmHg)	75

4. Respiratory Alkalosis

Respiratory alkalosis is the most common acid-base disorder in a critically ill patient. It is primarily caused by alveolar hyperventilation leading to decreased $PaCO_2$

$$\uparrow pH = pK^1 + \log \frac{base}{\downarrow acid}$$

Hypoxia due to acute pulmonary disease (e.g. pneumonia) or chronic pulmonary disease, sepsis and psychogenic hyperventilation are common causes of respiratory alkalosis.

Renal compensation to decreased arterial pCO_2 is decreased renal secretion of H^+. Consequently, bicarbonate is not generated in the kidneys. More importantly, even the filtered bicarbonate is not fully reabsorbed. Hence plasma HCO_3^- falls markedly which minimizes the change in blood pH:

$$pH = pK^1 + \log \frac{\downarrow base}{\downarrow acid}$$

A fairly typical pattern of acid-base and electrolytes in a patient with respiratory alkalosis is given below.

Na^+ (mEq/L)	135
K^+ (mEq/L)	3.2
HCO_3^- (mEq/L)	19
Cl^- (mEq/L)	105
pH	7.55
pCO_2 (mmHg)	22

Acid-base Analysis

A simple protocol to detect an acid-base abnormality in a patient is described in Fig. 30.1.

B. Mixed Acid-base Disorders

A patient may have more than one acid-base abnormality. The condition is called a mixed acid-base disorder. For example, a patient may have respiratory acidosis as well as metabolic acidosis or respiratory alkalosis as well as metabolic alkalosis. In view of the four primary acid-base disorders, six mixed acid-base disorders can be expected (Table 30.1).

The key to the diagnosis of mixed acid-base disorders is the clear understanding of the expected adaptations to the primary acid-base disturbances (Fig. 30.1.). If the acid-base values are outside the expected range, a mixed disorder should be suspected. Mixed acid-base disorders may be "benign" when the two primary disorders provide adaptations for each other, e.g. metabolic acidosis + respiratory alkalosis.

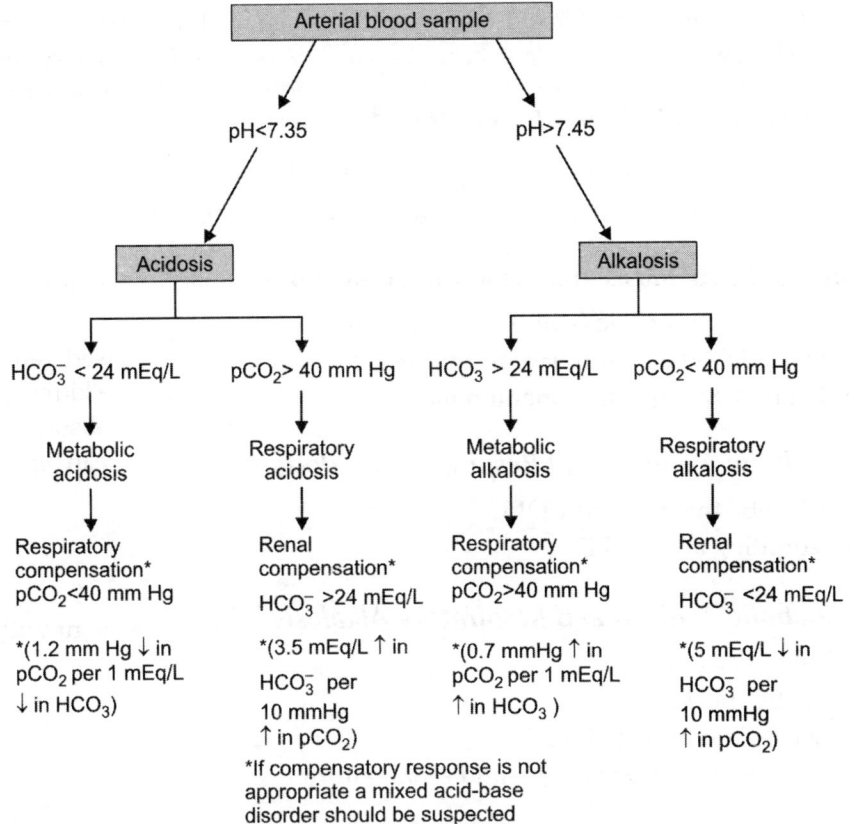

Fig. 30.1: Protocol to detect acid-base abnormality.

Some mixed acid-base disorders produce dangerous deviations in pH e.g. respiratory acidosis + metabolic acidosis, because the disorder that is hypoventilation would not allow the adaptive hyperventilation for metabolic acidosis. Moreover, low plasma bicarbonate caused by metabolic acidosis blocks the rise in plasma bicarbonate expected in respiratory acidosis.

Another important clue to the existence of a mixed acid-base disorder is the clinical setting, e.g. vomiting, use of diuretics, cardiac arrest, hypotensive shock or sepsis superimposed on COPD or renal failure.

Table 30.1 Typical chemical parameters in mixed acid-base disorders

	Na^+	K^+	Cl^-	HCO_3^-	Anion gap	pH	pCO_2
			mEq/L				mmHg
Metabolic acidosis + Metabolic alkalosis	140	4.0	90	25	25	7.4	40
Metabolic acidosis + High anion gap metabolic acidosis	140	5	115	5	20	7.10	17
Metabolic acidosis + Respiratory acidosis	140	5	100	15	25	7.10	50
Respiratory acidosis + Metabolic alkalosis	140	3	95	35	10	7.4	58
Metabolic acidosis + Respiratory alkalosis	140	4	105	10	25	7.45	15
Metabolic alkalosis + Respiratory alkalosis	140	3	100	25	15	7.60	26

Some common mixed acid-base disorders seen in clinical practice are given below.

Metabolic Acidosis and Respiratory Acidosis
- Patients of COPD who develop circulatory shock
- Patients with metabolic acidosis who develop respiratory failure

Metabolic Alkalosis and Respiratory Alkalosis
- Congestive cardiac failure and vomiting
- Diuretic therapy and hepatic failure
- Diuretic therapy and pneumonia

Metabolic Alkalosis and Respiratory Acidosis
- Diuretic therapy and COPD
- Vomiting and COPD

Metabolic Acidosis and Respiratory Alkalosis
- Salicylate overdose
- Septic shock
- Sepsis and renal failure
- Congestive cardiac failure and renal failure

Metabolic Alkalosis and Metabolic Acidosis
- Diuretic therapy and ketoacidosis
- Vomiting and renal failure
- Vomiting and lactic acidosis/ketoacidosis.

Further Reading

Androgue, NE; Madias ME. **Mixed acid base disorders**. In *the principles & practice of Nephrology*. Ed. Jacobson, HR, et al. St Louis; Mosby yearbook 1995: 953–962

Androgue, NE; Madias ME. **Management of life threatening acid-base disorders**. *N Engl J Med* 1998, 338: 24–34, 107–111.

Das, B. **Acid-base disorders**. *Indian J Anaes*. 2003; 47:373–379.

McNamara, J; Worthley, LI **Acid-base balance**: part II. **Pathophysiology** *Crit Care Resusc* 2001; 3: 188–201.

Walmsley, RN; White, GH. **Mixed acid-base disorders**.*Clin.Chem* 1985; 31: 321–325.

Index

Achalasia 63
Acid-base buffers 375
Acquired hemolytic anemia 19
Acromegaly 294
ACTH 292
Acute ischemic stroke 257
Acute renal failure 357
Acute renal injury 357
Acute tubular necrosis 360
Addisonian pernicious anemia 15
Adenohypophysis 288
Adrenal insufficiency 325
Adrenal steroidogenesis, regulation 317
Adult respiratory distress syndrome 224
Airway resistance 198
Alcohol liver disease 116
Alcoholic cirrhosis 118
Allergic inflammation 35
Ammonia metabolism 106
Anemia 10
  chronic diseases 13
  elderly population 21
  renal insufficiency 22
Anion gap 379
Anterior pituitary, hypothalamic control 288
Antidiuretic hormone 296
Antithyroid agents 306
Aortic regurgitation 144
Aortic stenosis 143
Aplastic anemia 20
Atherosclerosis 152
Atrial septal defect 146

Babinski sign 246
Bacterial overgrowth syndrome 90
Basophils 26
Bilirubin metabolism 109
Bleeding disorders 45
Blood glucose homeostasis 331

Blood pressure determinants 171
Blood pressure regulation 173
Bone remodeling 343
Bone 341
Bronchial asthma 203

Carbohydrate metabolism 105
Cardiac cycle 129
Cardiac output 160
Cardiogenic shock 188
Celiac disease 89
Cerebral
  blood flow 255
  circulation 253
  ischemia 256
Chronic bronchitis 206
Chronic obstructive pulmonary disease 205
Chronic pain syndrome 282
Chronic renal failure, stages 366
Circulatory shock 182
Clotting disorders 47
Coagulation 39
Cold shock 189
Coma 263
Congenital adrenal hyperplasia 324
Congenital spherocytosis 16
Congestive heart failure 162
Conn's syndrome 322
Coronary blood flow 150
Corticosteroid biosynthesis 316
Crohn's disease 95
Cushing disease 295
Cushing syndrome 322

Dead space 214
Deep venous thrombosis 49
Deglutition 59
Diabetes insipidus 298
Diabetes mellitus 333
Diabetic steatorrhea 91

Diarrhea 92
Diffusion capacity 221
Digestive enzymes 84
Disseminated intravascular
  coagulation 52
Dysphagia 62

Emphysema 208
Endogenous pain modulation 276
Eosinophils 25
Erythropoiesis 1
Erythropoietin 1
Escape phenomenon 321
Esophagus, endoscopy 59
Esophagus, functional anatomy 58

Fast, slow pain 271
Fetal steroid biosynthesis 316
Fibrinolytic system 42
Folic acid metabolism 9

G6PD deficiency anemia 17
Gastric acid secretion 74
Gastroesophageal reflux disease 68
Gate control hypothesis 277
Giantism 294
Glucocorticoids, actions 319
Gonadotropins 293
Graves' disease 309
Growth hormone 289
Growth, regulation of 299

Heart sounds 131
Helicobacter pylori 78
Hemoglobin A 2
Hemoglobin F 3
Hemoglobin S 3
Hemolytic anemia 15
Hemophilia 47
Hemostasis
  primary 38
  secondary 39
  tests of 43
Hepatic encephalitis 126
Hepatorenal syndrome 128
Hereditary spherocytosis 16
Hiatal hernia 65
Hirschsprung's disease 96
Hyperalgesia 276
Hyperprolactinemia 294

Hypertension 175
Hypertension, complications 178
Hypertension, pathogenesis 176
Hyperthyroidism 309
Hypertonia 248
Hyperventilation 218
Hypoglycemia unawareness 340
Hypoglycemia 339
Hypopituitarism 296
Hypothyroidism 310
Hypoventilatory syndrome 215
Hypovolemic shock 184

Infant respiratory distress syndrome 226
Inflammation, acute 28
Inflammation, chronic 36
Inflammatory bowel disease 94
Insulin 329
Insulin-like growth factors 289
Intracerebral hemorrhage 258
Inverse stretch reflex 245
Iodine deficiency 311
Iron deficiency anemia 11
Iron metabolism 3
Iron overload 6
Iron status 5
Irritable bowel syndrome 94
Islets of Langerhans 329

Lactose intolerance 87
Lipid metabolism 107
Liver
  cirrhosis 121
  function tests 111
  function 104
  structure 103
  ultrastructure 104
Lower esophageal sphincter 61
Lungs, defense mechanisms 196
Lymphocytes 26

M cells 86
Macrocytic normochromic anemia 14
Malabsorption symptoms 88
Malabsorption syndrome 87
Metabolic acidosis 380
Metabolic alkalosis 382
Microcytic hypochromic anemia 11

Index

Mineralocorticoids, actions 322
Mitral regurgitation 141
Mitral stenosis 139
Mixed acid base disorders 384
Monocytes 26
Motor activity, sensory information 241
Motor responses 240
Mucociliary clearance 197
Mucosal block hypothesis 4
Multiple organ failure syndrome 191
Murmurs 135
Muscle spindles 243
Myocardial infarction 156
Myocardial oxygen supply 151
Myxedema coma 314
Myxedema 312

Natural anticlotting mechanisms 41
Nelson's syndrome 295
Nonalcoholic fatty liver disease 120
Normocytic normochromic
    anemia 15, 20

Obstructive lung disease 202
Orthostatic hypotension 266
Osteitis fibrosa cystica 352
Osteoporosis 349
Oxygen
    therapy 229
    toxicity 231
    transport 228

Paget's disease 351
Pain
    chemical mediators 270
    effects 282
    management 284
    neuropathic 278
    nociceptive 269
    visceral 272
Pancreatitis
    acute 98
    alcoholic 99
    biliary 100
    chronic 100
Parathyroid hormone 344
Patent ductus arteriosus 148
Peptic ulcer 77
    stress 80

pH concept 375
pH regulation 377
Pheochromocytoma 328
Pituitary gland 286
Platelet plug 38
Polymorphonuclear neutrophils 24
Portal hypertension 123
Postgastrectomy syndrome 91
Postrenal ARF 364
Postural tachycardia syndrome 267
Prerenal ARF 357
Primary aldosteronism 322
Primary hemochromatosis 6
Prolactin 290
Protein metabolism 106
Purpura 46
Pyloric stenosis 82

Red cell indices 10
Referred pain 274
Regulation of muscle tone 257
Renal ARF 359
Respiration
    chemical control 213
    neural control 212
Respiratory acidosis 382
Respiratory alkalosis 384
Respiratory failure 222
Respiratory parenchyma 228
Restrictive lung disease 209
Reticular activating system 261
Reticulocytosis 2
Retrolental hyperplasia 231
Rickets 349
RIFLE criteria 365

Secondary hyperaldosteronism 323
Septic shock 188
Shift to the left 25
Shock, stages of 186
Short statute 302
SIADH 298
Sickle cell anemia 18
Sleep apnea syndrome 217
Small bowel syndrome 90
Small intestinal absorption 85
Small intestinal defense mechanisms 85
Spasticity 248
Stable angina 155

Stomach, motor function 76
Stomach, secretory function 74
Stress, peptic ulcer 80
Stretch reflex 244
Sympathoadrenal response 326
Syncope 264

Tall stature 302
Tendon jerks 245
Tetralogy of Fallot 149
Thalassemia 12
Thalassemia 19
Thrombosis 48
Thrombosis, arterial 48
Thyroid hormone actions 307
Thyroid hormone biosynthesis 304
Thyroid storm 310
Transfusional hemosiderosis 8
Tremor 248

Tropical sprue 89
TSH 293

Ulcerative colitis 94
UMN and LMN paralyses 251
Unexplained anemia 21
Unstable angina 156
Upper and lower motor neurons 242
Uremia 367
Urine formation 355

Valvular heart disease 139
Ventilation–perfusion ratio 221
Ventricular septal defect 147
Vitamin B_{12} metabolism 9
Vitamin D 345
Von Willibrand disease 47

Warm shock 189
Withdrawal reflex 245

Zollinger-Ellison syndrome 83

Reader's Notes

Reader's Notes

Reader's Notes

Reader's Notes

Reader's Notes

Reader's Notes